Passions, Persons, Psychotherapy, Politics

Andrew Samuels is one of the best known figures internationally in the fields of psychotherapy, Jungian analysis, relational psychoanalysis and counselling, and in academic studies in those areas. His work is a blend of the provocative and original together with the reliable and scholarly. His many books and papers figure prominently on reading lists in clinical and academic teaching contexts.

This self-selected collection, *Passions, Persons, Psychotherapy, Politics*, brings together some of Samuels' major writings at the interface of politics and therapy thinking. In this volume, he includes chapters on the market economy; prospects for eco-psychology and environmentalism; the role of the political Trickster, particularly the female Trickster; the father; relations between women and men; and his celebrated and radical critique of the Jungian idea of 'the feminine principle'. Clinical material consists of his work with parents and on the therapy relationship. The book concludes with his seminal and transparent work on Jung and anti-semitism and an intriguing account of the current trajectory of the Jungian field.

Samuels has written a highly personal and confessional introduction to the book. Each chapter also has its own topical introduction, written in a clear and informal style. There is also much that will challenge the long-held beliefs of many working in politics and in the social sciences. This unique collection of papers will be of interest to psychotherapists, Jungian analysts, psychoanalysts and counsellors – as well as those undertaking academic work in those areas.

Andrew Samuels has, for almost forty years, been evolving a unique clinical blend of post-Jungian, relational psychoanalytic and humanistic approaches to therapy work. He is recognised internationally as one of the leading commentators from a psychotherapeutic perspective on political and social problems. His work on the father, sexuality, spirituality and countertransference has also been widely appreciated. He is a past chair of the UK Council for Psychotherapy, a co-founder of Psychotherapists and Counsellors for Social Responsibility and of the Alliance for Counselling and Psychotherapy. He is Professor of Analytical Psychology at Essex University and holds visiting chairs at New York, London, Macau and Roehampton Universities. Andrew's many books have been translated into 19 languages. They include the groundbreaking *Jung and the Post-Jungians,* the indispensable *Critical Dictionary of Jungian Analysis*, his prescient account of pluralism in *The Plural Psyche* and his works on politics and therapy thinking – *The Political Psyche* and *Politics on the Couch*. www.andrewsamuels.com

World Library of Mental Health series

The *World Library of Mental Health* celebrates the important contributions to mental health made by leading experts in their individual fields. Each author has compiled a career-long collection of what they consider to be their finest pieces: extracts from books, journals, articles, major theoretical and practical contributions, and salient research findings.

For the first time ever the work of each contributor is presented in a single volume so readers can follow the themes and progress of their work and identify the contributions made to, and the development of, the fields themselves.

Each book in the series features a specially written introduction by the contributor giving an overview of his career, contextualizing his selection within the development of the field, and showing how his own thinking developed over time.

Rationality and Pluralism – The selected works of Windy Dryden
By Windy Dryden

The Price of Love – The selected works of Colin Murray Parkes
By Colin Murray Parkes

Attachments: Psychiatry, Psychotherapy, Psychoanalysis – The selected works of Jeremy Holmes
By Jeremy Holmes

Passions, Persons, Psychotherapy, Politics – The selected works of Andrew Samuels
By Andrew Samuels

Towards a Radical Redefinition of Psychology – The selected works of Miller Mair
Edited by David Winter and Nick Reed

Passions, Persons, Psychotherapy, Politics

The selected works of Andrew Samuels

Andrew Samuels

Routledge
Taylor & Francis Group
LONDON AND NEW YORK

First published 2015
by Routledge
2 Park Square, Milton Park, Abingdon, Oxon OX14 4RN

and by Routledge
605 Third Avenue, New York, NY 10017

First issued in paperback 2021

Routledge is an imprint of the Taylor & Francis Group, an informa business

Publisher's Note
The publisher has gone to great lengths to ensure the quality of this reprint but points out that some imperfections in the original copies may be apparent.

British Library Cataloguing in Publication Data
A catalogue record for this book is available from the British Library

Library of Congress Cataloging in Publication Data
Samuels, Andrew.
[Works. Selections]
Passions, persons, psychotherapy, politics : the selected works of Andrew Samuels / Andrew Samuels.
pages cm. — (World library of mental health)
ISBN 978-0-415-70792-3 (hardback)
1. Psychoanalysis and culture. 2. Psychoanalysis—Political aspects. 3. Political psychology. I. Title.
BF175.4.C84S257 2014
150.19'54—dc23
2014017674

ISBN 13: 978-1-138-81881-1 (pbk)
ISBN 13: 978-0-415-70792-3 (hbk)
ISBN 13: 978-1-315-76099-5 (ebk)

DOI: 10.4324/9781315760995

Typeset in Sabon
by RefineCatch Limited, Bungay, Suffolk

In memory of Fred Plaut (1913–2009)

> We're in this gig together, boy,
> So let's settle down and steal each other's song

CONTENTS

ACKNOWLEDGEMENTS

My books are replete with acknowledgements to dozens of individuals. In fact, those acknowledgements chart my personal, social, professional and academic trajectories over thirty years. So, rather than reproducing massive lists, I will confine myself to acknowledging the people directly concerned with this particular book.

My editor Kate Hawes and I have been working together for decades. I am her adviser in analytical psychology. Kate's and Routledge's commitment to analytical psychology, Jungian analysis and Jungian studies have helped to create, define and enhance the field. I have learned a lot from Kate about managing authors in one kind of emotional state or another – I wish I could manage myself better in this regard. Others at Routledge have been extremely helpful and I want to acknowledge Kirsten Buchanan, Sally Mesner Lyons and Natalie Larkin.

Friends have also encouraged me in this particular endeavour. Gottfried Heuer had been on at me for many years to let him publish a 'Collected Works of AS', and Chris Hauke had made similar noises about editing a selection. I hope that they are both hugely relieved and mightily disappointed (!) that the format of the series in which this book sits is one in which the authors select their own golden oldies.

Moira Duckworth and Martin Stone have been really supportive, always available in person, at the end of a phone or via text. Similarly, Tom Kirsch, Luigi Zoja, David Tacey, Chris Hauke, Gottfried Heuer, SoftSusie Orbach and Jessica Benjamin have offered containment and jollity as well as incitement to *kvetching* and lamentation.

I owe Sissy Lykou more than I can say. Without her encouragement and inspiration, I doubt I would (or could) have really roused myself and got into this project to the extent that I have done.

PERMISSIONS

By design, all of the chapters in this book have been published before in other books. I am grateful to Taylor & Francis for permission to use material from my books for Routledge – *Jung and the Post-Jungians* (1985) and *The Plural Psyche: Personality, Morality and the Father* (1989).

I am also grateful to Karnac Books for kind permission to use material from my book *Politics on the Couch: Citizenship and the Internal Life* (2001), first published by Karnac in 2007.

Finally, I am grateful to Cambridge University Press for permission to use my chapter from the *Cambridge Companion to Jung* (second edition, 2008), edited by Polly Young-Eisendrath and Terence Dawson.

Note on C. G. Jung's Collected Works

CW refers to the *Collected Works* of C. G. Jung, Ed. Herbert Read, Michael Fordham and Gerhard Adler, Trans. R. F. C. Hull (London: Routledge and Kegan Paul; Princeton, NJ: Princeton University Press, 1953–77). References, save where indicated, are by volume and paragraph number.

INTRODUCTION

Personal confesssions

Jung wrote that 'every psychology is a personal confession' and that remark guides the content of this introduction. I'd like to show why the themes in my work came to be there from a personal angle, and also to comment on them in an informal and conversational way.

To begin at the beginning, I have always struggled to find the vigorous to and fro in my image of my parents' marriage. I am not saying it was never there, only that I had an image of a conventional togetherness without much passion or risk taking. They were kind to each other but never went near (in my fantasy) the grotesque and divine experimentations I write about in the paper on the image of the parents in bed that forms Chapter 9 of this book.

I will talk about my mother in a moment. My father was a gentleman, and I mean this in two senses. First, that he was well-educated, had been through the war (ending up in a prisoner of war camp), and enjoyed a cultivated and comfortable lifestyle ranging from golf to classical music. But he was also, for me, what I came to call a 'dry' father (see Chapter 6), not giving out much erotic or aggressive playback – but a decent and polite man. In fact, I felt that he depended on me to provide a kind of excitement and, via my rebellious, bad and rejecting behaviour that is what I did.

My concern – even obsession – with relations between women and men stems, I believe, from this respectable but emotionally constrained background. I found it hard to buy into Jungian essentialist approaches to gender because they felt so limiting (see Chapter 7). And I have been strongly influenced by feminism so that what I wrote over the years about the relations between women and men (for example, Chapter 5) took some time to settle down to focus on men, which is what you would have expected me to write about given my interest in the father.

I am a competitive person, who delights in negotiation and bargaining, and I have become able to see that there is a principle of complementarity at work in life: some people are better than others at some things. But when it comes to other things, other people are more adept. These three principles lie at the heart of pluralism: competition, bargaining, complementarity. Pluralism gave me an opportunity to be aggressive and tolerant at the same time – and also to link the inner world with the social realm in psychological theory-making. Those three principles are relevant to many levels of experience, you see. I didn't include theoretical chapters on pluralism in this selection but you can see how the ideas work in practice with regard to moral process in Chapter 4. (Or you can look at my book *The Plural Psyche*.)

Although my classification of the schools of post-Jungian analytical psychology was worked out before I developed pluralism as a theory, it was the project that got me going. For those who do not know, in 1985 the Jungian analytical field was a mess, in terms of anyone being able to find their way around in it. There were huge differences in approach and things only held because each segment of the field claimed to derive something from its connection to Jung. I experienced it all differently from most of my friends and fellow students. I liked the argy-bargy and was able to see that what looked like totally inimical perspectives were in fact linked by their desire to go beyond Jung whilst retaining a critical connection to him. This meant that each of the revisionary tendencies (Developmental, Archetypal) could be seen as having a similar relation to the centre (Classical). (See Chapters 13 and 14.)

For a beginning analyst to write an overview of the field into which he had just arrived was, of course, an inflation. But I certainly made a name for myself. This leads me to comment a bit on my mother's influence on me. It was she who spotted, with her down to earth intuition and generally savvy approach to life, that writing could be a way for me to make my mark. She went on and on about this, and, unusually and amazingly, I listened even though I knew that my success was her stuff. It became clear to me that, although writing books on analysis and therapy tells us nothing about the writer's capacities as a healer, it was a way to move things along, to say the least.

This brings me to the not inconsiderable matter of my relationship, on all levels, to Tricksters in general and to Hermes in particular. What attracts me to the Trickster is his very lack of a political or psychological project. In fact, he lacks ambition *per se*! If he does good, it is entirely by accident. There can be little or no cleaning up. His primitivity makes him what he is. And 'he' is not only a 'he'. I do not really know why I was the first to spot the potential of the idea of the 'female Trickster'. When women writers took it up big time, my feminism (actually, my membership of the anti-sexist men's movement) meant I stepped aside. I now wish I had not because there is today so much idealistic, sentimental and romantic writing on the Trickster, especially the female version, that I yearn to re-enter the field and the fray. I think I will!

Hermes spoke to me, as to many analysts, because he linked the base, corrupt, grotesque aspects of the Trickster (dirty tricks in politics) with some kind of compulsive connection making. It remained murky and resistant to a wholly positive reading because the shadow of being an emissary of the Gods is that the messenger becomes (seeks to become?) more important than the message. So, behind my pluralistic tendency to pop up in many fields of psychotherapy beyond the post-Jungian one (humanistic psychology, body psychotherapy, relational psychoanalysis), there is, like there was for Hermes, a quest for power. (In this book, Tricksters and Hermes appear in Chapters 1, 2 and 9.)

I'll turn now to my writings on politics. Although decidedly progressive, with a leftist background and a history in community politics, my irascible personality led me to step outside the progressive circle from time to time. The result is the polemical (yet affectionate) piece on environmentalism from 1993 that you can read in Chapter 3. I always want to be both the outsider and the front runner, if I can manage it, and the critique of what has become ecopsychology fulfilled both of these desiderata rather well.

This desire to be outside the group that is already outside the mainstream is quite an intellectual and communicative problem for me. It means I am commenting critically on things that have still not yet been widely accepted. This was forcibly drawn to my attention when, deconstructing the idea of the Wounded Healer, arguing that this notion depotentiated the client, I realised that many people had not in fact got deeply into the Wounded Healer in the first place! Or, when arguing that contemporary academic attempts to see the individual always in a context or network missed the power of individual action in the political sphere, I realised that, for many readers and listeners, the idea of the individual as contingent was still not something they had integrated. I was going up against something that I felt personally was huge and had become reactionary but was not in fact perceived as such by many people.

Be that as it may, I don't think it was this rebellious nature and need to lead that motivated my controversial work on Jung and anti-semitism, which forms Chapters 11 and 12 of the book. If there was a personal background to this project, it was more to do with the plain fact of being Jewish in a community whose founder had written objectionable things about my people. There was also some kind of background wish to be more accepted as a contributor to academic, psychoanalytic and political discourses that was undermined by being seen as an adherent of the anti-semite Jung.

But it was the reactions to my early essays on the allegations of Jung's anti-semitism that really irked me. There was a closing of the Jungian ranks, a repetitious argument that Jung was only a man of his time, and even some pathologising of me as a Jew with a complex. Well, Jung was not a man of his time (as you can see in the following chapters) and it is those kinds of knee-jerk defences that represent our problem (the Jungians' problem) and not Jung's problem. Nevertheless, gradually, the Jungian community realised that apology and reparation was needed and the informal alliance of concerned people that emerged has done a pretty good job in this regard. Of course, for those who need a tribal enemy, this unfortunate legacy provides a marvellous base. Much work still needs to be done on Jung's racial attitudes and his theories and utterances about 'Africans', but I remain optimistic that this will come to pass.

What is not here

I took a personal editorial decision that, if this was to be a sort of Samuels Reader, it was not the place to introduce current works in progress but rather to work the backlist. So all the selections come from my four solo books up to 2013, plus a couple of commissioned pieces from authoritative anthologies. At the time of writing, I am working on three further books of new material and, *deo concedente*, these will appear in print in due course.

In spite of this self-discipline, I thought it would be interesting to set out what is likely to be in these yet to be published books because much of the material already exists in the form of academic papers. The reason why there has been a dearth of books from me since 2001 has been the need to publish in specific academic journals that fit the research 'profile' of my university department so as to earn funding. I am not alone in feeling uncomfortable working under this kind of lash but that is the sorry nature of academia in Britain today.

Anyway, here is a list of some of the things that occupy me at the moment:

I am continuing my work at *the interface of therapy thinking and political problems*. The themes that interest me are (i) the search for economic justice,

(ii) good-enough leadership and (iii) aggression and violence (I have written a paper entitled 'The value of aggression').

It seems to me that any progressive politics worth its salt must engage with *spirituality* in the broadest sense. In the process, both political and spiritual perspectives have to change. I think we can see this realignment beginning to fashion itself in many spheres and I think that psychotherapists can be good facilitators of new connections between the spiritual and the political – which are both *'more than personal'* after all.

The role of *the individual in politics* (which I touched on earlier) is beginning to loom larger in my mind. The catchphrase 'making a difference' (and its gloomy counterpart, 'activist burnout') is what I have in mind. But what kind of individual are we talking about? Does the individual who might make a difference have to be special in any way? And is the whole idea sensible (I mean the idea that an individual might make a difference)? I've found that *a hybrid of Jung and Albert Camus* gives a lot of insight into these complexities.

I have also gone on with my work on relationships to produce a rather ambitious piece on *promiscuity*, showing how there are political and spiritual aspects to consider as well as psychological ones. The work concludes with an onslaught on the hypocrisy of therapists when it comes to promiscuity, and a defence of homosexuality against projections onto it by heteronormative therapists.

Other topics that deserve inclusion in this list include:

- challenging the expansion of Western psychotherapy and analysis into 'frontier' areas – is this always a good thing?
- exploring questions of diversity and equality (inclusion and exclusion) in the therapy professions
- critiquing the notions of 'children' and 'the child'
- discussing of the limits of the relational approach to therapy – has the cutting edge become a cliché?
- reconfiguring the client as a healer
- exploring the secret politics of clinical supervision
- a range of ethical issues including the problem of sexual misconduct.

A note on how I became a Jungian analyst

I hope readers will not be disappointed by what follows, which is very far from being a full memoir or autobiography. Rather, it pretty much stops at the point I enter the Jungian professional community. Specifically, the personal events of my adult life are not covered – that is not what I wanted to write about in this concluding section of the introduction to my *Selected Papers*. It does get quite personal though.

I was born into a middle-class Jewish family in Liverpool in 1949. Three of my four grandparents were born in Britain or Ireland. The fourth, with whom I like to identify, came to Britain in 1912 from Poland. He was a dynamic and brilliant man who built up an outstanding collection of modern art. (I think he was a hugely problematic father for my own father.) The family business was what in Yiddish is called *schmatte* – inexpensive clothing (for women). Yet my father went to Cambridge to read history and my mother was studying medicine when she met my father and gave it up to get married. After the war, my father was, I think, too tired, ill and depressed to resist his fate and went into the family firm. He told me he hated every day of the 35 years he spent there. The family went into steep economic decline after a period of affluence.

I went to boarding school at the age of eight which I found very distressing and damaging. I regressed, becoming encopretic and enuretic, and wanted to be allowed home. I was not listened to. After a while, I found a niche as a 'brainy' boy and acquired the nickname 'Super Sam'. But I hated that preparatory school. I think my parents could not imagine it at the time and they seemed to me unable to challenge the school's insistence that all was well. In my late fifties I returned to the village in North Wales where the school had been and, to my surprise, in place of the memories of freezing mud and the absence of hot water for washing, there was a glorious sparkle on the sea and the mountains looked marvellous in the sunshine. So I saw very briefly something of what my parents might have seen. But, as I write this, the familiar feeling of fear and outrage comes upon me.

The next school, which was what we call in Britain a public school (meaning it, too, was private), was an emotional doddle after the fantastically rough and spartan conditions at the preparatory school. True, there was some bullying, due to the fact that there was a Jewish house in this school and, far from permitting a multicultural ethos, this incited anti-semitism. Adolescence hit me quite early and I rebelled against this second school and neglected my studies. However, I was rescued by one particular teacher who believed in me and recovered to the point where I got a scholarship to Oxford.

This teacher had been living and working in South Africa and he encouraged me to go there in the period between school and university. We were both in the Anti-Apartheid Movement. I ended up working for the Colonial Office in Swaziland and got secretly involved with the African National Congress. My work for the ANC was discovered and it landed me in prison in South Africa for a short while, where I was physically maltreated.

Eventually, I returned to take up the place at Oxford but just could not see the point. This was 1967 and some reading this may recall that we thought there was to be a revolution. Trotskyite politics and agitprop theatre became my interests and I dropped out of university to run a progressive theatre company. In those days, the Arts Council was generous with grants, especially if you got good reviews. The theatre company began to do more community work in hospitals and young offenders' institutions and I realised that I'd have to make a decision. As it happens, I was then headhunted for a job at the Royal Shakespeare Company but, in a moment that has shaped my life ever since, decided to go instead to South Wales where I worked in a youth and community project, doing drama with the kids (at least that was the plan).

Over time, I realised that I was more interested in what we would now call psychoanalytic psychotherapy or counselling and I wrote to all the trainings in London that existed then (there were three). The two psychoanalytic ones wrote back to say I was too young (I was 21–22 years old). The Jungians didn't reply at all! So I gave up and entered psychiatric social work training at the London School of Economics. One day, I was walking in Central London and stumbled across the street where the Society of Analytical Psychology had its office. I went in and was interviewed then and there. (I think they felt guilty at ignoring my letter.) So I went into training analysis in 1972.

It was even more complicated. My theatre background, with all the rehearsal tricks of the trade, made me quite suitable as an encounter group leader. Encounter groups were high-octane sort of therapy groups in the 1960s and early 1970s and I became apprenticed to an experienced leader under the auspices of a growth centre that was flourishing at the time. In the end, I realised I could not train to be both a Jungian analyst and an encounter group leader and made my decision. But I have been left with a serious appreciation for humanistic psychology.

As I said, I am going to leave this brief autobiographical note here. I could have written about how I became an academic at the University of Essex (a professor without a degree), or about my current involvement with relational psychoanalysis (a British Jungian on the board of the International Association for Relational Psychoanalysis), or about how I came to be the chair of the United Kingdom Council for Psychotherapy. I won't do more than mention some of the small groups I helped to found, all of them still in existence: Psychotherapists and Counsellors for Social Responsibility, Antidote, Alliance for Counselling and Psychotherapy, Confederation for Analytical Psychology. If anyone reading this wants to know more, you can contact me via my website (www.andrewsamuels.com). This is a highly interactive website featuring regular filmed 'rants' by me on diverse topics.

CHAPTER 1

THE MIRROR AND THE HAMMER

The politics of resacralization

Retrospective introduction

I wrote this as the first chapter of *The Political Psyche* in 1993. I wanted to challenge the distinctions that most people accepted – for example, between inner and outer worlds, or between therapy and political action. I was probably a bit too enthusiastic about the role that what I now call therapy thinking could play. But that could be seen as a laudable fault.

You see, Hillman and Venture had just produced a book called *We've Had a Hundred years of Psychotherapy and the World's getting Worse*. It contained a put down of the therapy project, as if all that was now needed was an engagement with social and political ills. I felt this book was misleading in that it totally ignored the long history of psychology and psychotherapy's engagement with the social and political world and I wanted to set my attempt to bring therapy thinking to bear in an accurate and respectful historical context (Freud, Jung, the humanistic pioneers).

I also wanted to set out the important paradox that you can't have personal growth and change in a sullied world, and you can't change the world if you don't change something in the people living in it.

I am really surprised at how little has changed! The things that worried and interested me herein – attitudes to the market economy, inequalities of wealth, social movements (more recently we have had Occupy), the feelings of disgust and alienation from politics, focus on the environment, the buried spirituality in many political ventures ('resacralization') – they all still prevail more than twenty years later. Therapy thinking has not really achieved much by way of improvement – but then nor has anything else. So the chapter seems to me to be anything but a relic; it is applicable in today's contexts as well.

The chapter also contains many definitions of terms, and hence is useful for teaching and study purposes.

Depth psychology and political transformation

This chapter is about the depth psychology of political processes, focusing on processes of non-violent political change. It is a contribution to the long-standing ambition of psychotherapy to develop a form of political and cultural analysis that would, in Freud's words, 'understand the riddles of the world.'[1] I will be trying to bring depth psychology as a whole, and the particular experience of clinical analysis, to bear on politics. An engagement of depth psychology with politics makes a contribution to social science, social theory and the other human sciences.[2] But the chapter is also oriented in the opposite direction: bringing an understanding of the political world to bear on the theories of depth psychology and the practices of clinical analysis, leading to a concern for humankind as well as an absorption in one's personal problems.

By 'politics' I mean the concerted arrangements and struggles within an institution, or in a single society, or between the countries of the world for the organization and distribution of resources and power, especially economic power. Politics concerns the way in which power is held or deployed by the state, by institutions, and by sectional interests to maintain survival, determine behavior, gain control over others and, more positively perhaps, enhance the quality of human life. Politics implies efforts to change or transform these arrangements and efforts to maintain them. Economic and political power includes control of processes of information and representation to serve the interests of the powerful as well as the use of physical force and possession of vital resources such as land, food, water or oil.

On a more personal level, there is a second kind of politics. Here, political power reflects struggles over agency, meaning the ability to choose freely whether to act and what action to take in a given situation. This is a feeling-level politics. But politics also refers to a crucial interplay between these two dimensions, between the private and public dimensions of power. There are connections between economic power and power as expressed on an intimate, domestic level. Power is a process or network as much as a stable factor. This version of political power is demonstrated experientially: in family organization, gender and race relations, and in religious and artistic assumptions as they affect the life of individuals.

Where the public and the private, the political and the personal, intersect or even meld there is a special role for depth psychology in relation to political change and transformation. The tragicomic crisis of our *fin de siècle* civilization incites us to challenge the boundaries that are conventionally accepted as existing between the external world and the internal world, between life and reflection, between extraversion and introversion, between doing and being, between politics and psychology, between the political development of the person and the psychological development of the person, between the fantasies of the political world and the politics of the fantasy world. Subjectivity and intersubjectivity have political roots; they are not as 'internal' as they seem.

The political tasks of modern democracy are similar to the psychological tasks of modern therapy and analysis. In both areas, there is a fight between consciousness, liberation and alterity on the one hand and suppression, repression and omnipotent beliefs in final truths on the other. Psychological and political processes share an uncertain outcome. Hence, the demarcation between the inner world of psychology and the outer world of politics has no permanent existence. The *Umwelt* is both inside and outside. This congruency of politics and depth psychology is demonstrated by the ubiquity of political metaphors that can depict personality: the 'government' signifies the ego, the 'citizens' signify constellations of object relations, social problems signify psychopathology. In this chapter, I do not in fact make use of notions such as 'the class system inside one's head', but I do draw conclusions from the existence of such notions about public referents of private matters.

From its beginnings, depth psychology has been interested in the world of politics. In his paper entitled 'The claims of psycho-analysis to the interest of the non-psychological sciences', written in 1913, Freud staked a claim for the proactive capacity of psychoanalysis

> to throw light on the origins of our great cultural institutions – on religion, morality, justice, and philosophy ... Our knowledge of the neurotic illnesses of individuals has been of much assistance to our understanding of the great social institutions.[3]

Jung made a similar point about the relationship of depth psychology and politics in a more reactive vein in 1946 in his preface to a collection of his essays on Nazi Germany:

> We are living in times of great disruption: political passions are aflame, internal upheavals have brought nations to the brink of chaos . . . This critical state of things has such a tremendous influence on the psychic life of the individual that the analyst ... feels the violence of its impact even in the quiet of his consulting room ... The psychologist cannot avoid coming to grips with contemporary history, even if his very soul shrinks from the political uproar, the lying propaganda, and the jarring speeches of the demagogues. We need not mention his duties as a citizen, which confront him with a similar task.[4]

At times, it seems that Freud and Jung were as interested in the broad sweep of cultural evolution and in an engagement with collective psychology as they were in their day-to-day work with patients. Certainly, there is a tension between their cultural and clinical projects and this is a tension that is still with their descendants today. In the last twenty-five years, we have witnessed the growth of psychoanalysis as an academic discipline, whether as a human, social or emancipatory science. The same is now beginning to happen in analytical psychology (inevitably, twenty-five years later). Of course, the origins of this intellectual movement go much further back to 'Freudian' writers like Harold Lasswell, Jürgen Habermas, Herbert Marcuse, Erich Fromm and Norman O. Brown, or to 'Jungians' like Mircea Eliade and Herbert Read.

The gulf between depth psychology in the academy and depth psychology in the clinic is at its widest in Britain and in the United States, but even in Europe we can see signs of a similar rift. Academic depth psychology might involve a close textual study of Freud's writings or comparative work that sets Freud alongside Heidegger or other important thinkers. Literary and film criticism, cultural and gender studies, psychohistory and psychobiography, sectors within anthropology, sociology and political studies – all may quite fairly be reckoned as aligned with academic depth psychology. Research into the outcome of psychotherapeutic treatment and diagnostic studies may also be understood as academic. Though academic depth psychology often seems more at home with an insertion into the political field than clinical depth psychology does, it lacks a vehicle for engaging with political issues in a pragmatic form while retaining a psychological orientation.

However, something new is rambling within the clinical world. In 1991, just before the Gulf War, a protest meeting was called in London by the Medical Campaign Against Nuclear Weapons and the Study Group on Psychosocial Issues in the Nuclear Age. It was held at the Institute of Psychoanalysis, a highly significant fact in itself, and psychoanalysts were prominent on the platform. What is more, over a quarter of the members of the British Psychoanalytical Society have joined a group called Psychoanalysts for the Prevention of Nuclear War.[5] In Britain, and all over the world, clinicians and some who have voluntarily given up clinical practice are arguing and writing about politics in a way that they did not just a few years ago.

It seems that the existence of a rupture between depth psychology in the consulting room and depth psychology in the political world is being challenged, if not exactly closed. One can tell that something significant *is* going on by the existence of fierce opposition to it from those who regard the clinical as an untouchable, privileged category, on the basis of its contribution to the alleviation of human suffering.[6]

Although I abhor that kind of clinical triumphalism, I do not suggest in this chapter that we should close all the consulting rooms. This is because I can see that clinical practice may be something other than a bastion of possessive individualism and narcissistic introspection. It is right to criticize myopic (and greedy) clinicians who cannot apperceive that their work has a political and cultural location and implication. But it is not right to indulge in simplistic thinking that would do away with the entire clinical project of depth psychology. *Without their connection to a clinical core, why should anyone listen to analysts at all?* The rejection of the clinical forecloses what is, for me, the central issue: the relations between the private and the public spheres of life. This foreclosure mimics the attitude of the most conservative, dyed-in-the-wool clinicians and mental health professionals. The high-profile apostates of therapy are as terrified of exploring the relations between the personal and the political as are the fanatical professional adherents of therapy.[7]

The patients who come to see analysts and therapists are playing a part in these debates. In Chapter 10 [of *The Political Psyche*, not included in this selection], I give the results of a questionnaire that was sent to analysts and psychotherapists in several countries. The questionnaire concerned political material brought to the consulting room, its prevalence, and how it is handled by the practitioner. From the survey, it seems clear that such material is being brought more frequently than before to the clinical setting, that the range of themes and problems covered is immense, that these do not invariably reflect the social situation or obvious preoccupations of the particular patient, and that practitioners are a bit puzzled as to how to interpret such material. *Through this survey, I have found that practitioners are more reluctant than I thought they would be to interpret political material in terms of the internal world of the patient.* I can confirm this puzzlement from my own experience. During the Gulf crisis of 1990–1, I was struck not only by how some patients employed war imagery to express their internal states (predicted by theory), but also by how some patients communicated what looked like inner world material when actually they had a deep desire to talk about the Gulf crisis (not predicted by theory).

Depth psychology's area of inquiry is moving on to make a new connection with the world of politics. However, I do not agree with the conceit that the unconscious itself has moved on and now resides outside the individual in the external world. The unconscious cannot be reified like that – and in any case who could doubt that the unconscious has always already been in the world as well as in the individual. The very idea of unconscious influence on action suggests that the unconscious itself influences the relations between the individual and the world. What has changed is our perception of what depth psychology can and should do. Maybe it is now the turn of the external world to receive the ministrations of the depth psychologists. Maybe it is the external world that now clamours for our attention, for there is certainly much political pain and disease 'out there' (as we say). But first we have to find out whether the political world *does* want something from depth psychology.

In spite of these developments, it has to be admitted that there is an intense reluctance in the non-psychological community to accept the many and varied ideas and suggestions concerning political matters that have been or are being offered by analysts of every persuasion. I do not believe this reluctance can all be put down to resistance. There is something quite offensive about reductive interpretations of complex sociopolitical problems in exclusively psychological terms. The tendency to pan-psychism on the part of some depth psychologists has led me to wonder if any adequate methodology and ethos actually exist to make an engagement of depth psychology with the public sphere possible.[8]

Depth psychology concerns a person's subjective experience of social and cultural structures, and that is valuable in itself. But in this chapter I want to ask: is there a special psychology of and for politics and culture? If so, what does the clinical practice of analysis and therapy with individuals or small groups contribute to the forming of such a psychology? And, conversely, I ask: what does a perspective taken from cultural or political analysis contribute to a clinical analysis of an individual or small therapy group? In what way is the personal political – and in what way is the political personal? Can these questions be answered without recourse to a totalizing politics, in a way that preserves and celebrates difference and diversity? A depth psychological approach to politics needs to be a humble one.

Depth psychology can help with these queries. In spite of claims that the age of psychology is over, we may be entering a period of cultural evolution in which it will become easier to work out the possible contribution of depth psychology to social science and politics. Modern social theory is concerned with identity, with difference, and with the relations between identity and difference. How am I wholly and unmistakably myself? How am I part of the mass, similar to or the same as others? These questions, which constitute the *cri de cœur* of what Anthony Giddens calls 'late modernity', shove us in the direction of psychology.[9] These are the pressing questions that the analytic patient brings to the consulting room – even in group therapy. And these are the crucial questions about that patient that the analyst has to contend with – to what extent can I encounter this person as a unique human being, to what extent must I react to him or her as a typical patient, to what extent as a combination of these? The political dimension of these psychological questions was summarized by Aristotle: 'Similars do not constitute a state.' Nor, we may add, do people with nothing at all in common.[10]

The characteristic of late modernity to try to make use of knowledge about itself can be recast as a struggle within our culture to become self-conscious; *our culture struggles to become psychological.* Moreover, the pervasive presence of *doubt*, even 'radical doubt', as a 'feature of modern critical reason' and as a 'general existential dimension of the contemporary social world', suggests that the psychology that is already being embraced by late modernity is depth psychology, the psychology of not knowing, of unknowing, of interpretation and reinterpretation.

The late modern (and, if you like, the postmodern) age has reorganized the categories of time, space and place, using technology to deliteralize and overcome them, permitting the exercise of power-at-a-distance. In its overturning of the laws of nature, the age itself more and more resembles the unconscious. The speedy and multilevelled tone of life at the close of the twentieth century means that we often do not know what it is that has hurt or disturbed us though we do know we have been hurt or disturbed. We may only know what it was after the event. Such 'deferred action', to use the standard mistranslation of Freud's *Nachträglichkeit,* means that we are condemned to afterwardness and retrospection, required to fashion our response to hurtful and disturbing social changes out of a backward-looking stance.[11] No wonder there has been an explosion of nostalgias.

Psychological reductionism

Here is an example of the difficulty with psychological reductionism to which I referred earlier. At a conference, a distinguished psychoanalyst referred to the revolutionary students in Paris in 1968 as 'functioning as a regressive group.'[12] Now, for a large group of students to be said to regress, there must be, in the speaker's mind, some sort of normative developmental starting point for them to regress to. The social group is supposed to have a babyhood, as it were. Similarly, the speaker must have had in mind the possibility of a healthier, progressive group process – what a more mature group of revolutionary students would have looked like. This 'regressive group of students' stunned nearly every intellectual in France and also fatally wounded Marxism. The regressive group was so effective that it forced an intelligentsia already intimately concerned with political issues to throw up its hands and realize the urgent need to retheorize politics. Not bad for a psychologically immature group. Be this as it may, my main point here is to emphasize that complex social and political phenomena do not conform to the individualistic, chronological, moralistic, pathologizing framework that is often applied in a mechanical way by depth psychological commentators.

The problem of reductionism does not stem from having a therapeutic *attitude* to the pathologies of culture as these are expressed in political issues. Rather, the problem stems from approaching an entire culture, or large chunks of it, *as if it were an individual or even as if it were a baby.* In this infantalization of culture, depth psychology deploys a version of personality development couched in judgmental terms to understand a collective cultural and political process. If we look in this manner for pathology in the culture, we will surely find it. If we are looking with a particular psychological theory in mind, then, lo and behold, the theory will explain the pathology. But this is a retrospective prophecy (to use a phrase of Freud's)[13] – twenty-twenty hindsight. In this psychological tautologizing there is really nothing much to get excited about. Too much depth psychological writing on the culture, my own included, has suffered from this kind of smug correctness when the 'material' proves the theoretical point. Of course it does! If we are interested in envy or greed, then we will find envy or greed in capitalistic organization. If we set out to demonstrate the presence of archetypal patterns, such as projection of the shadow, in the geopolitical relations of the superpowers, then, without a doubt, they will seem to leap out at us. But so often this is just more of the maddening rectitude of the analyst who has forgotten that we influence what we analyze. Psychological reflection on culture and politics needs to be muted; there is not as much 'aha!' as pioneers, such as the Frankfurt School, hoped for.

I am sure that this chapter cannot solve all the problems or answer all the questions I have mentioned. In the 1920s the Russian Futurist poet Vladimir Mayakovsky wrote that 'art is not a mirror to reflect the world, but a hammer with which to shape it.' I think depth psychology might try to reflect *and* shape the world, doing it as part of a multidisciplinary project, and in a mixture of styles ranging from exegetical sobriety to playfulness *to something quite frankly irrational.* In these diverse ways, we may find out more about the interplays between (a) personality development and social structure, (b) the private, intrapsychic world of an individual and the public, political system in which he or she is embedded, and (c) psychic reality and sociopolitical reality. The political world is today's uncanny (*Unheimlich*); something that was familiar (*heimisch*) has slipped out of the grasp of consciousness.

Psyche, culture and resacralization

It has never been more difficult to make a psychological analysis of politics for, in our day, every institution and element in culture is undergoing fragmentation and Balkanization. It has become harder and harder to see what political arrangements can hold societies together. Moments at which one apprehends a social unity have become as precious and vulnerable as those revelatory and mystical moments when one experiences a personal unity.

Increasingly, the fragility and disunity of our culture provokes a reaction arising out of a sense of the underlying oneness of the world – a holistic response. But, for me, the problem with the re-emergence in our day of cosmic visions of a unified world is that a sense of oneness tends to generate only one particular kind of truth. Moreover, proclaiming the indissoluble unity of a world soul may be little more than a *defensive* reaction to atomization. Advancing holism as if it were *the* solution is not an adequate critical response to the drama of cultural diversity. Holism founders on the sea of the discontinuities of life, for holism is secretly highly rational and ordered and cannot abide irrationality or a messiness in which its Truth has to coexist with lots of truths. A unified viewpoint has to find some kind of articulation with a diversity of viewpoints; this, holism finds difficult.

My approach here is not holistic. I want to take those anxiety-provoking ideas of cultural fragmentation, fracture and complexity, and re-imagine them as the very tools of the trade of psychological analysis of cultural political processes. Let us take our sense of fragmentation, fracture and complexity as *healing* as well as wounding to a sense of political and social empowerment. It follows that we have to try to engage with a diverse and fragmented culture by means of an analysis that sees through its own fantasy of homogeneity, is already itself diverse and fragmented, and seeks out complexity. Rousseau referred to 'the language of the heart' and I suppose that, in our day, we have to begin to speak the languages of the hearts.

Amidst the tragic anomie and baffling atomization, amidst the dreadful conformism of 'international' architecture, telecommunications and cuisine, amidst the sense of oppression and fear of a horrific future, amidst war itself, there is an equally fragmented, fractured and complex attempt at a *resacralization of the culture* going on. People have risen to the challenge and there are many diverse surface signs of resacralization: New Age or New Times thought, expressions of concern for the quality of life, green politics, feminism, demands for the rights of ethnic minorities, the human potential movement, liberation theology, gay activism, finding God in the new physics. I would even include trying to engage depth psychology with politics on this deliberately diverse list; I certainly do not want to leave myself out! It is suspicious that depth psychologists concerned with the public sphere have not paid much attention to *themselves* as a cultural phenomenon. I would go so far as to say that depth psychology itself may be regarded as one of the precursors of late twentieth-century resacralization. A depth psychologist has as a credo that he or she is 'in' whatever is being analyzed, whether patient, political problematic, or art work. I can readily understand objections to resacralization that find the linkage of depth psychology and fundamentalist religion difficult to stomach. It was hard for me, at first. But if one's goal is to track and speak up about such connections, then there is little alternative to leaving such shocking linkages out in the open. Perhaps the objections also have something to do with the differences between depth psychology and philosophy. While some philosophers might pay lip service to the impossibility of maintaining the observer/observed boundary, this often is not reflected in their experience-distant texts.

The groups and movements I have listed vary in the degree to which they seek fundamental changes in society as a whole; some of them have quite particular, sectional interests to pursue. Nevertheless, I see this heterogeneous phenomenon – resacralization – as held together by aspirational rather than socioeconomic ties. In fairness, I do not assume that only left-leaning, so-called progressive political and religious movements partake in resacralization. Born-again Christians, Islamic fundamentalists and the Lubavitch Jews are part of the same trend. In different forms, of course, resacralization is also a way to describe what has been happening in Eastern Europe and the former Soviet Union. Across the world, people have risen to the challenge of resacralization. It is the spiritual longings of ordinary people that have fuelled these movements – and perhaps all the more progressive political and cultural projects of the twentieth century. The resacralizing perspective recovers a sense of the religious verities but these are played through a changing world view less dependent on religious organization. The resacralizing ethic may be plebeian in its roots, but it is sublime in its aspirations.

Clearly I think that all these developments are extremely important. They may contain elements of a successful resolution of some of our most vexing dilemmas. *But I also think that, in their present form, they are at risk of failing* and the consequences of failure will be serious even for those who feel out of sympathy with many or all of the facets of resacralization.

As I said, I think these spontaneous movements are surface signs that there is something politically transformative going on. I want to suggest that resacralization is our contemporary attempt to shift a sense of holiness into the secular and material world. Let us look at holiness. The roots of holiness do not only lie in God or in a transpersonal realm. They also lie in humanity's *making* of holiness. We make holiness by the designation and construction of sacred spaces (which we call temples). We make holiness by the performance of sacred acts (such as sacrifice and repentance). I doubt that contemporary resacralization will ultimately glorify God or lead to a new religion. But, along the way, most aspects of human culture will be touched by this attempt to connect to a feeling level that we sense once existed but find has vanished from the modern world (hence resacralization). I think that, at the very least, this involves a search for a new ethical basis for society. In its preoccupation with the discovery of meaning, depth psychology has vectored in on the same search.

The notion that holiness is located in the material, social world is not a new one. For many, religious and non-religious alike, the world has long held a Chassidic gleam. Since my childhood, I have been fascinated by God's detailed instructions to the Children of Israel about how to build the Ark of the Covenant (not to mention the Tabernacle, or, earlier, Noah's Ark). In the divine detail of the construction, we see how ineffable holiness depends on every single joint, bevel, dimension, and the material used:

> And Bezaleel made the ark of shittim wood: two cubits and a half was the length of it, and a cubit and a half the breadth of it, and a cubit and a half the height of it. And he overlaid it with pure gold within and without, and made a crown of gold to it round about. And he cast for it four rings of gold, to be set by the four corners of it; even two rings upon the one side of it, and two rings upon the other side of it. And he made staves of shittim wood, and overlaid them with gold. And he put the staves into the rings by the side of the ark, to bear the ark.[14]

Bezaleel's name is hardly ever mentioned, not even in the film *Raiders of the Lost Ark*! Yet he is the collective image and cultural personification of resacralization, the contemporary drive to render the secular holy as a creative response to the fate of God.

This is why, for many, resacralization has indeed taken the form of a return to religion. This is sometimes established religion, sometimes archaic (or apparently archaic) religion. However, as a depth psychologist, I have to engage with resacralization in a different way. To do so, it is not essential to support or to believe in resacralization, and many do not. What is essential is to try to pick up on the psychology of what is happening in this particular piece of cultural process. I want to make something psychological, but not exclusively or excessively psychological, out of a host of social and political impressions. The idea is to bring something up and out that is *already* there – so these words of mine about resacralization are intended to be description, chronicle and interpretation, not sermon or advocacy, nor anything beyond an indirect contribution to resacralization itself. The parallel is with clinical analysis, in which the analyst can do no more than foster a process in which potentials within the patient are brought into consciousness.

One specific impression is of a growing collective sense of disgust, in both Western culture and the once-communist states, with the political world in whose making we have participated. Disgust is lurking alongside the shallowness and cruelty of much of modern life; our subjectivity is full of it. As Thomas Mann put it, 'Our capacity for disgust is in proportion to the intensity of our attachment to the things of this world.'[15] Disgust with our present politics leads us to aspire to a resacralized and reformed politics in which political openness and unpredictability lead to faith and hope rather than to fear and disgust. To achieve this, we need a new psychological valuing of the potential of political engagement itself. Involvement in the mess and confusion of the external world and passionate political commitment to that world are as psychologically valuable as an interior perspective or an intimate I–thou relationship. Political involvement *can* certainly be a means of avoiding personal conflicts or acting out such conflicts, leaving others to do the changing. But political involvement can surely also be a means of expressing what is best in humans, acknowledging the fact of our social being, that we are not the isolated, solipsistic monads that some psychological theories might lead us to believe we are.

A more evolved and realistic attitude to politics is something to work on in the consulting room, just as we work on more evolved and realistic attitudes to sexuality, spirituality and aggression. I will propose that analysts (and patients, too) begin to work out models that enable us to refer to a person's *innate political potential*, to his or her state of *political development*, and to the *apolitical level of the psyche*. In clinical practice, such a model would enable us to generate new readings of personal and collective *political imagery*. We may even find that there is *a politics of imagery* and that *countertransference and politics* are linked. Political imagery will be as fluid and unpredictable in its display of what is (or claims to be) positive and what is (or seems to be) negative as any other kind of imagery. Not all political imagery presents the worst case for humanity. For example, in Chapter 4 [of *The Political Psyche*] I attempt a psychological analysis of the imagery in Machiavelli's political thought to find out how an engagement with the political level of the psyche affects depth psychology and how depth psychology affects political theorizing. Here, I want once more to emphasize that *the core of my project is to move toward an end of the isolation of the consulting room, though not toward the end of clinical analysis itself*, and to work out the detail of a serious relationship between depth psychology and politics rather than huff and puff at the absence of such a relationship. (I discuss the role of the clinical project throughout *The Political Psyche*.)

Our culture (and not just our culture) is longing to atone for its social injustices and the sense of disgust it feels for them, longing to be able to think good thoughts about itself and rid itself of depressive preoccupation with its own destructiveness, longing for a resacralized politics. When depression infects a political system, the first victim is any capacity to find imaginative solutions to political problems. This is because depression leads to an awful literalism in which fantasy and actuality are hopelessly muddled. Collective fantasies of hate and aggression are taken literally, leading to depressive guilt (for example, over the possession of nuclear weapons) and mass delusional self-reproach. The problem is how to contain and integrate disgust on this scale without either repressing it or acting it out.[16]

On the political level, many are full of guilty contempt for capitalism (and for what passed for socialism in the East). But there is a lack of any cultural ritual by which reparation and repentance can be made. Lacking ritual and a symbolic language with which to express this unease and disgust, and the desire to atone, many resacralizers tend to make a split between the constructive and the cheating sides of capitalism and the market economy, preferring to see only the negative side. Perhaps in response, a group with a totally opposite ideology of support for capitalism and the market has emerged. If we do not do something about this split in our political culture, then, hard though it is to face, resacralization, so ardently sought by so many, will not take place; it will not work. To be specific: resacralization seems to be characterized by an attempt to construct a shadow-free politics in which the dark side is located somewhere else – in men, in whites, in the market, and so forth. Even when resacralizers do get involved with politics, it is a half-hearted involvement, distinguished, psychologically speaking, by a fear of getting dirty hands. I want to explore the damaging contents of this split.

On the *negative* side, there are fantasies of an apocalyptic end, whether by nuclear conflagration, an AIDS pandemic, or the greenhouse effect. All these are blamed on capitalism and the market economy. Certainly, these anxieties are rooted in reality and resacralizers are right to point this out. But taken as fantasies, they are the deepest signs of a self-punishing contempt for ourselves. Perhaps many people think we deserve to perish like this. On the *positive* side, there are other voices, not at all persuaded by the arguments of resacralizers, claiming to be 'realistic', extolling the virtues of capitalism and the workings of the market as the source of the material benefits that 'we' enjoy today and as the only economic system that seems to work.

Sometimes it seems that those involved in resacralization try to manage their disgust and guilt at the excesses of capitalism and the market economy by attempting to make reparation and repentance over literally – by making it up to the entire planet. There will be many good things to come out of the environmental movement but a prudish and facile environmentalism may not have enough psychological depth, enough connection to the dirt it seeks to cleanse, to ease the unease and even the disease in the culture. In Chapter 5 [of *The Political Psyche*], I consider whether there is a way to transform the dreams of environmentalists into pragmatic politics and hence make social realities out of them.

The market

This form of negative/positive split can be very clearly seen in relation to the market economy. Is the market economy a socially divisive rich man's charter, as even erstwhile supporters of it are beginning to say in Britain or the United States? Or is the market economy the road to freedom and dignity as many now seem to think in Eastern Europe and the former Soviet Union? Or is it the best available synthesis, a good compromise? Or – and this is the line I intend to take – is it both a negative and a positive phenomenon *at the same time,* with the negative and positive verdicts each having a distinct psychology of their own that resists synthesis and compromise? In this way of looking at the market economy, our negative and positive images of it are not split off from each other; indeed, they each guarantee the existence of the other for there will be no chance of realizing the positive features of the market economy *without* accepting the *simultaneous* presence of its negative features. It is relatively easy for a cultural critic to reject the Manichean, crude, psychologically primitive, split approach in which the market must be good or bad. But the approach that attempts a balanced view of the market is almost as problematic, psychologically speaking. In the so-called 'balanced' approach, which is supposed to 'heal' the split, there is a difficulty in integrating the undoubtedly unfair and ruthless features of free market economics, seeing as they *have to be* present for the benefits of the market to be available. Resacralizers need to come to terms with this. We are not talking of unfortunate by-products of the market; according to this psychological analysis, they are its *sine qua non* and cannot be ameliorated. We need to know more about the psychology of the market as a negative phenomenon *and* about the psychology of the market as a positive phenomenon. Both psychologies are relevant for resacralization. Resacralizers cannot stay pure, above, or outside the economic world. Disgust cannot be transcended to order; *there is no shadow-free politics.* Resacralization will have defeated itself as much as having been defeated by patriarchal exploitation and other reactionary forces.

Many sensitive and intelligent commentators have pointed out that the apparent triumph of capitalism is a moment for self-reflection. This is because market forces have already invaded or colonized most aspects of life. There is a need now to work on the development of a sense of community: caring, compassionate reaching out to the less well-off. But a sense of community that does not address the shadow of community – the totalitarian shadow of community – will be thin, dessicated, morally elevated classroom civics, and socially useless. We will not be able to limit or tame market forces unless we comprehend their psychological nature and the powerful imagery involved in such forces. To understand the market requires political imagination and imagination about politics. There is no either/or about politics; nor is there an average. Politics is certainly the art of speculating, calculating, secret agreements and pragmatic manoeuvering. But politics is also the art of making the world and the people in it better. There are *some* connections between these two distinct and separate images of politics that we should not ignore.

Our inability to stay in emotional contact with the psychologically distinct and separate images of the market makes it difficult to concentrate on the psychological issues of resacralization that are central to notions of economic and political change. Here, I am sure that *economics* can be a *psychological* focus. In Chapter 4 [of *The Political Psyche*], in order to concentrate on splits within the image of the market economy, I enlist the aid of the myth of Hermes to help us to hold onto both sides – positive and negative, enthusiasm and disgust – of our evaluation of the market economy. A political reworking of the myth of Hermes can provide a base for an approach that avoids the dangers of splitting *and* of trying to reach a supposedly balanced view. To the extent that there are opposite feelings in the air about the market, it is very hard, emotionally, to hold on to these as necessarily existing opposites without having recourse to either a schizoid, judgmental retreat or to glib sloganizing about accepting the bad with the good. As I said, we do need to know more about the psychology of the market as a positive phenomenon *and* about the psychology of the market as a negative phenomenon. Then, perhaps, we could move on to try to work out the psychology of the market without the introduction of the categories 'positive' and 'negative'.

For the moment, we do have to let 'positive' and 'negative' structure our psychological response to market economics. But there is a hidden gain in this. For maintaining an attitude of evaluation and judgment enables us to see to what extent the preceding ideas about attitudes to and images of the market are relevant outside Western, capitalistic culture.

It sometimes seems that the *Zeitgeist* in what was the Soviet Union and in Eastern Europe is quite different from that of the West. In the West, criticisms of the excesses of free market economics are beginning to surface in circles that had, hitherto, been gung ho for the market. For example, it seems that the long sentence passed on Michael Milken, the 'junk bond king', was 'widely seen as public retribution for the excesses of the 80s', resulting from 'public anger over the ethics of the age'.[17] Kevin Phillips, a one-time senior aide of President Reagan, published a bestselling book in 1990 entitled *The Politics of Rich and Poor* in which he prophesied the end of an ethical and political climate that permitted 'the triumph of upper America – an ostentatious celebration of wealth, the political ascendancy of the richest third of the population and a glorification of capitalism, free markets and finance.'[18]

In the East (and in many parts of the Third World), things seem to be going the other way. In progressive circles, the free market is hailed not only as the sole means to revive moribund economies, but also as a means to political and spiritual revival. However, I wonder if the two completely different political situations do not share some psychological features in common. Both kinds of society are fascinated, even obsessed by the market; the one eager now to condemn it, the other to praise and implement it. Both have the same difficulty in getting beyond a verdict that is either good or bad. Both seem to sense the limitations of the 'balanced' view. We see this in the former Soviet Union in the popular rejection of Gorbachev's idea of a 'third way' incorporating what was best in communism and in capitalism. We see it in the United States in the almost total disagreement about what can be done to ease the plight of the so-called underclass (including intense argument over whether such a grouping actually exists).[19] Crucially, in both West and East, modes of economic and political organization are seen nowadays as inseparable from psychological, ethical and spiritual themes. One Russian commentator had this to say: 'The main thing is for people to learn to be human. If we have bread and still become beasts, there will be no reason for us to live.'[20] Surface differences between Western and Eastern attitudes to the market mask a deeper psychological similarity.

Of course, we shall have to wait to see what, if anything, the psychosocial impact of a new Russian middle class will be.[21] But the psychological dimension is demonstrated in a comment made by a Russian political commentator in 1991: 'Our people are fed up with the free market without having lived in it for a single day.'[22]

I have not merely been proposing that our epoch *needs* resacralizing and encouraging people to do it. I am arguing that resacralization is already going on, and has a life of its own running underneath the development of technology and a hyper-rational way of life. As I said, I am trying to bring something to consciousness – to cultural consciousness – that is already there in culture. It is an analyst's way of making politics. And it is as an analyst that I have found myself thinking that, from a psychological point of view in which depth common denominators are given more weight than surface discrepancies, everything I have written about 'our' culture (meaning Western culture) is, paradoxically, *exemplified* by what has been happening in Eastern Europe since the late 1980s. The imagery from two differing contexts is not disconnected.

Numinous experience and sociopolitical criticism

I feel that split-inducing collective disgust would be moderated by a sense that culture can be transformed through a resacralized politics. The psychic energy locked up in disgust and cultural depression would be employed in a less masochistic way – in a more practical way, like Bezaleel's, with his sacred box. When considering such a political commitment, it is unavoidable that religious language and imagery, if not religion itself, will have a part to play. Here, the role played by the churches in the political changes of Eastern Europe should be borne in mind. One cannot imagine an expression of the more caring and compassionate side of liberal democracy without religious terms. We need to look again, more psychologically and more generously, at what we regard as sacred. Beneath and within the fractured surface of contemporary Western culture lies a protoreligious culture (and this is also shown clearly by events in Eastern Europe and in the emergence of liberation theology in Latin America). We can see the culture's attempts to resacralize itself in its extreme openness to numinous experience – not always along decorous lines, and including the ritually pagan: sexual experimentation, rock music, sports, food, fashion, money, collectible things. Maybe the best way to find the sacred today would be to submit and surrender to the apparently pagan.

However, political resacralization is not identical with religion or religious revival. In the latter case, there is usually or often a programme to be followed, a prescription, a recipe. What I perceive in resacralization is the marking out and making of a place – a social temple – in which something politically transformative can be born. The resacralizing place is also designed for self-reflection and the recovery of personal dignity.

In religious, mystical or holistic experiences, the individual is seized and controlled by something outside himself or herself that is possessed of a fascinating and awe-inspiring power. Such a power, in Jung's words, makes one feel 'its victim rather than its creator'.[23] This kind of experience was described by Rudolf Otto in *The Idea of the Holy* in 1917 as numinous experience. Otto was at pains to stress the paradox that, though the numinous experience was irrational, it could be analyzed rationally; an important point to remember concerning depth psychological analysis of politics. We can be rational about the irrational and honour both dimensions while so doing; we can be secular and social about the holy and the sacred. Nevertheless, the irrational *is* irrational. Otto, in fine German academic style, lists his criteria for the irrational:

> Pure fact in contrast to law, the empirical in contrast to reason, the contingent in contrast to the necessary, the psychological in contrast to transcendental fact, that which is known *a posteriori* in contrast to that which is determinable *a priori;* power, will, and arbitrary choice in contrast to reason, knowledge, and determination by value; impulse, instinct, and the obscure forces of the subconscious in contrast to insight, reflection, and intelligible plan; mystical depths and stirrings in the soul, surmise, presentiment, intuition, prophecy and finally the 'occult' powers also; or, in general, the uneasy stress and universal fermentation of the time, with its groping after the thing never yet heard or seen in poetry or the plastic arts – all these and many more may claim the names 'non-rational', 'irrational'.[24]

It is remarkable that Otto, the author of one of the most influential works on religious psychology and the psychology of religion, publishing in the revolutionary year of 1917, should perceive in the 'uneasy stress and universal fermentation of the time' a groping not for a rational system as a form of panacea (such as Marxism) but for the nub of the irrational itself – the *numen.* I want to take this statement of Otto's as an account not only of the raw material of a psychological analysis of political process, but also of the orientation of the political analyst. It is a kind of clarion call to pay attention to what seems absurd and trivial, as well as to what seems dignified and profound. What is 'deep' (as in 'depth' psychology) may be on the surface.

Reacting to Otto has led me to muse on the styles or, perhaps more accurately, the tropes of depth psychology in its attempt to do cultural and political analysis. We need to introduce the irrational into our discourse on politics: measures of exaggeration, grotesquerie, vulgarity and broad comedy, making a social critique out of these just as the unconscious itself sometimes manages to. For example, the wild and compelling imagery of aggressive fantasy eventually promotes concern for other people. The hidden social *telos* of aggressive fantasy, the covert function it serves, the thing that it is secretly for, is the fostering of an emergence of concern. Without my base and sordid aggressive fantasies in the direction of another, there would be less need for concern about him or her on my part.

Similarly, the seductive and shifting fantasies of sexual selfhood that I call 'gender confusions' respond to a political and prospective reading, leading to a far more positive and welcoming evaluation than the one usually given by analysts. In the future, we will all become even more confused about gender. Provided we stay close to the confusion and the confused experience and do not try for an instant escape by 'androgyny' or flee into 'gender certainty', and provided we keep our judgmental tendencies under control, then the earthy challenge to the established order represented by gender confusions may move onto an ever more practical, collective, political level. (See Chapter 7 [of *The Political Psyche*] for a further discussion of gender confusion.[25])

As I see it, the tasks of depth psychologists who seek to engage with the political are to locate the enormous psychic energy that is presently locked up in collective and subjective self-disgust, and to try to release the energy so that it becomes available for political renewal. If depth psychology is to make a contribution on a political level to the processes of resacralization of which it is already an unconscious part, it must surely continue to engage with the irrational and numinous aspects of life. Depth psychology can attempt to work these into a social and political analysis of culture. But this fantastic and original project cannot always be carried on within a rational or moral framework. A politics of transformation can hardly be totally rational. However, working with the irrational and the amoral is the forte of depth psychology. In Donald Williams's words: 'The greatest possibilities for wisdom in the psyche come from its immediate aliveness to new, current and contemporary sources that take advantage of its innate adaptability and resourcefulness.'[26]

To be sure, as I mentioned, this brings up matters of style and, at the same time, something more than style is involved. For what looks like a matter of style is also relevant to the concrete contribution depth psychology can make to the social sciences, especially politics. It may be that it is the general areas of interest that depth psychology covers that earn it the right to be taken seriously by social scientists, as Ian Craib has suggested. He saw the central features of depth psychology as (a) its concern with the irrational, (b) its focus on emotions, (c) its apprehension of the complexity of personality, and (d) its concern for creativity (including, in Craib's listing, religion and artistic production) and for morality.[27] Depth psychology reaches the parts of human nature other disciplines, such as sociology, do not reach: 'The complexity and conflict of people's emotional lives, . . . the profound ambiguities of motivation and meaning, . . . the strange and often difficult relationships we have with our bodies.'[28]

I want to take this clarion call of Ian Craib's and rotate it through 180 degrees. The central features of depth psychology, meaning the areas it has staked a claim for in the knowledge-battle, may also be the ways and styles in which it should make its contribution to social science. Not only saying something *about* irrationality, emotion, personality, creativity, morality – but saying something *with and through* these thematics, and with and through dream, fantasy and passion. The style of a depth psychological contribution to an understanding of political process should be congruent with what depth psychology has habitually done, while not reducing one field to the other. We should focus on a particular political problem in terms of its irrational aspects, the emotions (and hence the images) it engenders in our subjective experience of the problem, the complexity of the issue as it impacts on people's evolving personal lives, and the ways in which what is going on speak of the fostering or negating of human creativity and moral sensibility.

This idea is strengthened by noting that many of the criticisms of attempts to link depth psychology to social and political issues have settled on the oversystematized, hyper-rational, mechanical nature of these 'applications'. In particular, the project of combining Freud and Marx to create a politics of the subject(ive) has degenerated into an obsession with Freud – the man and his texts – and a preoccupation with the work of Jacques Lacan that, for many, has cut psychoanalysis off from those very features of itself that could make a distinctive contribution to social science (as listed, for example, by Craib, above). While these failings are not going to be totally absent from my book [*The Political Psyche*], I have tried to be aware of them. Hopefully, this enables me to ask:

Can social theory truly respond to the challenge of telling us who we are as subjects and what our place in cultural process might be *without* its taking account of a realm of interiority? This, in turn, leads to exploration of the various criticisms of depth psychological accounts of subjectivity that have been mounted.

Before concluding the chapter, I want briefly to make some distinctions about the ways I am using the overlapping terms 'subjectivity' and 'the personal' and how these relate to 'the irrational'. *Subjectivity* is a perspective on things that tends toward direct experience of them and an evaluative response fashioned out of direct experience, however illusory that might be from a philosophical standpoint. The sensation of direct experience remains even when the intellect is aware that one experiences things through ideological filters and that subjective experience is itself culturally and politically constructed. In addition, I see the body as a prime source (and recipient) of subjective experience and of subjectivity.

I regard *the personal* as being implicated in the identity/difference theme that I referred to earlier in the chapter. This implies a sense of boundary, however permeable ('skin-ego'), and hence a potential for relationship. The narrative and mythology of people's lives contribute to their sense of what is personal of and for them.

The irrational can scarcely be comprehended without reference to its spouse: rationality. Moreover, what is and is not considered irrational is highly variable according to personal, historical and cultural features. However, when attempting to factor subjectivity and the personal into political discourse, there is little doubt that a sense of irrationality will (and ought to be) generated from time to time.

These distinctions are the background to the 180-degree turn I proposed earlier in which the central concerns of depth psychology are revisioned as the tools with which to make an analysis of a political problem: irrationality, subjectivity, the personal dimension, and a focus on creativity and morality.

As I said, the way in which depth psychology engages with political themes is both a matter of style and, at the same time, something more. On the stylistic and on other levels, I return in *The Political Psyche* to the topic at many moments – a sign that I find myself unable to reach a conclusion about the balance between rational and irrational elements in my text. Perhaps what is needed at the present time is a more generous conception of what is 'serious' and 'scholarly' in writing. Maybe we are on the verge of a revolution in our understanding of what constitutes scholarly, academic and intellectual writing, based on the realization that many apparently discursive texts in the human sciences are full of rhetoric. An antithesis between scholarly and imaginative writing can itself be an obstacle to the success of a text in either mode.

Sometimes depth psychologists will seek to accomplish their political tasks irrationally, making use of the least rational psychological function: intuition. Intuition provides a person with a subjective sense of where something is going, of what the possibilities are, without depending on conscious knowledge or empirical proof (though, hopefully, without downgrading these). Hence, intuition moderates the vicissitudes of *Nachträglichkeit,* the deferring of action that, in social terms, condemns us to study the impact of political change only retrospectively, only when it is too late. Though intuition may tend toward prophetic or oracular pronouncement, it also has the capacity to weave empathy, compassion and imagination into social theorizing. Crucially, intuition is required for the conversion of subjective response into sociopolitical criticism.

Notes

1 Sigmund Freud, 'Post-scriptum to a discussion on lay analysis'. *SE* 27: 235. *SE* refers to The Standard Edition of the *Complete Psychological Works of Sigmund Freud*, 24 vols, ed. and trans. James Strachey et al (London: Hogarth Press and The Institute of Psycho-Analysis, 1953–73). References are given by volume and page numbers.
2 The term 'human sciences' derives from Wilhelm Dilthey's distinction between *Naturwissenschaften* and *Geisteswissenschaften*. Dilthey placed psychology among the human sciences. See Michael Ermarth, *Wilhelm Dilthey: The Critique of Historical Reason* (Chicago: Chicago University Press, 1978).
3 Sigmund Freud, 'The claims of psycho-analysis to scientific interest'. *SE* 13: 185–6.
4 C. G. Jung, Preface to *Essays on Contemporary Events*. *CW* 10: p. 11. *CW* refers to the *Collected Works* of C. G. Jung, ed. Herbert Read, Michael Fordham and Gerhard Adler, Trans. R. F. C. Hull (London: Routledge and Kegan Paul; Princeton, NJ: Princeton University Press, 1953–77). References, save where indicated (as in this note), are by volume and paragraph number.
5 Jane Temperley, 'Psychoanalysis and the threat of nuclear war'. In *Crises of the Self: Further Essays on Psychoanalysis and Politics*, ed. Barry Richards (London: Free Association Books, 1989), p. 259.
6 This attitude was exemplified in some of the (often rather abusive) responses I received to the questionnaire on political material brought into the consulting room (see Chapter 10 [of *The Political Psyche*] for a report on this international survey).
7 See Jeffrey Masson, *Against Therapy* (London: Collins, 1989) and James Hillman, 'The yellowing of the work'. In *Personal and Archetypal Dynamics in the Analytical Relationship* (Proceedings of the Eleventh International Congress for Analytical Psychology), ed. Mary Ann Mattoon (Einsiedeln, Switzerland: Daimon Verlag, 1991). Hillman has also expressed his views in numerous newspaper interviews and in James Hillman and Michael Ventura, *We've had a Hundred Years of Psychotherapy and the World's Getting Worse* (San Francisco: Harper, 1992).
8 I am thinking of embarrassing 'psychoanalytic' books like Leo Abse, *Margaret, Daughter of Beatrice* (London: Cape, 1989). In this work, the author, a Labour Member of Parliament, 'analyzes' Mrs Thatcher. From more professional sources, I am thinking of remarks made during the Gulf War about the phallic symbolism of cruise missiles, etc.
9 Anthony Giddens, *Modernity and Self-Identity: Self and Society in the Late Modem Age* (Cambridge: Polity Press, 1991).
10 Ibid., pp. 181–5.
11 For accounts of the difficulty in translating *Nachträglichkeit* into English and other languages see the whole issue of the *International Review of PsychoAnalysis, 18*: 3 (1991).
12 This was at the 1990 conference of the International Association for the History of Psychoanalysis in London.
13 Freud's phrase was contained in a letter to Wilhelm Fleiss. See *The Complete Letters of Sigmund Freud to Wilhelm Fleiss 1887–1904*, ed. Jeffrey Masson (Cambridge, MA and London: Harvard University Press, 1985), p. 320.
14 Exodus 37: 1–5.
15 Thomas Mann, *Confessions of Felix Krull, Confidence Man*. Trans. Denver Lindley (Harmondsworth: Penguin, 1958).
16 See Andrew Samuels, *The Plural Psyche: Personality, Morality and the Father* (London and New York: Routledge, 1989), pp. 194–215. In that chapter, entitled 'Original morality in a depressed culture', I make connections between depression and unimaginative approaches to political problems.
17 *The Times*, November 22, 1990.
18 Kevin Phillips, *The Politics of Rich and Poor: Wealth and the American Electorate in the Reagan Aftermath* (New York: Random House, 1990), p. xvii.
19 For a statement of the main details of the 'underclass' theory see Charles Murray, 'Underclass' in *Family Portraits*, eds. Digby Anderson and Graham Dawson (London: Social Affairs Unit, 1990). For a critique of the theory see Sue Monk, *Escaping the Underclass* (London: National Council for One Parent Families, 1990). The debate

has been extensively reported, see Anna Coote, 'Mother and father of a battle' (*The Guardian,* September 26, 1990) and Sarah Boseley, 'Trauma that can last a lifetime' (*The Guardian,* January 31, 1990). It seems clear that the debate has been raging in Britain and the United States. My position is that the 'underclass' theory is fuelled as much by moral panic engendered by a threat posed to 'normality' by single-parent families as by anything else.

20 *The Times,* November 15, 1991.

21 The problem was addressed in dramatic form in Tariq Ali and Howard Brenton, *Moscow Gold* (London: Nick Hem Books, 1990).

22 *The Times,* November 15, 1991.

23 C. G. Jung, *Psychology and Religion.* CW 11: 6.

24 Rudolf Otto, *The Idea of the Holy.* Trans. James Harvey (Oxford and London: Oxford University Press, 1923), p. 58.

25 See also Andrew Samuels, *The Plural Psyche,* Chapters 4–6, especially Chapter 6, 'Beyond the feminine principle', in which I discuss problems with equating anatomy and psychology critique essentialisms purporting to be based on archetypal theory.

26 Donald Williams, Review of David Barash, *The Hare and the Tortoise: Culture, Biology and Human Nature. San Francisco Jung Institute Library Journal, 8*: 1 (1988), p. 27.

27 Ian Craib, *Psychoanalysis and Social Theory: The Limits of Sociology* (London and New York: Harvester Wheatsheaf, 1989), pp. 7–11.

28 Ibid., pp. 2–3.

CHAPTER 2

THE LION AND THE FOX

Morality, Trickster and political transformation

Retrospective introduction

This chapter also comes from *The Political Psyche* in 1993. In it, I set out my stall for the significance of the Trickster for a renaissance of politics. The three main examples are Machiavelli, the Winnebago Trickster and Hermes. All of these are massaged into an account of how imagination and a special kind of socially conscious grandiosity and refusal to accept 'reality' as consensually defined could have utility and benevolence. I don't assume that all political Tricksters are male, as you will see.

I continued the quest, started in the previous chapter, to see if there was a working of the market economy and of capitalism itself that would satisfy me. So I entered as deeply as I could into the psychological complexities of the market economy.

This led me to return to a key theme from a previous book (*The Plural Psyche* of 1989) which concerned the importance of bargaining and negotiating at all levels of human existence. I feel that there is a marriage of idealism and sticking to the nitty-gritty in the notion of bargaining, at least as I conceived of it.

The chapter was actually first drafted in 1989 as the Iron Curtain was coming down all over Europe. Yet, again, I don't find what I wrote dated if applied to the Arab Spring of 2011–13. Nor is the concern to find a version of capitalism that does not show all the cruelties and sadism of the one that we have. A doomed quest, perhaps? I think I would say that this remains an open question.

Morality and Machiavelli

In the previous chapter, I mentioned the importance of paying attention to political imagery. I now want to move on to a psychological analysis of the imagery in the political thought of Niccolò Machiavelli. The idea is to explore what an engagement with politics does to psychology and what psychology can bring to political theorizing. Machiavelli is important for us precisely because he does not look like a modern resacralizer. There is no deep ecology in Machiavelli's Prince, no upbeat spiritual optimism, not a lot of femininity or feminine consciousness. He's a meat eater, isn't he? He can be dishonest, unreliable, impure, worldly – and, perhaps because of these things, he is very effective in the worlds of psychology and politics alike. What we find in Machiavelli is the kind of bleak realism and sense of civic duty that sees things through. If only resacralization could tap into Machiavellian energies . . .

In Machiavelli's short book *The Prince,* written in 1513–14, we find a psychological analysis of the political process. Machiavelli blends wanton subversiveness, subtly buried morality and relentless imagination. It is possible for us to encounter his encounter with the political culture of his time, seeing 'the Prince' as a metaphor for a certain kind of political psychology, or psychological approach to politics.

We can make psychology in a Machiavellian way, think Machiavellian thoughts, see with a Machiavellian eye. The opprobrium heaped on Machiavelli's head for nearly five hundred years is also something to muse about. Depth psychologists, such as Freud or Jung, also stir up similar reactions when they bring their psychological theories to bear on the political and social scene. As with Machiavelli's writings, what depth psychologists have to say often appears to subvert every generally held decency. But it is the peculiar quality of the subversiveness found in an apparently reactionary thinker that is the compelling quality in Machiavelli's writings. The subversiveness is not contrived or adolescent but argued out rather logically.

The prince is a person who is subject to history and, above all, to Fortune. His job is to make sure that Fortune does not mar his attempts to write his own script, be a successful ruler and achieve glory. So, at the same time as noting that the prince is a contingent and constrained person, Machiavelli emphasizes that the prince also has creative autonomy. His future, and that of his people, is bound up with how comprehensively he can create his own Fortune.

In classical political theory and also in the new Renaissance humanism, the prince's task was to develop in himself the four cardinal virtues: wisdom, justice, courage and moderation. In addition, there were many other virtues which the prince was also supposed to possess. The phrase 'honesty is the best policy' summarizes the tenor of this way of thinking about politics. In *The Prince,* Machiavelli completely rejects these virtues. His *virtù* is that the prince should follow the dictates of necessity. The rejection of humanistic political morality is given dramatic and precise imagistic form: the prince should follow the fox and the lion. Not God, not the inner voice; the prince should learn from animals:

> A prince is forced to know how to act like a beast. He should learn from the fox and the lion; because the lion is defenseless against traps and a fox is defenseless against wolves. Therefore one must be a fox in order to recognize traps, and a lion to frighten off wolves. Those who simply act like lions are stupid . . . Those who have known best how to imitate the fox have come off best. But one must know how to color one's actions and to be a great liar and deceiver.[1]

Machiavelli is not content simply to ignore humanism; he does not seem much troubled by Christian morality either. The prince is never admonished to take care lest he be judged in the afterlife and the usual Christian virtues of forgiveness and gentleness are explicitly ruled out: the prince should punish his enemies instantly and with public ruthlessness. The ideology to be found here is the deliberate rejection of ideology. I mean that there is a rejection of ideology as a rational system, a reliable and predictable way of getting through the chanciness of the world. However, Machiavelli is not advocating a patternless mode of behaviour for the prince. Nor is a conception and recognition of human moral capacity missing from Machiavelli's outlook: the prince's morality should, above all, be of a flexible nature; he is required to *choose* to be evil, to be evil in spite of himself:

> And so he should have a flexible disposition, varying as fortune and circumstance dictate . . . He should not deviate from what is good, if that is possible, but he should know how to do evil, if that is necessary.

The act of choice, of temporarily suppressing the dove in favour of the hawk, takes us onto a subtle moral plane. Problems of choice lie at the heart of political and moral philosophies. Being 'Machiavellian' means more than being ruthless or always allowing ends to justify means.

In modern psychological language, what Machiavelli is doing is making an ideology and a morality out of the shadow, out of those aspects of human psychology that we would rather disown. Most political theory seeks to combat and deal with the shadow.[2] Machiavelli's approach is to embrace the shadow and go *with* its energies rather than against them. This is what we today find so difficult – to accept that even resacralizers have motives such as greed and the desire for power:

> One can make this generalization about men: they are ungrateful, fickle, liars, and deceivers, they shun danger and are greedy for profit; while you treat them well, they are yours . . . when you are in danger they turn against you. A prince who has come to depend entirely on promises and has taken no other precautions ensures his own ruin . . . The bond of love is one which men, wretched creatures that they are, break when it is to their advantage to do so; but fear is strengthened by a dread of punishment which is always effective.

To adopt this as a *conscious* base for government was truly revolutionary, at least in the West. For Machiavelli, political actions are enclosed in a conception of human psychology. The message for cultural and political analysis is clear: a perception of what people are like precedes a conception of political change. Perhaps we cannot follow Machiavelli in his bleak generalization as to what human nature is. Maybe he is wrong, or his view is one-sided and incomplete in leaving out the positive side of human potential. But Machiavelli is right to place psychology at the heart of the political process. One reason why I have been drawn to Machiavelli is his eschewal of easy answers. Nowhere in his work is there anything that resembles a modern psychodynamic medicine, such as genitality or individuation or the depressive position, which is claimed to 'cure' the political system of its psychopathology. Machiavelli's stand here is to take no stand, to go with the flow of what we usually reject or cannot face, to stay with the dirt rather than try to make gold out of it. Remaining disillusioned about the possibility of political and cultural transformation is a hard path to take. But the point for political and cultural analysis is that Machiavelli is dealing with what is possible and also with what is the case – that is, politics – and doing this from a psychologically realistic point of view. Hence, he has a realistic chance of changing things.

Paradoxically, Machiavelli's realistic angle on political morality leads us to the legendary figure of the Trickster. When we explored Machiavelli's morality, we noted that 'if a prince wants to maintain his role he must learn how not to be virtuous, and to make use of this or not according to need'. The prince, it seems, must overcome his innate virtue. However, at the same time as being bad, he must not *appear* to be bad:

> A prince should be so prudent that he knows how to escape the evil reputation attached to those vices which could lose him his state . . . To those seeing and hearing him, he should appear a man of compassion, a man of good faith, a man of integrity, a kind and religious man . . . Everyone sees what you appear to be, few experience what you really are.

It's a trick, you see. Perhaps it needs to be made clear that this is not Satanic, nor perverse, not Machiavelli taking evil as his good, nor foul as fair. For this unavoidable tricksterism lies at the heart of the *political.* By exploring the psychology of Trickster, I intend to test the insight about links between the Trickster and political processes. The aim is to gain a deeper understanding of the depth psychology of political process in general and the depth psychology of political change in particular. What have we done to ourselves by evacuating the shadow from accounts of political motivation and by shunning the Trickster in politics?

Politics and the trickster

Trickster figures and stories appear in many cultures, as has only quite recently become accepted. For the Greeks, the arch-Trickster was Hermes, with his tendency to play jokes, to lie, to cheat, to steal, to deny reality, and to engage in grandiose fantasy. (We will be turning to Hermes in the next section of the chapter.) Genuine Tricksters, from Coyote in North America to Ananse or Eshu in West Africa, follow that pattern, undermining the prevailing organization of power and even the perceived structure of reality itself. Tricksters can certainly be seen as personifications of primary process activity, challenging and disregarding the laws of time, space and place. Rather, let us speculate about why Trickster mounts this challenge. He does it *precisely to test the limits of those laws,* the bounds of their applicability, and, hence, the possibility of altering them. At the moment we say this, the political referents of the Trickster are revealed. Challenging the limits of laws, their applicability and the possibility of altering them – and doing this in an ideological climate that is hostile to such a challenge – is *the* classic progressive political project. Claiming the Trickster for politics might seem like the most crass over-interpretation. But if Trickster's political theorizing can retain his own capacity for shock and irony then no more than a little damage will have been done to him. Later in the chapter, when I try to imagine what the female Trickster looks like, I think I play a trick on Trickster, which should make him happier.[3]

In the Middle Ages, carnivals began to take their present form and there would usually be a portrayal of some disturbance in the hierarchy. For example, an unsuitable person, such as a child or the village idiot, would be dressed up as the bishop. In fairy tales, we find figures like Tom Thumb parodying our usual conception of the hero. Tyl Eulenspiegel and Pulcinella have similar attributes. Parapsychology is full of tricky poltergeists who strain the boundaries of what we take for reality by living out the dramas of the unconscious itself. Sometimes, animals represent the Trickster (Machiavelli's fox is a good example). According to Jung, many aspects of God's behavior in the Old Testament show Trickserish features, as does Zeus's behavior in Greek mythology.[4] When the world doesn't conform to expectations, when Sod's or Murphy's law prevails, when things get jinxed, when the Emperor, though not the small boy, is deceived by his own vanity, when tummy rumbles uncomfortably punctuate a silence, when we laugh at the clown – Trickster is present.

The question of Trickster's sex radiates undecidability. His representations are not conventionally male in either an anatomical or a behavioral sense. But he is not a straightforward hermaphrodite either. Moreover, to refer to Trickster as bisexual is already to make far too definite a statement, while the term 'polymorphous perversion' leads us to regard Trickster as either a baby or a damaged grown-up. The one thing that *can* be said about most, if not all, traditional images of Trickster is that they are not usually presented as female and that there is an emphasis on phallic prowess in Trickster stories. One common theme involves Trickster cuckolding an earnest, respectable husband. For example, the West African Trickster Ananse manages to trick Akwasi so that Akwasi ends up actually ordering Ananse to make love to his wife Aso.

I find myself wondering where the images of the female or proto-female Trickster are to be found. I do not think that Trickster as a 'he' is irrelevant to women's issues (in fact, I think the opposite), and feminist scholarship has demonstrated that the absence of things female from a discourse is rarely of no significance. So, throughout this chapter, I weave into my text a search for the figure that I will continue to refer to as the 'female Trickster' even though I am aware that she will be no more an ordinary woman than the male (or proto-male) Trickster is an ordinary man.

One of the most studied Trickster stories is the Trickster Cycle of the North American Winnebago Native Americans, brought together by Paul Radin in 1956 at a time when the ubiquity of the Trickster figure was first being recognized.[5] The Winnebago Trickster lacks even rudimentary body unity: his intestines are outside his body, his penis is autonomous, enormously long, sometimes kept in a box, sometimes wrapped round his abdomen, each hand regards the other as a mortal enemy (like Dr Strangelove in Kubrick's film). Trickster's odyssey is a picaresque one – organized episodically, full of fortunes, misfortunes, violent attempts at punishment and surprisingly resilient opportunism on the part of the protagonist who survives his mishaps. In picaresque fiction, all the characters suffer greatly as they play out the tensions between unaccommodated man and a hostile society and the fact that the picaroon or scoundrel is usually of low birth adds to that tension. Trickster's suffering is itself an occasion for new Tricksterism, and further resourcefulness.

One episode of the Winnebago Trickster Cycle will illustrate the kind of thing that happens. Trickster has sent his penis into a tree to punish a chipmunk who has been teasing him. When he withdraws, he finds that only a small piece of the penis is left. He gets hold of the chipmunk and tears him open . . .

> There, to his horror, he discovered his penis all gnawed up. 'Oh, my, of what a wonderful organ he has deprived me! But why do I speak thus? I will make objects out of the pieces for human beings to use.' Then he took the end of his penis, the part that has no foreskin, and declared, 'This is what human beings will call the lily-of-the-lake.' This he threw into a lake nearby. Then he took the other pieces declaring in turn: 'This the people will call potatoes; this the people will call turnips; this the people will call artichokes; this the people will call ground-beans; . . . this the people will call rice.' All these pieces he threw into the water. Finally he took the end of his penis and declared, 'This the people will call the pond-lily.' He was referring to the square part of the end of his penis.

> What was left of his penis was not very long. When, at last, he started off again, he left behind the box in which he had until then kept his penis coiled up.
>
> And this is the reason our penis has its present shape. It is because of these happenings that the penis is short. Had the chipmunk not gnawed off Trickster's penis our penis would have the appearance that Trickster's first had. It was so large that he had to carry it on his back. Now it would not have been good had our penis remained like that and the chipmunk was created for the precise purposes of performing this particular act. Thus it is said.[6]

Well – is Trickster really the creator of lilies, potatoes and so on? Or is he the creator only of an illusion that he is? Is he a kind of Adam, an original man, whose morphology determined ours? Or is he the prototype of the infant, who has to work out a fantastic explanation of the origins and limitations of the body which he or she inhabits? The passage certainly supports Jung's view that during a cycle of such stories 'the marks of deepest unconsciousness fall away from [Trickster]; instead of acting in a brutal, savage, stupid and senseless fashion the Trickster's behaviour . . . becomes quite useful and sensible. The devaluation of his earlier unconsciousness is apparent even in the myth.'[7] It would seem that involving the Trickster in political discourse does not injure the Trickster. What does it do to our conception of politics?

Given the conventionally moralistic nature of most depth psychological analysis of politics, the Trickster, like Machiavelli, often gets a bad press as symbolizing the antisocial personality. Trickster's mendaciousness and self-deception are placed in the foreground, obscuring his transformative and generative aspects and, in particular, masking the way in which Trickster acts as a sort of yardstick and spur to consciousness. Sometimes people take a rather patronizing attitude, one that is full of knowing laughter at Trickster's antics, evacuating their political pointedness. Of course, a sense of humour is necessary when relating to Trickster but not for the purpose of depotentiating him.

If we try to interpret the Winnebago Trickster Cycle from a conventional psychodynamic angle, the main themes are the absence of a coherent body schema (the mobile penis), projection and splitting (for example, of aggression into the chipmunk) and pathological grandiosity (Trickster as Creator). However, if we recover our sense of irony and suspend judgment for the moment, then these themes lead to certain psychological questions which can be seen to have a political flavour – such as the following:

Do the erotogenic zones ever constitute a fixed body schema? Human sexual attraction seems to rest on the interdependence and even interchangeability of the zones: a kiss on the mouth, a cute bottom of either sex, big breasts, a well-stuffed wallet. Similarly, is a split object always so pathological? I wonder whether it is always as necessary or desirable for splits to be healed, for loving and aggressive impulses to be brought together, as psychodynamic theory usually suggests? Or is Trickster's so-called primitive fantasy of a split-off object worthy of positive consideration? Finally, what about Trickster's grandiosity? After Kohut's revaluing of grandiosity, how can grandiosity be omitted from any account of human creativity?[8]

These questions are of interest to analysts and therapists for they contribute to a revision of what constitutes developmental maturity. But, as I suggested earlier, there is a *political* reading to be made of these psychological questions. For, in revaluing the psychology of Trickster, we revalue the politics of Trickster, maybe even revalue politics itself. Those boring psychodynamic questions about body schema, projection and splitting and grandiosity have themselves had fascinating *political* consequences in our own time.

If the bodily zones can be quite healthily muddled, then no established order is safe, anything can be muddled: the personal can be political, the fixity of gender roles probed, tyranny challenged (if not always overthrown). If love and hate do not always have to be linked in so-called normal ambivalence, then there is a place for both community spirit and ruthless selfishness. They do not have to be seen as cancelling each other out. If grandiosity is respected and taken seriously, then what is condemned by the wise old man (*senex*) as immature (*puer*-like) fantasies of global solutions to the world's problems can be reframed as an excursion into practical politics.[9] We can see that it is not really the grandiosity of such solutions that is the problem, as is so often thought; it is *lack* of grandiosity that makes for political compliance. Watching the Rumanian revolution on TV in December 1989 (which is when I wrote the first draft of this chapter), watching unarmed workers and students refuse to leave the streets, getting shot while the army fought the *Securitate* (security police), drove the point home: that grandiosity of aim can be the healthy ground of realizable ambition. Unhappily, the Rumanian people will have further need of their grandiose courage. Trickster's denial of mortality is a political statement, for the fear of death plays a part in maintaining the political *status quo*; it is feared that any change will lead to the elimination of life itself. The need to accept the inevitability of death makes one think of the corollary need to celebrate life when one has it. This means a passionate yet socially responsible engagement with the erotic and sensual dimensions of life, art, religion, tradition, the life of the intellect, and play. Grey is not the only colour.

I am arguing that the genuine Trickster should not be omitted from a psychology of the political. I want us to stop accusing others of being Tricksters, using the term only in a derogatory sense when applied to politics. The Trickster is compatible with order and organization on the one hand, and with chaos and fluidity on the other. Trickster's order is created *through* chaos; his stabilizing influence on human culture (lilies, potatoes) is an outcrop of his destabilizing influence. Is Trickster the first chaos theorist? Recently, the Trickster has even been given a role in management – the need for ambiguity and paradox, for dissonance in place of coherence, decentralization in place of coordination have all been recognized. What is more, as John Beebe has pointed out, we should be very careful about *not* trusting Trickster. If, as usual, we don't trust him, then he will trick and betray us in an unexpected way and turn out to be absolutely worthy of confidence and trust.[10] This facet of Trickster maybe explains why so many fathers, in myth and family, are trustworthy/untrustworthy Tricksters. (We will encounter the politics of the Trickster father in Chapters 6 and 7 [of *The Political Psyche*].)

We should not look to the Trickster for signs of individuation, achievement of the depressive position, maintenance of firm boundaries, or consistency. I am all too well aware of what he cannot do. But I am trying to develop a depth psychology of politics in which we are not hamstrung by rigid orthodoxies. We tend to accept without question that what seems the most psychologically mature will turn out to be the most socially useful and true, and to assume that this kind of balanced insight is what constitutes a psychological contribution to politics. Trickster challenges this assumption. Nevertheless, many may want to know whether a political apprehension of Trickster means that anything goes in politics, that every view, no matter how irrational, should be given equal weight, that political tolerance of subjective responses should be infinite, that there is no political morality.

I think that political morality incorporates a ceaseless dynamic between a passionately expressed, codified, legally sanctioned set of principles and certitudes (original morality) and a more open, flexible, improvised, tolerant kind of morality that is basically code-free (moral imagination). These two aspects of political morality are both present in varying degrees in any political system and it is important to resist the temptation to see one of them as somehow more advanced, rising from the ashes of the other. Certitude and improvisation are *equally* valuable and, even assessed from a conventional psychodynamic perspective, they are equally mature. It is easy to see that a political morality based exclusively on improvisation would be too slippery by far and would contribute to a climate in which anything goes. But a political morality based exclusively on principle, law and certitude would be equally problematic (in psychological language, equally 'primitive'). To begin with, laws are not politically effective on their own; legal codes reflect and depend on the distribution of wealth and power. Moreover, political principle easily becomes ossified and used to gain control over others. Finally, codified political and moral prohibitions do not always work, as the prevalence of theft or adultery demonstrates.

Trickster *is* aware of the existence of moral and political certitudes but they do not constitute his particular trajectory. If you think about it, in moral process exceptions are the rule. There is a Taoist saying: 'The reason why one does not wear a leather coat in summer is not to spare the coat but because it is too warm. The reason one does not use a fan in winter is not disdain for fans but because it is too cool.'[11] Yes, there are fundamental truths (even Truths with a capital letter T), but for each diverse context there is a separate and diverse fundamental truth. Trickster's political morality is anything but phallogocentric.

Even if orthodox political and moral principles are the windmills against which Trickster tilts, he does not deny them their existence as he tries to undermine them. Can the serious, respectable world of economic, political, and psychological theory and organization extend the same emotionally complex generosity toward the Trickster?

I accept that Trickster's discourse may seem like garbage to some readers. Yet his refusal to say definitively that *this* is the only reality (for example, an unjust social and economic system) and *this* is Utopian fantasy (for example, reform or revolution) is in itself a profound political statement.

During the Gulf War in 1991, the image of Trickster kept cropping up, usually in relation to Saddam Hussein.[12] While I think it is significant that people are sensitive to the Trickster's presence when things are changing or transforming, I want to say that Saddam Hussein was *not* a Trickster. And, in keeping with my overall thesis, I would add that the leaders of the coalition were not Tricksters. For tricksters do not cheat and lie as part of a programme; they are not tricky to advance policies; they do not have goals as such. They just lie and cheat because that is how they are and who they are.

Citizens in most countries are faced with leaders who lie and cheat as part of a programme and to advance policy. Here in the West, we have to learn from the experiences of the dissidents of Eastern Europe and the former Soviet Union who developed a profound cynicism that enabled them to read between the lines. We need to acquire this skill urgently.

The Trickster exists in political culture but he or she is not acknowledged therein and hence is not theorized about. Hence, instead of Trickster's admixture of fantasy, practical ingenuity and transformation, we get a kind of repressed and distorted trickster (that's Saddam Hussein as Trickster, bribery and corruption, dirty tricks).

It certainly is not a question of needing more Trickster if more Trickster means more violence, more bribery and corruption, more dirty tricks. It is a question of an integration of a more complete – less repressed and distorted – version of Trickster, and at a deeper level. This would be an integration of the irregular psychology of Trickster into the regular psychology of political theorizing. Just as I have tried to revalue subjectivity in political discourse, I do not want to leave the Trickster on the level of unlicensed stalls selling rural produce by the side of the road in city centres, to use an image familiar in countries as disparate as Russia and Brazil. I do not want to sideline the Trickster like that. After all, the 'black economy' or 'parallel economy' plays a huge part in the socioeconomic life of developing countries. On the basis of official figures, everyone in a country like Somalia should have starved to death during the 1980s, so low was the official per capita income. Yet at the same time, new taxis regularly appeared on the streets of Mogadishu and sales of petrol increased every year. Somalia's measured and stagnating official economy could be seen as an appendage of an unmeasured and dynamic informal economy. The success of informal economies all over the world requires a new kind of psychological explanation or interpretation of economic behaviour, one that is informed by the experience of functioning in a black or parallel economy. This is where Trickster comes in, so different from conventional, psychodynamic explanations or interpretations of economic behaviour. Psychodynamic understandings are, perhaps, the equivalent of the economic literature on the Third World written 'from above' by the World Bank and similar institutions.

If we are to integrate the Trickster into political discourse, then we have to explore why he is on the scene in the first place – what is Trickster's *telos,* Trickster's goal? Surely this is more than the promotion of devious and corrupt political practices? Anyway, I am going to try to show that it is.

Hermes and the market economy

Hermes is a Trickster of a different order than the Winnebago Trickster and we grasp something more specific about power politics from his myth. We grasp something about capitalism, the market economy and relations between capitalism and the market because, in a sense, Hermes helps us to rescue the idea of the market from capitalism. Hermes is certainly deceitful and criminal, but, as we will see in the myth, the accent is equally on his constructive and transformative nature. After all, Hermes is a god: guide of souls to the underworld, the divinity of olive cultivation, athletics, boundaries, commerce, and messenger of the gods. Hermes stands as a liminal presence, on the threshold or boundary of depth psychology and politics, of psychic reality and social reality, of the personal and the political. Hermes also articulates a relationship between the Trickster and the market economy – that particular political phenomenon causing confusion, idealization and splitting across the late twentieth-century world. In Chapter 1, struggling to get a depth psychological angle on resacralization, we saw that a split in the image of the market economy lessened the chances of converting dream into pragmatic politics. Most resacralizing movements are too one-sided in their evaluation of the market economy and this one-sidedness is also to be found in the enthusiasms of the gung-ho free marketeers. In short, there is a psychological problem with our politics and it is a problem to do with opposites – opposite evaluations of the market. Nobody actually *advocates* a one-sided view but, as we saw, taking an average does not help us because we miss out on the quite specific and suggestive psychologies of the market as negative and the market as positive. Merely holding those opposites in mind strikes me as far too passive, which is why I want to work out a means of developing each side separately, thus permitting ongoing interplay between them.

The tale of Hermes is, in many ways, the pattern of our particular socio-economic epoch which, like him, is a shape-shifter with numerous names to match its myriad presentations: late capitalism, late-late capitalism, post-capitalism, post-Fordism, the information culture (Hermes as messenger), post-industrialism, post-modernism, late modernity and so forth.

In the myth, we hear of the deceit and lying of Hermes. This inspires associations to the ruthlessness of economic inequality, stock market fraud and insider trading. We also hear of the capacity of Hermes to bargain and negotiate in a compassionate and related style. That inspires associations to the need of any political culture to avoid oligarchic hegemony and gross injustice. Let's consider each of these in turn, trying to hold on to them in imagination. Then we can let the two sides of Hermes come together. This is the first step in an approach to those crude splits in our image of the market economy that could ruin the prospects for resacralization. As I suggested earlier, there is a necessity to overcome *both* schizoid tendencies to make an either/or split between positive and negative assessments *and* the temptation to reach an uncritical synthesis. If we can manage that, then we can establish a credible psychological analysis of economic themes that are not usually approached by depth psychologists. This is a tragic lack when one considers the colonial and neocolonial connections between economics, economic inequality and war. We have to try to address the underlying psychology, the depth psychology, of our political compulsions. Can we introduce a depth psychological dimension into a questioning of our dependence on existing levels of consumption, personal mobility and comfort?

Difficulties with images of the market economy are of central concern in both West and East as both struggle with their confused reactions to the market economy. In the rich countries of the West, we have to face that, in spite of growing disgust, we are still caught in a collective love affair with a rotten social order and an unfeeling culture. We made our commitment to this order of things a long time ago and however much we may know intellectually that it does not work for us on the ethical level, however much we may know about the psychodynamics of greed and envy, we cannot seem to break our tie to our lover: economic inequality.[13] It is a deep guilt over the undeniable fact of our love of economic inequality that takes us to the cheating heart of global capitalism, the partner we refuse to leave, having never really chosen, remaining locked in an enigmatic relationship whose tensions drive us crazy.

Perhaps we should now take a closer look at the mythic patterns of this dilemma. Myths open issues up when they are understood as expressive of mutable external and social forces rather than of immutable internal patterns. Joseph Campbell regarded this aspect of myths as 'social dreams'[14] and I would add that myths may also be cultivated as political fantasies that have, over time, shown themselves capable of surviving the inevitable violence done to them by appropriating them for all kinds of purposes. Their ambiguity is their strength. Nevertheless, those who adopt a hyper-kosher academic approach to myth – for example, one that insists on knowing the precise social origin of a myth on grounds of cultural relativity, or constituting a refusal to listen to a source fatally flawed by its patriarchal roots – are not going to be well pleased with what follows. But, even if myths depend on ideology they are not the same as ideology. Myths alter and new ones come into being; as the historian Ludmilla Jordanova puts it, 'as stories about human doings they are overtly powerful and emotionally dense. In this respect they differ from ideologies . . . Hence, to speak in terms of myth need not imply an ahistoricity of any kind, because myths are perpetually put to work in different, historically shifting ways.' Jordanova argues against the suspicion that exists in academic circles of 'anything not rooted in particular circumstances [and] historical specificity'.[15]

As far as interpretation is concerned, myths do not normally admit of an unchallenged reading. They are characterized by 'density and complexity, imaginative depth and universal appeal . . . Myths are on the one hand good stories, on the other hand bearers of important messages about life in general and life-within-society in particular.'[16]

In *The Homeric Hymn to Hermes,* on the first day of his life, Hermes leaps up to look for meat. Pausing only to kill a turtle and fashion a lyre from its shell, he steals fifty head of cattle from the herd of Apollo, his half-brother. Hermes drives the cattle backward so that their tracks seem to point away from his stables. According to the *Homeric Hymn,* Hermes was the inventor of fire and he roasts two of the animals he has stolen and makes a sacrifice of this meat to the other gods.

Understandably, Apollo is very upset that his cattle have been taken and quickly works out what must have happened. Charles Boer's brilliant modern translation[17] conveys his agitation: 'Listen kid, /lying in your cradle, /tell me where my cows are, /and quick!/We're going to fight this out/and it won't be very pretty!' Hermes is innocence itself – how could a milk-sucking baby do such a thing and, as he says, after all, 'I was just born yesterday.' Doesn't fool Apollo, though: 'You trickster, /you sharpie, /the way you talk/I bet you have broken into a lot of expensive homes /in nights past.' In humorous vein still, Apollo prophesies that Hermes will come to a bad end. Hermes sticks to his guns and goes on denying the theft. The two Gods present themselves before Zeus. Apollo accuses, Hermes declares himself not guilty. But, to Zeus, all is clear and, with a laugh, he orders the two Gods to try to sort out their differences.

We shall be returning to the narrative of the *Homeric Hymn.* Let us now react psychologically to the story so far and reflect on its political implications.

The myth amplifies my earlier remarks about our devotion to the economic realities of capitalism, how we seem to want – really want – inequality, cheating and injustice between individuals, groups, nations and regions. The fact that there is no reference in the *Homeric Hymn* to Hermes actually eating the meat makes me think of the non-productive nature of the capital markets. They feed no one directly and yet accumulate wealth invisibly and inequitably.

What is the depth psychology of economic inequality? I mean something more than its psychodynamics. If we free ourselves from interpretations that depend on the psychology of the individual, then we can say that economic inequality maintains the social structures of desire. The baby Hermes covets Apollo's cattle even when he can only suck at the breast – he has no truck with psychodynamic narratives of infancy. That he does not eat the meat tells us that the cathexis, the emotional investment, is on the wanting and on the sense of incompleteness. Such a sense of incompleteness is by no means a wholly negative phenomenon for it acts as a spur to constructive activity. However, the nagging and gnawing in Hermes's spiritual stomach, which our epoch surely can recognize, are settled only when, by acquisition, by takeover, by theft, he gets into a relation with another.

Some might argue that tricksterism cannot constitute a type of relating. But it is clear that Hermes's magical introjection of food is more than just a phase or passage on the road to 'true' internalization. Economic inequality itself is tied up with a devotion to primitive magic, amorality and even criminality, all of which belong to the introjective attitude: it's there, I want it, I don't want to ask for it, I'll take it.

Apollo really responds to Hermes and, as we will see, things deepen between the two brothers. Hermes gets Apollo's attention and this, too, is part of the psychology of economic inequality. Not only stirring up envy, but really being seen, and even mirrored.

Our devotion to the differences displayed by means of economic inequality has something to do with space for symbolization. What I mean is that the wealthier the individual, family, clan, class, nation, region, the greater the space for symbolization seems to be. One can afford movies, the theatre, opera, eating in restaurants, driving in automobiles, and even personal analysis. These are activities which secure and provide the space for symbolization. Of course, this display of differentiation is illusory. I am not saying that the space is really taken advantage of. I am certainly not saying that the well-off are enjoying richer inner lives or that the richer countries are spiritually richer. But the illusion that they are is hypnotic. In economic inequality, there are located personal and national hopes for the richness of the symbolic life. We believe this emotionally even though we know intellectually that such richness cannot be bought by women, men, corporations or governments.

Another factor in economic inequality that makes this condition psychologically attractive to us is the fantasy that the other does not amount to much, particularly if he or she has less money. The poor other does not count. Hermes does not worry about Apollo's reaction or even think about Apollo at all when he steals the cattle. If one's space for symbolization expands, it can eliminate the other's space for symbolization, and hence can eliminate the other, or seem to. Economic inequality does away with the anxieties of alterity, of having to relate to people who are psychologically other; it encourages fantasies of insulation and isolation. Rich people do not necessarily have rich consciences. Another Taoist saying is apt here: 'If you are not satisfied with yourself, even if you have a whole continent for your house with all its people for your servants, this will not be enough to support you.'[18]

We see the link between economic inequality and emotional isolation in the modern legends of Howard Hughes and Paul Getty – and also in the *Homeric Hymn* when, after the theft, Hermes elects to spend the night alone, kicking dust over his fire and generally covering up. The fantasy plan is of concealing the crime altogether so that its perpetrator can walk away. In Hermes's case, and here he truly does represent the unconscious motivation of the modern business tycoon, he walks home to his mother. He tells her of his plans to be the most successful capitalist ever: 'I'm capable certainly/to be thief number one.'

So far, we have been looking at one part of the Hermes story. We saw the myth as a psychological patterning of the unjust and inequitable aspects of market economy capitalism. The myth illumined our investment in such corruption. Yet the rest of the myth brings out that there is another side. For there is more in humanity that a collective love of a rotten world order and an unfeeling culture. There is also in humanity a collective love of a healthy world order and a commitment to a just culture concerned with alterity and the wellbeing of all its members. *There is absolutely no contradiction.* Both exist side-by-side at the same time, and in permanent competition with each other. Both sets of human traits are patterned in the Hermes story. I want to state my argument once more: in our age, in both the capitalist West and the once communist East, it is very hard to go beyond our split emotional attitude to the market economy.

What follows next in the Hermes story may be taken as a metaphor for the kind of constructive and creative relationship the market supports rather well. The I–Thou aspects of market relations between people or peoples are revealed alongside the ruthless aspects, compassion functioning alongside competition.

We return to the narrative of *The Homeric Hymn to Hermes* at the point where Zeus tells Apollo and Hermes to come to terms. Zeus has made it impossible for Hermes to conceal the theft any longer. Apollo, reunited with forty-eight head, decides to tie Hermes up, perhaps as a prelude to further punishment. To the Sun God's amazement, the thongs he has placed round Hermes's ankles suddenly extend to tie up all the cattle! (This trick of Hermes's can be compared with Trickster's use of his penis in the Winnebago Cycle of stories.) To placate his older brother, Hermes then plays a tune on his lyre. Apollo is quite transfixed by its beauty, which is unlike any music known before. At this point, Apollo relents. He states his intention to make Hermes his protégé. Apollo will be a kind of theatrical agent for Hermes. He will be an impresario for his musical gifts. Apollo promises Hermes the roles of soul-guide and messenger of the gods. But, in the pecking order, Hermes will most certainly be *under* Apollo. Apollo wants the kind of deal Colonel Parker struck with Elvis Presley. The god of capitalism is to be a wage slave.

Hermes's response to this offer is to come up with a revolutionary counter-suggestion: he will give the lyre to Apollo, if Apollo will give him the cattle. Hermes also takes Apollo up on the job of soul-guide and messenger. *They make a bargain* – the first bargain – and the imaginative implications for the market economy, for liberal democracy and for global politics are immense. Exchange and mutuality are now highlighted by the myth; Hermes the Trickster makes a constructive contribution to political thought. It may be objected that there is plenty of deal-making around, perhaps too much. Yes, there is too much deal-making outside of alterity, outside of relationship. Admitting Hermes to cultural consciousness at least gives the potential for related deals.

Apollo installs Hermes as 'being in charge of/exchanges among men/on the nourishing earth'. Being no fool, Apollo also makes Hermes swear an oath not to steal anything from him again. Hermes does so and Apollo gives him the caduceus, the famous staff of the messenger. In this transaction, neither god is altered; gods do not change. It was a bargain not a transformation but the point is that it would not have occurred without the earlier cheating, stealing and lying. Apollo remains the oracular god. Hermes remains the liminal god, the Trickster god, moving freely between Olympus and the earth, helping the gods (saving Zeus's life once in a battle with the giants), lubricating the orgy of trade he has set in motion. But, as the *Homeric Hymn* soberly reminds us, 'even though he helps a few people, /he cheats an endless number'.

Hermes and social theory

Both sides of our image and evaluation of the market economy have equal existence and equally significant psychologies. As we have seen, to be able to develop two distinct though limited psychologies of the market economy means something different from striving for a conjunction, synthesis or balance of them. What is required is a profound emotional recognition of the ineluctably negative aspects of the market that cannot be done away with or averaged out. They will always exist and flourish alongside and in competition with more positive aspects and we need to know more about them – especially if we seek to combat them. We cannot even begin to identify the positives of the market without identifying, working through and coming to terms with the negatives of it. A synthesis is by no means the only psychological or political option available to us. For, in a synthesis of our split image of the market economy, the psychological specificity of *either* its cheating *or* its constructive aspects is lost. *We cannot just dispense with the problems of the psychology of theft because we want to enjoy the fruits of the psychology of bargaining.* There is a psychological co-existence, acceptance of which opens up the possibility of exploring the social and political realities of these sibling economic modes and of transforming their relationship. That is why, earlier, I stressed the need to integrate the Trickster into our conception of the political. He steals for sure – but he also transforms the political scene by his souk-like skills.

The political significance of the female trickster

It is important not to idealize the bargaining process. To begin with, Apollo and Hermes do not cease to eye each other cautiously. Moreover, there are many different styles of bargaining. Bargaining should not be seen as something pertinent only to men and money. One can conceive of a negotiatory approach to knowledge and, maybe, this is something that, for reasons of acculturation and socialization, women in Western countries do anyway. Certainly, even if the evidence exists only on an anecdotal level, the capacity of women to bargain and derive pleasure from it in a commercial setting seems to have been established. It is possible to take the idea of bargaining to the point where bargains are struck with reality itself – and this would include social reality. It may be that it is in this kind of bargaining that we will find the missing female Trickster. Or is it that life for women is always already constituted within Trickster's discourse as the only way to flourish within a male-dominated socioeconomic system?

This point is strengthened by an understanding of Trickster stories as depictions of what social life ('real' life) is like for the people who enjoy the story. Trickster's capacity to make us laugh is a depiction of the tragicomic cast of life itself, his or her undermining of pomposity and received wisdom a depiction of what we would all like to do to parental figures, his or her sexual and gustatory excess a depiction of how to follow a certain kind of bliss, his or her economic and mercantile ingenuity a depiction of what is required to keep one's head above water. Put like this, the Trickster can be seen as exemplifying what Eliade called 'the mythology of the human condition'.[19] Now, to the extent that women's condition has not been written into accounts of the human condition, the female Trickster remains *terra incognita* (though she is beginning to appear in movies). My hunch is that her emergence will be in the economic sphere and her methods will be those of the politics I have been sketching out: subjectivity and refusal to accept social reality as the only reality there is.

I can think of one political enterprise, undertaken exclusively by women, which demonstrates the female Trickster in political action. The Mothers of the Plaza de Mayo in Buenos Aires assembled in the plaza each day during the period of 1976–82 to protest at the 'disappearance' of their children at the hands of unofficial elements directly connected with the military dictatorship in Argentina. It has been estimated that at least 6,000 and maybe as many as 20,000 persons, mostly under the age of forty, 'disappeared' during this time. As Jean Bethke Elshtain has shown, the Mothers politicized the collective, cultural images of motherhood that were central to Argentinian family and public life. The Mothers were extraordinarily effective – in my view – because they tapped into a Tricksterish format for their political intervention.[20]

The Mothers did not reject the dignified, stately, caring, elemental role assigned to maternal women in Argentinian culture. But they expanded upon, parodied and utterly transformed that role in a Tricksterish way. The trick was to ensure that their mobilization of a mass positive, maternal transference to themselves, in Argentina and abroad, was never interfered with by the premature or careless revelation of the degree of radicalization and politicization that had taken place among them. The trick, the masquerade, was to use the Holy Mother to destabilize the junta.

The Mothers wore traditional scarves on which the names of their children and the dates of the 'disappearance' were embroidered – a striking example of what Rozsika Parker has called 'the subversive stitch'.[21] The Mothers presented themselves as sacrificial victims and as the victims of sacrifice, deploying traditional maternalism for decidedly non-traditional ends. And, crucially, they did all this in a public place. The gender solidarity of the Mothers constituted a Tricksterish kind of organizational sophistication. The Mothers were not overtly involved in politics at all but, as Elshtain points out, 'staying "above" politics may well be a way of *doing* politics that is far more effective than entering the arena on established terms'.[22] The Mothers were both faithful and unfaithful to the traditional image of the mother in their country. Yet their Tricksterish achievement was to politicize that tradition and, ultimately, the image of Woman in Argentinian society was affected and – who knows? – may have been transformed.

It is important not to approach the bargaining process with a jaundiced eye, with the prejudices of old-style socialism or new-style eco-politics. The purpose of these psychological reflections on the market is to do something to tame and temper the power of the market *by facing up to its negative features and seeing what we can do with them,* rather than fulminating against them. Whether this leads to the 'social market' concept of European social democrats, or to a 'socialized market' as proposed by some socialists,[23] or to a concept of the market with a more psychological tone, remains to be seen. Facing the negative features of the market enables us to celebrate its positive features and its variegated potentials. I am not saying that what is unmarketable does not exist or has no value and I am aware of the possibility that a market tyranny may have developed in Western and other cultures. But it is the very possibility of a tyrannical global market that, from a psychological angle, should make us hesitate before indulging in knee-jerk protest about the market *per se.* Something potentially (or actually) so powerful as to become a global ideology with practical implications for everyone on the planet must also be regarded as the most concentrated and dynamic source of creative energy that we possess on the social level.

I am not one of those who think that socialism is dead but, in company with many others, I recognize that we have to try to think in terms of there being a plurality of socialisms, each resisting the hegemonistic impulses of the other brands, but all somehow linked. As Karl Kautsky put it in 1918, 'Socialism as such is not our goal, which is rather the abolition of every kind of exploitation or oppression, be it directed against a class, a party, a sex, or a race.'[24] To achieve these ends, I agree with those who argue that socialist thought has to engage with what is implied by the market. It seems to me that socialism is already moving on to do just that. Hence, what is needed (if anything at all is needed) from depth psychologists is a contribution concerning the depth psychology of the market. Depth psychological critiques of the market should expose what R. W. Johnson called the 'warmed-over wishfulness of so many on the left'.[25]

I have not suggested that we 'chose' capitalism but rather that people are invested in certain ways in maintaining economic inequality. Nor have I assumed that, in a bargaining or negotiating situation, everyone starts from the same place. The psychosocial consequences of the destruction of free collective bargaining in the United States, Britain and elsewhere have been immense. But it is amazing how often current left-wing texts, for instance in the British journal *New Left Review,* return to the question of the 'socialized market', meaning some way of factoring compassion, social justice and alterity into market economics.

Unfortunately, no body of knowledge exists that gives a satisfactory and satisfying account of the relations between, for instance, a class-based analysis of social and economic conditions and an unconscious, phantasy-based analysis of the internal world. My text displays what will be, for some readers, an almost relentless concentration on economics, if not in the language that some old-fashioned socialists would have preferred me to use. As I said earlier, this has been a Hermetic attempt to recover the idea of the market from capitalism and make a contribution to notions of a socialized market. My Tricksterish expansion of what we take as 'the political' was informed by the realization that there is a fundamental interdependence of the market (or the markets) and politics (or the political).

Perhaps the left will have to be content with a more modest role in relation to this interdependence of the markets and the political. As Jürgen Habermas put it, socialism will become 'the radically reformist self-criticism of a capitalist society which, in the form of constitutional democracy with universal suffrage and a welfare state, has developed not only weaknesses but also strengths'.[26]

Depth psychology offers a new gloss on the protests about the triumph of the market that are beginning to emerge. Some of these protests emanate from Eastern Europe, supposedly the seat of the market's triumph. One Rumanian commentator claimed that the market economy was a 'big hoax'.[27] Growing foreign debt arising from the marketization of the economy and from the built-in inequities of the East–West trade structures slewed the whole system in the West's favour. These developments caused great instability and unhappiness in the society concerned – 'the initiation of the technological revolution actually goes against the interests of the working class . . . the market generates a large middle class that gets all the goodies.'[28] Here we are most certainly confronted with the economic and psychological products of the negative side of the market. However, the psychology of the negative side of the market is not a stagnant psychology – it is too orthodox to restrict the expectation of psychological movement to positive psychologies. We can work out some rather pragmatic political ideas on the basis of the negative depth psychology of the market. The global market has created a global community composed of all those communities that are suffering because of the negative aspects of the market – its social injustices, wastage of talent, privileging of the already wealthy and its general political pathology. The global poor are linked by a common set of experiences whether these are in debt-laden Latin America with its vast fetid cities, declining rust-belt communities in Europe and the United States, or the starving in the Horn of Africa. I wonder if it is possible that a political consciousness born out of global poverty, out of the negative psychology of the market, will emerge in the next quarter-century. This would be a 'poor' politics, characterized by a psychological orientation, for the psyche itself can only be commodified with the greatest difficulty. If, as I will argue in Chapter 9 [of *The Political Psyche*], the psyche can be construed as an autonomous source of social change and movement, then *its active presence in poor politics, blended into subjective political discourse, may spawn modes of organization and production that we are not at present familiar with.*

There is a human level to be considered here. For, alongside the desire to make a good deal, the bargaining process supports and fosters compassion for the other, without whom there would be no bargaining possible. As Montesquieu put it, 'Wherever the ways of men are gentle, there is commerce, and wherever there is commerce, the ways of men are gentle.'[29] The bargaining process can be exhilarating and fun, even sexy – and the eroticism of the negotiatory process is an important part of its psychological viability and peace-making potential.

The relevance of these ideas about negotiation and bargaining for the resolution of warlike conflict was ably summarized during the Gulf War of 1991 by my then four-year-old son. I do not recall him hearing me speak about it but one day he said: 'Daddy, I want to tell you something. A bargain. A bargain is all standing round in a circle and asking if we can stop fighting.' I am not sure I can fully explain why bargaining, too, cannot be split off from stealing, cheating and lying. But that seems to be the way it is in the collective psyche.

A collective psychology that is infused with a tricky but related mercantile spirit may help a society to avoid tyranny and enjoy an active and diverse political and social life. Competition and bargaining are ways of resolving conflict as well as generating it. But they do not close down options; that is why I stress the emancipatory potential of doing deals. Bargaining is an alternative to potlatch – the explosive evacuation of personal wealth undertaken by the Northwestern Native Americans. The world does not have easy access to such surpluses. Bargaining is different from the distribution of gifts.

These comments on the process of bargaining and its political psychology should not obscure the fact that the two bargainers in the myth have very different standpoints and political philosophies. Apollo stands for order, harmony, hierarchy and the unavoidable knowledge of the oracle. Hermes stands for Tricksterism, revolution, panic and intuitive knowledge. Apollo stands for the deep *status quo*. Hermes stands for its subversion. The political tension between Apollo and Hermes will always be culturally significant.

The image of the two brother-gods bargaining makes me wonder how a society should seek to achieve a greater degree of economic equality. To what extent should a society demand of its members that they accept responsibility for the economic well-being of others? Depth psychologists rarely address the questions that arise from an inequitable distribution of wealth. Therefore we do not know very much about the depth psychological implications of seeking a more equitable distribution. Bargaining between 'haves' and 'have-nots' might seem to have only one outcome were it not for the possibility of the apparently weaker uniting together, and maybe even taking extra-constitutional action, a form of poor politics. The image of bargaining is, therefore, not an unrealistic basis for a rectification of economic injustice.

That there is injustice is not in doubt. In countries like Brazil, less than 20 per cent of the population is covered by minimum wage legislation and general conditions, along with the real disposable income of 70 per cent of the population, are worsening year by year. In 1961, it was estimated that 38 per cent were malnourished and the estimate for 1991 from the same source is almost 70 per cent. There are 14.5 million disabled people in Brazil (almost 10 per cent of the population) and somewhere in the region of 10 million abandoned children. (It is these abandoned children who are being exterminated by vigilante hit squads formed by disaffected police officers as a horrendous response to the soaring crime rate.)

In Britain, the poorest million of the population have suffered a decline in real living standards of at least 10 per cent and, in some cases, as much as 15 per cent since 1980. (The lowest paid tenth of British families saw their real income decline by 7 per cent in the same period. In the United States, the average after-tax income of the poorest 10 per cent of the population declined by 10.5 per cent in the period 1977–87.)[30] I do not want to claim an equivalence for conditions in Britain and America and conditions in Brazil – after all, in Britain infant mortality rates continue to decline while in Brazil the opposite is true. But there is one particular socioeconomic pattern that does seem common to Britain, the United States and Brazil (and can also be observed in the evolving once-communist countries such as the former Soviet Union).

This pattern, in which the gap between rich and poor gets larger, leading to an ever-increasing concentration of wealth, was exemplified in the United States in the 1980s. It is this polarization that should be highlighted when we talk of economic inequality – not just the material gap between rich and poor but their *relative* wealth, meaning the scale of income differences within a society. The point is that, in recent years in many countries, after a certain level of economic development is reached, and this does not seem to be a particularly advanced level, all subsequent reward goes to the section of the population that already possesses a disproportionate share of resources, thereby increasing their political power. It follows that increasing productivity beyond a certain point benefits fewer people than would be expected. Worldwide, it is this particular economic configuration that has been reached and many countries are at a point where trickle-down prosperity ceases to occur to any great extent.

Some recent research shows that income distribution, the gap between haves and have-nots, is the most important determinant of health standards in the developed world (and I can see little reason why the same arguments should not be valid for a country like Brazil).[31] The research highlights the psychological aspects of economic inequality which will be deleterious in terms of self-esteem.[32] That, in turn, means that the poor will be less able to develop a sense of agency and hence be less effective on a political level. Not forgetting the simple point that living in poverty is incredibly stressful.

In the *Wealth of Nations,* Adam Smith explored how competition can work in favour of the less powerful, provided that competition is permitted to exist. For example, if manufacturers raise their prices too high, a chance is created for one of them to make an increased profit by selling at a lower price. In this way, competition acts as a kind of regulator upon selfishness. Adam Smith's attitude to self-interest was very even-handed. He observed that self-interest was *the* primary economic motivation but, Machiavelli-like, he never said that self-interest was a virtue. He saw competition as a means of transforming a socially destructive aspect of human behaviour into something more benevolent and useful. In the Parable of the Talents, the good servant *trades* with the money – he does not merely save it. This suggests not only the well-known linkage of religion and capitalism, but also an emphasis upon outcome and utility.

Recapitulation

As I have been saying, questions of economics are at the heart of psychological engagement with processes of political change, especially nonviolent political change. The problematic of a more equal distribution of wealth has everything to do with the power relations within a single society, or in the world as a whole, and hence with its political organization. But political reorganization, in its turn, cannot be cut off from whatever psychological processes of resacralization might be taking place.

There is a process of resacralization going on in Western culture, and the same is true of Eastern Europe and the Soviet Union as well as the Third World, though the surface signs may be different in different societies. Those who seek to link depth psychology with politics should admit that they too are caught up in a resacralizing process. Resacralization is essentially a secularization of the holy, following the pattern of Bezaleel, master craftsman of the Ark of the Covenant. But resacralization is threatened by a massive split in our image of and attitude towards the market economy. Disgust with ourselves, and confusion about the inequalities of world capitalism and the market economy fuel the urgency of addressing the split if resacralization is going to occur. Machiavelli addresses many of these issues in *The Prince*. Here we find that the essence of politics is to know how to be evil when necessary, without anyone thinking you are evil: a trick. Machiavelli's politicization of the shadow led us to the Trickster and his role in processes of political change. Hermes is a special kind of Trickster and exploring the Hermes myth helps us with our splits and confusions about capitalism and the market economy. Hermes speaks for both the inequitable, unjust, cheating side and the creative, transformative, compassionate side of the market. Hermes is a passageway to a depth psychological engagement with the political dynamics of the economic system.

Returning to the connecting tissue between depth psychology and politics, I want to add that it would be a pity and a mistake to restrict the political significance of Hermes to the impersonal, collective, global levels of political and economic theory and organization. There is also a pressing, personal and individual level. By engaging with Hermes, we also have to engage with the warring sides of our Hermes-selves: on the one hand, our fraud, our criminality, our belief in magic, our love of economic inequality, our own depression-inducing violence; on the other hand, our capacity for exchange, integrity, relatedness, flexibility, our own love of dignity and freedom, our desire to reject coercion and bullying, our skill at making peace.[33]

Notes

1 I have used the George Bull translation of *The Prince* (Harmondsworth: Penguin, 1961).

2 See 'shadow' in Andrew Samuels, Bani Shorter and Fred Plaut, *A Critical Dictionary of Jungian Analysis* (London and New York: Routledge, 1986): '"The thing a person has no wish to be" (Jung, *CW* 16: 470) . . . Over and over again Jung emphasizes that we all have a shadow, that everything substantial casts a shadow, that ego stands to shadow as light to shade, that it is the shadow that makes us human . . . Jung professed to deal with the shadow in a way different from the Freudian approach which he said he found limited. Recognising that the shadow is a living part of the personality and that it "wants to live with it" in some form . . . involves coming to terms with the instincts and how their expression has been subject to control by the collective . . . In other words, it is impossible to eradicate shadow; hence the term most frequently employed by analytical psychologists for the process of shadow confrontation in analysis is "coming to terms with the shadow."'

3 Problems met when writing about the Trickster are described by John Beebe, 'The Trickster in the arts', *San Francisco Jung Institute Library Journal*, 2: 2 (1981).

4 See John Beebe, 'Trickster' and William Willeford, *The Fool and His Sceptre* (Evanston, IL: Northwestern University Press, 1969).

5 Paul Radin, *The Trickster: A Study in North American Mythology* (New York: Schocken, 1972). First published in 1956.

6 Ibid, p. 39.

7 C. G. Jung, 'On the psychology of the Trickster figure'. *CW* 9: 477. *CW* refers to the *Collected Works* of C. G. Jung, ed. Herbert Read, Michael Fordham and Gerhard Adler, Trans. R. F. C. Hull (London: Routledge and Kegan Paul; Princeton, NJ: Princeton University Press, 1953–77).

8 Heinz Kohut, *The Analysis of the Self* and *The Restoration of the Self* (New York: International Universities Press, 1971 and 1977).

9 See '*puer aeternus*' and '*senex*' in Andrew Samuels et al., *Critical Dictionary.* These are not developmental terms – you can have babies with senex-type qualities of wisdom, moderation, etc. and we all know older people who are *puers* or *puellas*.

10 John Beebe, 'Trickster', p. 39: 'The Trickster manipulates the other men to the point that even their lack of confidence in him is betrayed.'

11 Thomas Cleary (ed. and trans.), *The Tao of Politics: Lessons of the Masters of Huainan* (Boston, MA: Shambhala, 1990). For a fuller version of my account of moral process see Andrew Samuels, *The Plural Psyche: Personality, Morality and the Father* (London and New York: Routledge), Chapter 11.

12 *The Times,* January 25, 1991. Headline: 'Saddam's box of tricks a match for Powell's hi-tech tools.' The Iraqis were making use of subterfuge and camouflage.

13 According to the British Office of National Statistics report *Social Trends 1991,* half the money earned in Britain goes to the richest fifth of all households. The poorest fifth get 2 per cent of the nation's wealth. The gap between rich and poor has widened since 1977: the poorest fifth have had their proportion of the total income halved, while the richest fifth have seen theirs increase by 16 per cent. Allowing for taxes and benefits, the richest fifth get 44 per cent of the total national income, up from 37 per cent in 1977. In 1989, the richest 1 per cent of the population owned 18 per cent of the wealth, up from 17 per cent the year before. The richest half of the population owns 94 per cent of the wealth.

The children of unskilled workers in Britain are twice as likely to die in their first year as those of professional parents. Unskilled manual workers are twice as likely as professionals to suffer from long-term heart disease, digestive problems and nervous complaints.

Similar figures for the United States may be found in Kevin Phillips, *The Politics of Rich and Poor: Wealth and the American Electorate in the Reagan Aftermath* (New York: Random House, 1990).

14 Personal communication, November 1986.

15 Ludmilla Jordanova, *Sexual Visions: Images of Gender in Science and Medicine between the Eighteenth and Twentieth Centuries* (London and New York: Harvester Wheatsheaf, 1989), p. 9.

16 G. S. Kirk, *The Nature of Greek Myths* (Harmondsworth: Penguin, 1974). Quoted in Ludmilla Jordanova, op. cit., p. 182. Hans Blumenburg writes that myths are characterized by a combination of a 'high degree of constancy' and a 'pronounced capacity for marginal variation'. So 'myths are not like "holy texts", which cannot be altered by one iota' (quoted in Drucilla Cornell, 'The doubly prized world: Myth, allegory and the feminine', *Cornell Law Review, 75*: 3 (1990).

17 All quotations are taken from the translation by Charles Boer, *The Homeric Hymns* (Dallas: Spring Publications, 1979).

18 Thomas Cleary, *The Tao of Politics.*

19 Mircea Eliade, *The Quest: History and Meaning in Religion* (Chicago, IL: Chicago University Press, 1969), p. 157.

20 Jean Bethke Elshtain, 'The passion of the "Mothers of the Disappeared" in Argentina', *New Oxford Review,* January–February 1992.

21 Rozsika Parker, *The Subversive Stitch: Embroidery and the Making of the Feminine* (London: Women's Press, 1984; New York: Routledge, 1990).

22 Jean Bethke Elshtain, 'The passion of the "Mothers"', p. 10.

23 See *New Left Review, 185* (1991).
24 Quoted in Robin Blackburn, 'Socialism after the crash', *New Left Review, 185* (1991).
25 R. W. Johnson, Review of C. Lemke and G. Marks (eds.), *The Crisis of Socialism in Europe* (Durham, NC: Duke University Press, 1991). In *London Review of Books*, March 12, 1992.
26 Quoted in Steven Lukes, Review of Robin Blackburn (ed.), *After the Fall: The Failure of Communism and the Future of Socialism* (London: Verso, 1992). In *New Statesman and Society*, March 6, 1992.
27 *The Guardian*, July 2, 1991.
28 Ibid.
29 Charles Louis de Secondat Montesquieu, *The Spirit of Laws* (London: Fontana, 1973).
30 Source: Report of the United Nations Development Program (UNDP) 1992. The report states that the gap between rich and poor countries has doubled in the last thirty years and the richest fifth receive 150 times the annual income of the poorest fifth. The report concludes that this is a recipe for global social unrest.
31 Richard Wilkinson, 'Inequality is bad for your health'. Summary of research, *The Guardian*, June 12, 1991.
32 Ibid.
33 Frans de Waal, *Peacemaking Among Primates* (Cambridge, MA: Harvard University Press, 1989).

CHAPTER 3

AGAINST NATURE

Retrospective introduction

This chapter from *The Political Psyche* got me into a lot of trouble because people didn't recognize it was written from a viewpoint that actually supported the environmental movement. I felt that there was a dangerous idealization of nature going on. I utilized a nineteenth-century French novel (*Against Nature*) and a late twentieth-century 'enivonmental' novel to make salient points about a change of tone (at the very least) in environmental discourse. I stand by what I wrote but it was not in fact effective for we still have the same problem as the following story illustrates.

At an ecopsychology conference in 2009, I gave a workshop also entitled 'Against nature'. In it, I put the point I'd first made in 1993 in *The Political Psyche*. If environmentalists (as we called them then) want to be effective then they need to stop blaming people for ruining the world or turning a blind eye to its ruination. Fantasies of being destructive and of destroying that which one loves and needs lie at the heart of depressive anxiety; and depressive anxiety involves paralysis of action and will. Ergo, we need to find other ways to get the political result.

I argued that ecopsychology fails to celebrate the urban and the cosmopolitan, fails to understand that artifice is natural for humans. In order to deepen this thought experientially, in the workshop, I distributed sample phials of many perfumes that Selfridges very kindly gave me. In pairs and threes, participants used the perfumes, applied them to each other, and compared notes. It was a smelly old exercise and a lot of fun.

Before the exercise, I asked who in the audience of around seventy-five eco-psychologists wore perfume or its male equivalents. Only one said that she did. Who read fashion magazines in which perfumes are widely advertized. None, though one person said guiltily that she did it in the dentist's waiting room. I said that this showed why environmentalism would fail and why ecopsychology had truncated itself. For those in the room – I arrogantly excepted myself! – had got completely cut off from ordinary life. I am as frightened of the destruction of the planet as many people in the ecopsychology world, I think. But I am also convinced that, if you look in the right way, there is much of value in the fripperies of fashion and consumerism and it is elitist to deny that. Depth lying hidden on the surface (to use words from Margaret Atwood's novel *Surfacing*).

In this chapter, I discuss environmentalism and ask: must the environmental movement fail? I suggest it will fail unless it becomes more conscious of the authoritarianism and depression within it, and the idealization of nature is somehow moderated.

Criticisms of the authoritarianism of the environmental movement, referring to its 'eco-terrorism', could wreck it by playing into the hands of entrenched industrial and financial institutions.[1] I think we should begin by admitting that there is a degree of accuracy in such criticisms. For there is a hidden authoritarianism in much of the new environmental politics which are the latest manifestation of the Enlightenment belief in perfectibility. Whether this takes the form of a downgrading of humanity to the level of fauna (or flora) or the issuing of a whole set of edicts about what is 'good', the tendency is clear to see. And already a backlash is going on. I think that environmentalist authoritarianism stems from a deeply buried misanthropy and, unless challenged, will itself turn out to be secretly and horrendously destructive. In Jungian terms, this is the shadow of the environmental movement and it would be helpful to become more conscious of it. Then the advantages of the unquenchable human thirst for a better world can be enjoyed – for only things of substance cast a shadow.

Casting an analyst's eye over the information and education material put out by organizations like Greenpeace and Friends of the Earth, I am struck by the one-sided portrait of humanity that is presented. Certainly, there is much to feel guilty about, much thoughtlessness and destructive behaviour to be owned, much acquiescence in horrid developments to be confessed. But the unremitting litany of humanity's destructiveness may not be the way to spur movement in a more creative direction. The result of too much self-disgust may be the cultivation of a deadening cultural depression that would interfere with environmental action. This is because fantasies of being all-bad and all-destructive usually lie at the heart of depressive illness. Therefore environmentalists should try to avoid any presentation of ideas about the environment that reflects humanity in an exclusively harsh light.

Instead, they might also celebrate what careful tending of the earth there has been over millennia. They might reaffirm the goodness, gentleness and aesthetic sensibility of humanity's artificial, cultural productions – our buildings, cities, art works and so forth. As an instance of what I am talking about, I think of the continuity to be found in the relations between humans and the environment in England. There is a sense in which the landscape itself has been made and remade over time as each succeeding generation leaves its mark. Emphasizing this cultural layering means that a more positive estimation of our environmental potential is brought into being.

It is vital not to represent environmentalism as a concern of the privileged classes, cut off from wider issues of social justice. To begin with, we have already seen that the greening of politics is going to be painful, both within Western societies and in terms of the relations between the developed and the undeveloped worlds. A whole host of moral decisions arises when we in the industrially advanced countries call for limits on deforestation in poor countries or advocate their controlling of their birth rates. We need an educational programme that faces people with these decisions and choices rather than letting them be made for them by experts who will offer protection from the moral implications of what is being done. Otherwise we will end up with a new Western hegemony: we will be OK but the poor of the earth will be even worse off.

What is more, we must not look to things like changes in consumer spending patterns to bring about improvement. Are we to say that when the going gets tough the greens go shopping? If substantive issues of social justice are not addressed then we *will* just be doing a landscaping job.

The question of economic redistribution within advanced societies is going to have to be addressed. If the polluters are to pay, then prices will rise enormously. The knock-on effects will be dramatic and many goods that we take for granted will be priced out of reach. *I want to suggest that this is a marvellous opportunity!* We are going to have to think about how we live and about how resources are distributed within our more advanced societies – and this will mean challenging the awesome power structures that exist. The problems confronting the world force a critical engagement with the banks, the multinational corporations, the IMF and with governments.

Calls for a return to traditional forms of homeworking or the setting up of *ersatz* agrarian-style communities should be treated with caution. For, in such situations, the lot of women has been and would continue to be an unhappy one. Instead, we should think of greening the cities we already have, making them safer and more pleasant for the groups they oppress – women, children, the elderly. For it has never been demonstrated that agrarian, parochial life is inherently superior to urban, cosmopolitan life. Advocating the tearing down of cities so as to foster the triumph of nature would be the way of a Khmer Vert.

Our young people will see through any educational campaign that idealizes nature, leaving out its frightening, harsh and bloody aspects and our ambivalence toward it. Such a campaign would resemble those commissioned portraits of the eighteenth century in which the lady of the manor is pictured dressed up as a milkmaid. The effect was to make nature an acceptable decorative element in the salons of the rich. Nature is itself not 'natural' but a culturally constructed idea. Moreover, the environmental movement still has to work on a balance between its 'anthropocentric' middle-of-the-roaders and its extreme wing – sometimes called 'ecologism'. Are we doing this for ourselves, for our own benefit and that of our children and other humans? Or is that simply a new gloss on the old exploitative attitude to nature? Should we not be acting for the benefit of an entire planetary organism? Battle lines are even now being drawn up between green extremists and the rest of the community, including 'ordinary' environmentalists. The argument that trees and rivers have rights needs to be assessed so that we can distinguish between its potential to inspire action and its gross oversimplifications. Does the HIV virus have 'rights'? Is it ethical to destroy dams or insert into trees spikes that injure loggers?

In this chapter, I will question some of the underlying assumptions and practices of the modern environmental movement by exploring the tensions between nature and artifice revealed by a critical comparison of two very different yet somehow complementary novels that seem to mark out this particular patch of psychological, cultural and socioeconomic territory. The novels are Margaret Atwood's *Surfacing* (1972)[2] and J.-K. Huysmans's *Against Nature* (*A Rebours,* 1884).[3] The interplay between Huysmans's hymn to artifice and Atwood's celebration of a woman's journey to a profound encounter with nature turns out to have political and social resonances. In addition, I suggest that in *Surfacing* we have a beautiful account of the progress of a female Trickster. I hope that the results of making this juxtaposition of two unrelated novels will justify the transgression of ordinary academic norms. Certainly, these are very different books. But they both engage with the idea of nature, they both present definite though complicated visions of sexuality, and they were both written at times when the relations between humanity and industrialism, and between women and men, were displaying rapid changes. Atwood was writing at the beginning of contemporary feminism, during the Nixon era with the Vietnam War in progress. Huysmans was working in the ferment of Paris in the 1880s, a time when the functions and forms of art were undergoing the most radical revision. Yet Huysmans, whom one would have thought of as the quintessential Artist (with a capital A), spent his entire working life in a government office and, in retirement, attempted to join a Trappist monastery. I hope the books can indeed bear the burden I am placing upon them. However, this chapter is more than a literary critique of two novels.

I assume that readers are broadly familiar with the current debate associated with environmentalism: the possibility of global warming, deforestation and species depletion, damaging of the ozone layer, acid rain and other pollutions, the limits to growth, the need for sustainable growth, the debate about population limitation, the general decay of urban civilization. I assume, too, an awareness of the gap in wealth between the industrially advanced countries and the developing countries, with the latter group heavily in debt to the former and often economically dominated by global corporations based in the industrially advanced countries. The tensions between the two kinds of country have also been written about so often that, allowing for differences of opinion, most readers will be aware that many developing countries assert their own right to the technological and industrial features that provide the consumers of the developed world with all their goodies. It is all very well for the industrially advanced countries to worry about pollution or deforestation in the developing countries but there is a certain irony in the fact that those who protest about what is happening to the rain forests of Amazonia themselves live in countries that consume a disproportionate amount of the earth's resources. In 1986 the United States was the only country to vote against the Declaration on the Right to Development passed in the General Assembly of the United Nations, and at the Earth Summit of 1992 the United States was also out of step with the rest of the world.

I am sure I am not the only one to be bewildered by the competing claims of groups of scientists that the situation is very grave indeed, or that it is grave but not disastrous, or that the warnings of planetary collapse are greatly exaggerated. It was partly to think my way through a thicket of information that I began the work that now forms this chapter.[4, 5]

Surfacing

Surfacing is presented in the first person. The anonymous narrator is returning to the northern bushlands of Canada because she has been informed of the mysterious disappearance of her father. She is a city-based commercial artist who has lost touch with her family and has not been 'home' for many years. Some time previously, she has left her marriage and child, and is travelling with three companions: a couple, Dave and Anna, and her lover, Joe. Dave and Joe are supposedly making a film in a *cinema verité* style. The four are depicted, not uncritically but also with humour, as creatures of the late 1960s or early 1970s, with the typical linguistic affectations and cobbled-together values of the middle-class rebels of that era. However, the novel's repeated mention of 'Americans' is not simply to be taken literally. 'Americans' are signifiers of all that is crass, destructive of natural beauty and threatening. This is a particularly Canadian referent, connected to Atwood's concern over the fate of Canadian culture and letters shown in another book of hers also published in 1972 – a book of literary criticism entitled *Survival*.[6] Moreover, as we saw, today's environmentalism has to deal with its own literal and metaphorical 'Americans'.

Drawing a blank at the homestead of an old farmer who was the narrator's father's best friend, the group of companions take a boat to the isolated cabin on an island in the lake in which the narrator had lived with her mother and father (her mother is dead). At the cabin, there is still no clue about what has happened to her father but, instead of returning to the city, the group decides to stay on for a further week, a decision which the narrator at first does not like. She organizes the others so that they can live relatively comfortably in the deliberately simple domestic arrangements her father has chosen. She takes them on blueberry-picking and fishing trips and, in general, acts as a kind of wilderness guide for the other three.

All the while, she is studying her mother's photograph albums and the scrap-books she and her brother had assembled. She is swamped by memories. Then she finds some drawings that her father has made. These are crude representations of human-like, exotic creatures. She concludes from the drawings, and his comments on them, that her father had gone mad. She is forced to change this view when she finds a letter from an anthropologist regarding material her father had collected and sent to him on ancient Indian rock paintings in the locality. The drawings must be of these paintings. She realizes by now that her father is probably dead but is impelled to make use of a map she has found that seems to indicate the where-abouts of the rock paintings.

She goes out onto the lake and dives beneath the surface, for the map shows that some of the paintings are under water due to a rise in the surface level of the lake. There she finds not a rock drawing, but her father's body, weighed down by his heavy camera. However, in the shock of that moment, she confuses his swollen and waterlogged body with the foetus she had aborted many years before when her then lover, her teacher and about the same age as her father, convinced her to get rid of the baby:

> It was there but it wasn't a painting, it wasn't on the rock. It was below me, drifting toward me from the furthest level where there was no life, a dark oval trailing limbs. It was blurred but it had eyes, they were open, it was something I knew about, a dead thing, it was dead . . . it was in a bottle curled up, staring out at me like a cat pickled; it had huge jelly eyes and fins instead of hands, fish gills. I couldn't let it out, it was dead already, it had drowned in air.

Following this catalytic experience, the narrator begins a *nekyia,* a kind of descent,[7] in which she seeks to reverse her acculturation and attain a state of merger with nature. She persuades Joe to impregnate her, but does it in a way marked out as a meaningful ritual, an initiation rite.

> We go over the ground, feet and skin bare; the moon is rising, in the greygreen light his body gleams and the trunks of trees, the white ovals of his eyes. He walks as though blind, blundering into the shadow clumps, toes stubbing, he has not yet learned to see in the dark. My tentacled feet and free hand scent out the way . . .
>
> I lie down, keeping the moon on my left hand and the absent sun on my right. He kneels, he is shivering, the leaves under and around us are damp from

> the dew, or is it the lake, soaking up through the rock and sand, we are near the shore, the small waves riffle. He needs to grow more fur.

By now the narrator has disappeared from the sight of her companions who return to the city in frustration. Acting on implicit knowledge that she is on some kind of significant journey, the narrator sinks into, embraces and identifies with the earth and its animals, with *nature.*

> Something has happened to my eyes, my feet are released, they alternate, several inches from the ground. I'm ice-clear, transparent, my bones and the child inside me showing through the green webs of my flesh, the ribs are shadows, the muscles jelly, the trees are like this too, they shimmer, their cores glow through the wood and bark.
>
> The forest leaps upward, enormous, the way it was before they cut it, columns of sunlight frozen; the boulders float, melt, everything is made of water, even the rocks. In one of the languages there are no nouns, only verbs held for a longer moment.
>
> The animals have no need for speech, why talk when you are a word. I lean against a tree, I am a tree leaning. I break out again into the bright sun and crumple, head against the ground. I am not an animal or a tree, I am the thing in which the trees and animals move and grow, I am a place.

Right at the end of *Surfacing,* Joe returns on his own to look for her and, like an inquisitive but cautious beast, she watches him from the trees. The frame freezes.

Perhaps more than any other single artistic production of the past twenty-five years, *Surfacing* deepened and highlighted questions about the cultural and psychological linkages of women and nature.[8] These questions have mainly been taken up in two contradictory ways. First, as referring us to a power and knowledge of nature held exclusively by women, based on their reproductive and nurturing capacities. Thus, women are the true guardians of nature, creatures of the earth goddesses, emblems and purveyors of all that is fecund.[9] The second view is that the equation of women and nature is one of the main processes that bind women into their oppressed place in patriarchal culture. For, as the subjugation of nature by (male) science proceeds, the subjugation of women, equated with nature, will proceed in parallel. *Surfacing* appears, superficially, to come down on the side of the first viewpoint, supporting and celebrating a twinning of woman and nature. But, as we will see, it is not as straightforward as that and *Surfacing* is not at all an essentialist tract.

It is interesting that, in the intense debate between feminist circles over these issues that were and are highlighted by *Surfacing,* there has been (quite rightly, in my view) very little space for the facile line beloved of the rote Jungians that at-oneness with nature is a 'feminine' capacity or quality, meaning a femininity capable of being developed internally by any woman or man. This metaphorical femininity is not the theme of *Surfacing,* nor the basis of what has been termed 'eco-feminism' – the perspective that sees correspondences between a despoiled planet and the exploited and ravished female body.[10] The equation of women and nature, whether taken as an indication of female potential and female gifts, or as an indicator of culturally driven female inferiority, cannot be split off from flesh-and-blood women.

Of course, there are many layers in a polysemous novel like *Surfacing* and, as Francine du Plessix Gray says, 'Atwood's genius rises above these debates.'[11]

However, I do not agree with du Plessix Gray that the novel has to be taken as a religious quest or as the working out of a female religious vision or, as other critics have claimed, as part of a typical, 'Jungian', 'individuation' process, following the 'archetypal' stages of a (or the) shamanic journey.[12] Undoubtedly, the narrator does go through a transformative process in which psychologically heightened exposure to the material world of her childhood functions so as to transcend the materiality of that childhood and, indeed, the materiality of the physical world itself. But this is quite specifically a transformation downward: down into the lake, down into the animal world, down (if you will) into the unconscious. This journey downward involves the narrator in nothing less than a transcendence of her human body:

> The footprints are there, side by side in the mud. My breath quickens, it was true, I saw it. But the prints are too small, they have toes; I place my feet in them and find they are my own. I am part of the landscape, I could be anything, a tree, a deer skeleton, a rock.

Transcending the body, and doing it downward not upward toward spiritual planes, implies a transcendence of ego-consciousness itself, or rather an assumption of a kind of 'natural' consciousness, a fathomless Nature consciousness – so that there is a paradox of total unconsciousness acting as a phantasmagoric *consciousness*. It is a paradox we have met before, when we met the Trickster who challenges the habitual division: below, matter; above, spirit.

Let us review the particular features of the narrator's transformations: the downward moves to an embrace with inferiority, the absolute bodily fluidity, the naive but magical omnipotence, the unconsciousness that is revealed as a treasure chest of natural consciousness, even the ambiguous ending of the book (will she, can she go to Joe or not?). Taking all of these features into account, I suggest that we are indeed in the realm of the female Trickster. As I noted in the previous chapter, in our culture the female Trickster lacks texts, lacks recognition, and yet one senses her readiness to be texted, to be recognized, if only for a millisecond.

The oft-discussed equation of women and nature now takes on yet another set of implications. It ceases to be a question posed in terms either of the celebration of women or of the subjugation of women. The equation of women and nature, taken on the level of the female Trickster, viewed as a trick, is revealed as having as its goal or *telos* nothing less than the social transformation of women. In Atwood's words:

> [The Americans] can't be trusted. They'll mistake me for a human being, a naked woman wrapped in a blanket: possibly that's what they've come here for, if it's running around loose, ownerless, why not take it. They won't be able to tell what I really am. But if they guess my true form, identity, they will shoot me or bludgeon in my skull and hang me up by the feet from a tree.

This is a trick because a woman who is by now not a woman but really an animal is pretending to be a woman lest in her true form she be treated as an animal by American men who have come to hunt in the Canadian wilderness. The female narrator of *Surfacing* quite literally 'drops out'. Ceasing to be a woman, she cannot be subjugated *like* nature because she *is* nature. But, to the extent that nature threatens people, especially men like Joe, or Americans, as a woman still she acquires nature's deathly powers – woman as 'Ice Woman', to use a phrase from

Atwood's other book, *Survival*. But we know it is still an illusion, because men still have the 'real' power, the socioeconomic power, the political power. It is no accident that, in the carefully crafted ghost story that is *Surfacing*, Atwood assigns all the pioneering skills – fishing, fire-making, tracking – to a female.

Reflecting upon the image of the female Trickster as agent of political change, especially of change in our attitudes to and dealings with the environment, offers an opportunity to break away from those three problems I mentioned at the beginning of the chapter: authoritarianism, depression and an idealization of nature. Environmentalism is itself subjected to a critique modelled on the upside-downness of the Trickster.

The trick is to use the most eternal, the most 'natural' formulation but to orientate that usage in the direction of social change. The eternal points up the mutable. Atwood is neither extolling woman as nature nor critiquing the notion: she is using it to reinforce a political project. The power of nature is, as we say, harnessed – but under a different aegis than that of phallogocentric industrialism controlled by 'Americans'. Tricksters push the logic of a particular piece of cultural oppression to the point where it implodes. We saw the same thing in the emancipatory effectiveness of the Mothers of the Plaza de Mayo, and we will witness the same capacity in des Esseintes, hero of Huysmans's novel *Against Nature*.

I must emphasize that my claim that *Surfacing* refers to a female Trickster and her socially transformative potential is not intended to depreciate its version of female potency. Quite the reverse. For, as we saw in the previous chapter, there is a neglected political capacity in Tricksters of whatever sex to transform passion and dream into the germ of a pragmatic political programme. The female Trickster's impressionistic manifesto deploys what seems to be an intrapsychic identification with nature as a template for changes in a different but related area of reality, namely the sociopolitical realm. Here, Atwood's concern with the survival of Canadian letters in the face of American cultural imperialism needs to be brought back into the picture. The relationship between the novel *Surfacing* and the critical work *Survival* is an extraordinarily complex one, not least in Atwood's own mind. But I think it is justifiable, at least in imagination, to propose that the female Trickster narrator of *Surfacing* is part of a response to the political problem of cultural and environmental survival depicted in *Survival*. In her critical book, Atwood points up the difference between 'nature as woman' and 'woman as nature'. As one who is both poet and novelist, she tells us that prose writers incline towards 'woman as nature', thereby confirming, if in code, that it is *women* on whom she wishes to focus in the prose work *Surfacing*.[13] Hence, perhaps, these lines:

> This above all, to refuse to be a victim. Unless I can do that I can do nothing, I have to recant, give up the old belief that I am powerless and because of it nothing I can do will ever hurt anyone. A lie which was always more disastrous than the truth would have been.

Nature and anxiety

Woman as nature makes many of us anxious. Yet, on the cultural level, the equation of woman and nature may itself be seen as a *response* to anxiety. In his seminal book, *Man and the Natural World*, Keith Thomas argued that the snowball of industrialism, Enlightenment and modernity created a profound anxiety in

European cultural consciousness, to the point of neurosis, over what was being done by civilized humans to the natural world.[14] Between 1500 and 1800, massive doubts emerged over the changes brought about by science and technology in the ways the natural world was perceived. There were many expressions of this counter-cultural sentiment. Theologians altered their notions about the relations between humanity and the rest of creation so as to gentle those relations and accommodate a certain decentering of humanity. Naturalists tried to understand and classify other species in non-anthropomorphic terms, thereby respecting their separate existence. Scientists explored links between humans and animals. Moral philosophers urged kindness to animals. In the city, the land came to be regarded as a thing of beauty, fit for contemplation, not as a useful resource. In sum, by 1800, people had responded to the anxiety engendered by the brutalizing path on which the world seemed embarked. The list of cultural and intellectual developments I have cited is evidence of the anxiety-driven shift in consciousness.

Today's concerns over the limits to growth, animal welfare and the fate of the environment may be regarded as descended from these earlier expressions of cultural anxiety. Yet we should temper our admiration for those who could not stomach 'progress'. They did not actually stop its march. Today, animal experimentation and factory farming have to coexist with the supreme idealization of the animal: the child's toy furry animal. As Thomas says, these cuddly creatures 'enshrine the values by which society as a whole cannot afford to live' – an observation he extends to include nature parks and conservation areas.[15]

The revolution in consciousness that Thomas writes about constituted a kind of underground resistance to what was being done to the natural world. This resistance went beyond a reaction to the ruination of nature. The perception of slaves, non-Europeans, children and women also underwent profound changes. As far as women were concerned, the form that liberal anxiety about modernity's denigration of women took was of an oppressive (and convenient) idealization that restricted women to private and domestic roles. The idealization of women and the idealization of nature share similar roots in cultural history in the West: they are both reaction formations. But women and nature remain deeply threatening because the idealizations of them are based on such flimsy and anxiety-ridden foundations. Hence the swiftness with which the image of the 'natural' woman moves from one who soothes a crying child or makes beds neatly into one who, transparent and web-footed, gazes at the man she commanded to fertilize her from behind a screen of trees.

So the cult of the countryside has this she-demon at its heart. Gaia[16] tips over into the Terrible Mother and the proud, human illusion of serving as Gaia's physicians is replaced by the starker reality of our being her slavish attendants, her Cabiri.[17]

Against nature

Any difficulty with summarizing the plot of *Surfacing* fades into insignificance compared with having to summarize the plot of *Against Nature*.

Duc Jean Floressas des Esseintes admits that he suffers from 'une névrose', a neurosis. At the age of thirty – Atwood was thirty-three when she wrote *Surfacing* – des Esseintes, the scion of a degenerated aristocratic family, decides to leave the debauched, big-city life of Paris and retreat to a 'desert equipped with all modern conveniences, a snugly heated ark on dry land in which he might take refuge from the incessant deluge of human stupidity.' We are told that

> try what he might, he could not shake off the overpowering tedium which weighed upon him. In desperation he had recourse to the perilous caresses of the professional virtuosos, but the only effect was to impair his health and exacerbate his nerves.

Even prior to his move, des Esseintes has a reputation as an eccentric. For example, he gave the by now notorious 'black banquet', a dinner modelled on a funeral feast:

> The dining room, draped in black, opened out into a garden metamorphosed for the occasion, the paths being strewn with charcoal, the ornamental pond edged with black basalt and filled with ink, the shrubberies replanted with cypresses and pines. The dinner itself was served on a black cloth adorned with baskets of violets and scabious; candelabra shed an eerie green light over the table and tapers flickered in the chandeliers.
>
> While a hidden orchestra played funeral marches, the guests were waited on by naked negresses wearing only slippers and stockings in cloth of silver embroidered with tears.
>
> Dining off black-bordered plates, the company had enjoyed turtle soup, Russian rye bread, ripe olives from Turkey, caviare, mullet botargo, black puddings from Frankfurt . . .
>
> On the invitations, which were similar to those sent out before more solemn obsequies, this dinner was described as a funeral banquet in memory of the host's virility, lately but only temporarily deceased.

By the way, thinking of those invitations, Huysmans made up des Esseintes's name from railway timetables to avoid the possibility of being sued for libel.

Having constructed his retreat, des Esseintes sets out to lead a life devoted to the experience of the highest forms of artifice and artificiality. Using the finest and most expensive materials, he builds for himself a replica of a monk's cell in which he will sleep. The point is that great expense is employed to create the *appearance* of humble poverty. Des Esseintes also constructs what he calls his 'mouth organ', a machine that dispenses liqueurs in tiny quantities, thus permitting a kind of blending to go on within the blender's own mouth:

> The organ was then open. The stops labelled 'flute', 'horn', and 'vox angelica' were pulled out, ready for use. Des Esseintes would drink a drop here, another there, playing internal symphonies to himself, and providing his palate with sensations analogous to those which music dispenses to the ear.
>
> Indeed, each and every liqueur, in his opinion, corresponded in taste with the sound of a particular instrument . . .
>
> Once these principles had been established . . . he even succeeded in transferring specific pieces of music to his palate . . .

Surrounding himself with exotic hot-house flowers, specially chosen for giving the appearance of being artificial flowers, des Esseintes spends many hours blending perfumes, seeking to reproduce, by artificial means, exact replicas of natural odours: 'One aspect of the art of perfumery fascinated him more than any other, and that was the degree of accuracy it was possible to reach in imitating the real thing.'

If des Esseintes wants to travel to London, he does not actually go there. He constructs a room on gimbals that reproduces artificially the rolling motions of the cross-Channel ferry and he has his servants make splashing sounds with barrels of salt water outside the window, using fans to waft in the salty smell. He travels to Paris so as to eat English food in an English restaurant, claiming that this is as 'real' as doing it in London. He wears a fur coat in hot weather, forcing himself to shiver, admires the convolutions of Decadent Latin poetry, adores the play of gorgeous colours on his walls and praises the marvels of modern manufacture above all the works of nature in a passage which is surely the ideological heart of the book:

> Nature, he used to say, has had her day; she has finally and utterly exhausted the patience of sensitive observers by the revolting uniformity of her landscapes and skyscapes . . . In fact, there is not a single one of her inventions, deemed so subtle and sublime, that human ingenuity cannot manufacture . . .
>
> There can be no shadow of doubt that with her never-ending platitudes the old crone has by now exhausted the good-humoured admiration of all true artists, and the time has surely come for artifice to take her place whenever possible.
>
> After all, to take what among all her works is considered to be the most exquisite, what among all her creations is deemed to possess the most perfect and original beauty – to wit, woman – has not man, for his part, by his own efforts, produced an animate yet artificial creature that is every bit as good from the point of view of plastic beauty? Does there exist, anywhere on this earth, a being conceived in the throes of motherhood who is more dazzlingly, more outstandingly beautiful than the two locomotives recently put into service on the Northern Railway?

I have given what must necessarily be a partial list of the things des Esseintes gets up to in the privacy of his own home. Perhaps the *pièce de resistance* is des Esseintes's adoption of a system of rectal feeding by means of peptone enemas. He fantasizes about all manner of delicious meals that might be consumed in this way. Thus, by artifice, basic biology is transcended.

How are we to understand des Esseintes's story, one hundred years later? We have our own *mal de siècle* with which to contend. Certainly, he acts with a directed energy quite foreign to his enervated and dilapidated physical state. He acts strongly so that his weaknesses may be pursued – the enemas were actually recommended by his doctor as a last resort for his drastically failing health. Des Esseintes, as I understand him, is merely doing something *natural* by creating an *artificial culture* for himself; for making culture is 'natural' for humans. Huysmans's genius is to hold a mirror up to ourselves, to disabuse us of the notion that we can separate nature from culture – and, thinking thoughts that hark back to *Surfacing,* to disabuse us of the notion that we can clearly separate so-called feminine (i.e. natural) and so-called masculine (i.e. cultural) capacities.

For sure, des Esseintes is not made happy by his experiment. Torn by vicious nightmares, he contemplates a return to the Catholic church. In the ecclesiastic yearnings of des Esseintes, the Trickster artificer expresses his religious instinct – just as 'I', the narrator in *Surfacing,* apparently on a religious quest, expressed her Trickster self.

Des Esseintes bears a message for our epoch about the ambivalence towards and fear of nature that no environmentalism can disguise. His neurosis is not merely a personal condition but a symbol of a collective malaise. Des Esseintes is both terrified of the body and seemingly quite at home with its febrile gestures. His mouth organ and his perfumery show that, within his own self-designated limits, he remains a perfectly sensual man. Moreover, throughout *Against Nature,* in his diatribes against nature, do we not hear des Esseintes calling out for some kind of connection to her? In his manipulated, artificial delights do we not perceive a recognition that no direct experience of nature is possible? (Nor direct experience of anything else, for that matter.) Nature is an artificial entity, a constructed phenomenon, existing in the hearts and brains of human beings. And here, does not des Esseintes anticipate Jung's idea that everything that exists exists first in psychic reality? Or, in a more modern vein, is not *Against Nature* an anticipation of the virtual reality of the computer game and a screen-bound, theme park culture? *Nature can be improved on by means of culture.*

Like Margaret Atwood, Huysmans cannot resist the move (almost a 'natural' move, it seems) from an engagement with nature to an engagement with the social – though, for Huysmans, artifice serves as the essential mediator. What could be more *engagé,* not to say *enragé,* than these lines from *Against Nature*?

> Under the pretext of encouraging liberty and progress, society has discovered yet another means of aggravating man's wretched lot, by dragging him from his home, rigging him out in a ridiculous costume, putting specially designed weapons into his hands, and reducing him to the same degrading slavery from which the negroes were released out of pity – and all this to put him in a position to kill his neighbour without risking the scaffold, as ordinary murderers do who operate single-handed, without uniforms, and with quieter, poorer weapons.

But Huysmans wouldn't be Huysmans and des Esseintes wouldn't be des Esseintes if these anti-war sentiments were not immediately followed by this remarkable *non sequitur.*

> Ah! If in the name of pity the futile business of procreation was ever to be abolished, the time had surely come to do it.

Flexible specialization

Viewed imaginatively, des Esseintes stands as a kind of economic and technological pioneer rather than an omnipotent narcissistic type seeking to control nature. His 'work' is carried out at home, not in office, factory or field. He makes constant use of technology – the mouth organ, the perfume-making apparatus, the room on gimbals, the syringe for rectal feeding. Following trends in development economics, des Esseintes uses technology that can be characterized as 'appropriate technology', operating on a small scale and with regard to environmental and social costs.[18] From the standpoint of the 1990s, it is hard at first to share des Esseintes's enthusiasm for technology, yet, in spite of ecologistic alterations in cultural consciousness, we in the West remain committed to and dependent on technology. Technology is, for us, a part of nature. Des Esseintes seems to know just which technology or, more accurately, which level of technology to apply to his consciously chosen tasks. In this sense, he can act as an imaginal bridge between a perspective that would restrict appropriate (or intermediate) technology to developing countries and one that could sense that the same pragmatic, modest approach might have applicability in the industrially advanced countries.

Another concept, also taken from development economics, which finds symbolization in des Esseintes's activities, and even in his personality, is that of 'flexible specialization'.[19] When I first heard this term, I thought immediately of human psychology because the capacity to perform many separate tasks according to the quite specific dictates of consciousness is characteristic of our species. In fact, the theories of flexible specialization are a response to the limitations of models of industrialism founded on mass production. In mass production, purpose-built machines are used by semi-skilled workers to produce standardized products. Standardization of the product permits economies of scale and helps to maximize profits. Flexible specialization, on the other hand, requires a combination of craft skill and flexible equipment – maybe electronics-based machinery that can be reprogrammed. As Kurt Hoffman and Raphael Kaplinsky put it, we are at a transitional point between the eras of 'machinofacture' and 'systemofacture'.[20] It may be that we are entering an era of technological Darwinism. It is important, for the developing countries *and* the industrially advanced countries, that flexible specialization kill off mass production because flexible specialization could then come into its own as the globally appropriate approach to technology for the last decade of the century.

That this should happen is important when we consider the possibility that environmentally linked conflicts may well erupt in the developing world in the near future – for example, conflicts over scarce supplies of water or large-scale migrations caused by desertification. The Gulf War of 1991 may also have been a precursor of other resource wars.

However, none of this will mean anything, and we run the risk of staying on a des Esseintes level of practicality, if we do not address the contemporary form of slavery represented by international debt. Developing economies need emancipating from the burden of debt and this will be facilitated by changes in mindset in the industrially advanced countries. The debts of the Third World were not incurred – are not being incurred – under a system of rules of fair play. Flexible specialization and appropriate technology may produce export-led growth, but the foreign currency never reaches the producers. If we consider a development problem such as the feminization of poverty, the trend in which women's economic lot often worsens as the wealth of their community increases, then the disaster that is going on right now is a deathly disaster for women and children.[21] The human rights of women and children are integral to effective and sustainable development. People have some 'right to development', no matter how artificial or against nature that turns out to be. Even the arch-dandy, esthete of esthetes, hyper-misogynist Duc Jean Floressas des Esseintes would agree (at least I think he would).

Spectrum

Let me review some of the links between *Surfacing* and *Against Nature* that I have been conjuring into existence. First, there is the interplay in both novels between Trickster and the person on a religious quest. Second, there is a searching examination in both novels of the relations between culture and nature, leading to all manner of destabilizations of our habitual diagrams of these relations. Third, in both novels the protagonists explore the possibility of a transcendence of the body. Fourth, there is in both novels an explicit search, by means of excess, whether natural excess or artificial excess, for a more fruitful relation to nature. As far as I can tell from empathic identification with both writers, the result should not interfere with the fullest possible living out of an unbalanced, supposedly one-sided position: 'I am a place' says Atwood's narrator; 'But I just don't enjoy the pleasures other people enjoy' says des Esseintes. Fifth and last, both writers are concerned with the relation between depth and the surface, the particular depth to be found on the surface, when surfacing; the unnatural depth of the environment.

What I have been trying to do is to construct a spectrum of responses to environmentalism out of the narratives, imageries, and underlying ethoses of the two novels *Surfacing* and *Against Nature.* What happens if we allow Atwood's narrator and des Esseintes to have a baby? What if des Esseintes were the father instead of Joe? What would *that* baby be like?

Environmentalism and education

Unlike Margaret Atwood, I have had to combine in one piece imaginative, fantasy thinking and pragmatic, directed thinking. What follows is both a depth psychological contribution to the many debates about environmentalism and an attempt to answer the question with which I ended the previous section: what *would* the baby look like?

The ideogram that is born out of this joint presentation of fantasy thinking and pragmatic thinking is that of *change.* Maybe the image of change always underpinned my argument already. One message of the environmental movement has been that we must change the way that we live and this will have to be done on the basis of changes in the ways we apprehend our relation to nature. It is hard to say succinctly whether the environmental movement is truly 'for' or secretly 'against' change. In the sense that environmentalism represents an opposition to the forms of social organization established in the industrially advanced countries in the past two centuries, the environmental movement supports a change. But in the sense that environmentalists, along with everyone else, have not caught up in consciousness with the techno-industrial revolutions of the past two hundred years, and are rooted in a pre-industrial cultural matrix, environmentalism may be seen as being against the very changes that have already happened. Hence, environmentalism may be regarded as deeply conservative. (It is a good example of the operation of *Nachträglichkeit* on the cultural level.)

But the key question, in all its school debating society naivety, remains: does, or can, human nature change? We saw how Atwood developed the eternal to point up the mutable. Des Esseintes does artificially what comes to us naturally by creating a new micro-culture. Oscar Wilde, profoundly influenced by Huysmans, wrote in his tract 'The soul of man under socialism' that 'the only thing we know about human nature is that it changes. Change is the one quality we can predict of it . . . The systems that fail are those that rely on the permanency of human nature, and not on its growth and development.'[22]

I think that what our thinking and feeling lacks most is a unit – I mean a unit of size and space – which is a comfortable one to have in mind when discussing environmental concerns. The temptation is to propose the world itself (as in the Gaia theory) or, at the other extreme, to focus on the bottle bank in one's own neighbourhood. We are, after all, embarking on nothing less than an exploration of the psychology of the earth, of what in Britain is called soil and Americans call dirt. How does the very ground on which you stand, on which you grew up, contribute to who you are?[23]

Not a conclusion

There can be no conclusion to a chapter such as this one. I am aware of its dissonances and jerkiness. The making of pragmatic suggestions when confronted with insoluble problems is itself an act of faith; there is an undecidability that cannot be denied. So the move on which I want to end is to salute the conception, or rather the construction, of a new kind of actor, an environmental actor with an environmentally attuned political consciousness.[24] Atwood's words from the closing passage of *Surfacing* chime with this:

> I bring with me from the distant past five nights ago the time-traveller, the primaeval one who will have to learn, shape of a goldfish now in my belly, undergoing its watery changes. Word furrows potential in its proto-brain, untravelled paths. No god and perhaps not real, even that is uncertain; I can't know yet, it's too early.

Or, in des Esseintes's words, at the end of a meditation on the evil triviality of the power held by the bourgeoisie whose only interest is the accumulation of wealth:

> Well, crumble then, society! Perish, old world!

Notes

1 See *The Times,* May 6, 1992.
2 Margaret Atwood, *Surfacing* (London: Virago, 1972).
3 J.-K. Huysmans, *Against Nature.* Trans. Robert Baldick (Harmondsworth: Penguin, 1959. Originally *A Rebours,* 1884).
4 See note 13 to Chapter 2 for statistics.
5 See note 30 to Chapter 2 for statistics.
6 Margaret Atwood, *Survival: A Thematic Guide to Canadian Literature* (Toronto: Anansi Press, 1972).
7 A *nekyia* is a form of temporary regression in which a person makes contact with his or her internal world at the expense of a loss of contact with external reality. In myth and legend, this is represented by a journey downward into darkness -the 'night sea journey'. According to Jung, regression is 'not necessarily a retrograde step in the sense of a backwards development, but rather represents a necessary phase of development. The individual is, however, not consciously aware that he is developing; he feels himself to be in a compulsive situation that resembles a nearly infantile state or even an embryonic condition within the womb. It is only if he remains stuck in this condition that we can speak of involution or degeneration.' In 'On psychic energy'. *CW* 8: 67–78.
8 For an account of the woman equals nature theme see Ludmilla Jordanova, *Sexual Visions: Images of Gender in Science and Medicine between the Eighteenth and Twentieth Centuries* (London and New York: Harvester Wheatsheaf, 1989).
9 See Anne Baring and Jules Cashford, *The Myth of the Goddess: Evolution of an Image* (London: Viking, 1991).
10 See Andrew Dobson, *Green Political Thought* (London: Harper Collins, 1990), pp. 201–2.
11 Francine du Plessix Gray, Introduction to Margaret Atwood, *Surfacing,* p. 6.
12 For example George Woodcock, *Surfacing, A Reader's Guide* (Toronto: General Paperbacks, 1991).
13 Margaret Atwood, *Survival,* pp. 202–4.
14 Keith Thomas, *Man and the Natural World: Changing Attitudes in England 1500–1800* (London: Allen Lane, 1983).
15 Ibid., p. 301.
16 See James Lovelock, *Gaia: A New Look at Life on Earth* (Oxford: Oxford University Press, 1982).

17 Cabiri were dwarf-like, phallic creatures who served the Great Mother goddess, especially in her guise as the Terrible Mother. They could be dangerous to her opponents.

18 Raphael Kaplinsky, *The Economies of Small* (London: Intermediate Technology Press, 1990).

19 Kurt Hoffman and Raphael Kaplinsky, *Driving Force: The Global Restructuring of Technology, Labor, and Investment in the Automobile and Components Industries* (Boulder, CO: Westview Press, 1988), pp. 36–40.

20 Ibid. (1978), pp. 64–9.

21 See Gertrude Goldberg and Eleanor Kren (eds.), *The Feminization of Poverty: Only in America?* (Westport, CT: Greenwood Press, 1991). Amartya Sen argues that we are dealing with a case of millions of 'missing women'. Given equivalent health care, nutrition, etc., women will live longer than men. The fact that, in the Third World, they do not live longer than men shows that they are not getting equivalent levels of health care, nutrition, etc. Hence, on an institutional level, the feminization of poverty in the Third World, and maybe in the industrially advanced nations as well, is a kind of murder. See Amartya Sen, 'Women's survival as a development problem', *Bulletin of the American Academy of Arts and Sciences, 43:* 2 (1989).

22 Oscar Wilde, 'The soul of man under socialism'. In *Complete Works of Oscar Wilde* (London: Book Club Associates, 1978), p. 1010.

23 See W. G. Hoskins, *English Landscapes: How to Read the Man-Made Scenery of England* (London: British Broadcasting Corporation, 1973) and John Barrell, *The Dark Side of the Landscape: The Rural Poor in English Painting 1730–1840* (Cambridge: Cambridge University Press, 1980).

24 I have in mind that an 'environmental actor' would move to central stage, ceasing to be part of what Bataille calls 'the heterogeneous'. See Georges Bataille, *Visions of Excess: Selected Writings 1927–1939* (Minneapolis, MN: University of Minnesota Press, 1985).

CHAPTER 4

ORIGINAL MORALITY IN A DEPRESSED CULTURE

Retrospective introduction

This was published in *The Plural Psyche* in 1989 but was in fact written for a big international conference in still-divided Berlin in 1986 at the height of the Cold War. I wanted to try to understand what the psychological inhibitors were on disarmament because the world felt at genuine risk of nuclear war.

There are two main themes: first, what I called 'moral process' and second, the impact of depression on our capacity for creative and positive action in the political as well as the personal field.

The idea that there is a basic ineluctable moral sensibility (original morality) in humans seems supported by science and social science these days. At the time, it was a bit more controversial a perspective. But the concomitant idea that there was some kind of valuable moral relativism to consider (moral imagination) still unsettles people. Nevertheless, my vision was of these two components of moral process in a ceaseless and tense dynamic relationship. I didn't come down totally on the side of moral imagination. Of black and white thinking, I wrote that these are valuable primary colours.

The analysis of cultural depression rests on something that has continued to be a main interest of mine: the vicissitudes of aggression. In this chapter, I range from anxious fear of aggression tipping into violence via nuclear conflagration to valuing the role of aggressive fantasy in individuation for women.

This chapter is about morality, imagination, depression and aggression, and I introduce the nuclear situation as a kind of case illustration. The chapter is written in a mixture of familiar and unfamiliar language. This is because unmediated psychodynamics seem to me an unsatisfactory basis for an analysis of culture unless a wider orientation is added, one that embraces the collective features in a cultural situation. So a link is made with a particular approach to moral process that I have developed. Links of that kind, and what we do with them, constitute the beginnings of working out a methodology to aid the integration of psyche's dynamics, the institutions of depth psychology, and the public sphere. Such an integration reflects the preoccupations of the first chapter [of *The Plural Psyche*] and anticipates the content of the final chapter.

Women and men are moral creatures. Psychology, ethology and the arts all attest to this. Yet, as confrontation with the problem of nuclear weapons shows, our fundamental sense of morality does not guarantee ethical behaviour either in relationship to ourselves, or to others, or to the general environment. On its own this moral sense is inadequate; there has to be some dialogue and interplay with a different kind of morality. This second morality – equally inborn, easy to recognize but hard to define accurately – generates tolerance, forgiveness, openness and an ingenious approach to problems. I want to call it *moral imagination* and to distinguish it from the first, fundamental, ineluctable morality that, in its certitude, I would like to designate *original morality.* The reference to original sin is deliberate.

In this chapter, I suggest that, while these two moralities differ, there is a crucial link and articulation between them. Original morality employed on its own has a tragic outcome. Yet it is the home base to which prodigal moral imagination constantly returns. Without the grounding in certitude that original morality supplies, moral imagination is too evasive by far.

We need not judge between the two moralities, branding one as schizoid and the other as mature and concerned, for original morality is not all blood and bone. Nor does one kind of morality adhere to the ego and the other to soul, for both subsist in each of these. Original morality does not *develop* into moral imagination, so I shall not be talking of the need to make individual a collective moral code or render personal an archetypal superego. Original morality ('sense') and moral imagination ('sensibility') are equally 'archetypal'. Hence, both have to become personal and express themselves in human relationships at all stages of life. Original morality and moral imagination are 'equals'; neither is superior to the other, nor divine.

Throughout the chapter, a personal matrix for moral process is assumed, in particular that provided by the infant–mother relationship that would, at any one time, display a mix of original morality and moral imagination in some proportion. However, as previously remarked, the argument is not primarily concerned with moral development as such; it is claimed that a baby can demonstrate moral imagination (e.g. when experiencing frustration) and an adult, original morality (e.g. when judging the behaviour of others). Similarly, in the paranoid-schizoid position, we may see moral imagination and, in the depressive position, original morality (see below for further discussion of this point). Original morality and moral imagination are not stages of moral development in Kohlberg's sense (1968), nor is the former 'masculine' and the latter 'feminine' in Gilligan's (1982) usage (and see Sayers 1986: 19–20 for a convincing refutation of Gilligan's thesis).

What will emerge, I hope, is an anatomy of morality in its own terms rather than in the languages of myth or of the psychology of the individual. Then some communication among all of these may be fostered. The intention is to do more than aim towards a synthesis that would simply set two moral viewpoints side by side and then transcend their differences in a calm and superior manner. The pluralistic tension within morality between certainty and improvisation cannot be resolved as easily as that.

Positing these two moralities may illuminate some of those perennial conundrums about destructiveness, wickedness and the shadow with special reference to the nuclear situation. These may be recast so that such dark riddles are seen as reflecting a clash of moralities rather than a struggle between morality and immorality or between conscience and evil or between ego and shadow. Morality itself contains a paradox and is a conflicted ideogram; the split resides in our moral perception, not between our moral side and our baser aspects.

If we could allow original morality its dialogue with moral imagination, maintaining the contact between them, and do this easily and reliably, there would be no need for this chapter. But what often happens is that we get hooked up on one or the other of original morality and moral imagination. If the former, then our approach to problems that cry out for choices to be made will be 'by the book', correct, stolid and safe, reliable – but missing out on the nuances of the situation. If we are hooked on moral imagination, our one-sidedness will have a different tone: bags of ingenuity and so-called 'flexibility', responsiveness to the uniqueness of the situation – but without any real grounding, conviction, or moral muscle. To make any headway at all when things are tough and complicated, we need the blend of certainty and improvisation that I have been describing. Moral imagination enables us effectively to use original morality; original morality guarantees the depth and authenticity of moral imagination. I will show how it is *depression,* functioning on a personal basis and on a cultural level, that is one of the main obstacles to the development of morality in its fullest sense. Depressive dynamics align with and support those of original morality and I will present depression as a kind of philosophy whose ideological stance is set against the reciprocity of original morality and moral imagination.

But first we should look at what is involved in a term such as original morality.

Original morality

Jung pointed out that morality emanates from within; it is a daimon, a voice that we have in us from the start. He was referring to our 'moral nature', of course, and not to precise moral formulations (Jung 1953: para. 30). At times, according to Jung, the moral aspect of man constitutes one of the primal pathways or canals along which, in metaphorical terms, libido may flow, equal in its fundamental status to biology and the spirit (Jung 1960: paras. 100–13). Conscience, then, is not a product of education or parental instruction; if it comes from anywhere, it comes from God. Jung's focus was on the split that may develop between personal ethics and the collective moral code. Jung's use of 'moral' and 'ethical' in relation to conscience is idiosyncratic and confusing (Jung 1964: paras. 825–57). Given that ethics, as a branch of philosophy, concerns itself with justification, codification and assessment of moral principle, an 'ethical' conscience would suggest one more in tune with the values and norms of the day, the exact opposite of Jung's usage. Morality, viewed philosophically, is a term that defines a broad but well-known area of human behaviour and ideation. However, Jung writes as a psychologist not a philosopher and it is clear what he is getting at; we shall return to this later. What I'd like to add to Jung's recognition that morality has its own force and drive is an attempt to go further into its dynamics, without presupposing the kind of conflict he described as being at the heart of the formation of conscience (cf. Jacoby 1985: 165–9).

In contemporary psychoanalysis, we see similar claims being made for some kind of innate moral sense. One of Klein's contributions was to raise the possibility of the superego being an innate factor. This idea then forms a theoretical base for Winnicott's insistence that children have an innate sense of guilt and hence are not born amoral (Davis and Wallbridge 1981: 72). Milner also suggests that we stop seeing morality solely as something implanted in children by parents and society (Milner 1977: 67). These psychoanalysts are not overlooking either the key role of parents and family in superego development, or the fact that what is rewarded by the cultural collective as moral, and hence what is punished as criminal, changes over time (nowadays one is not even hung for a sheep). What they *are* doing is pointing up the existence of a primal moral sense – original morality, in my phrase.

To my mind, Freud foreshadowed this view. One reading of his thinking about the superego suggests that he, too, was interested in seeing morality as a part of human make-up. All depends on what might be meant by words like 'archaic' when used in relation to the superego. Sometimes (e.g. Freud 1916–17: 370–1) such a word implies 'phylogenetic' and not merely 'traditional', and inhibitions upon instinctual activity are seen as 'organic' (Freud 1905: 176). Then there is an innate disposition for the self-preservative instincts to become more 'social'. The superego itself may be thought of as a vehicle for the transmission of culture, hence an omnipresent factor, neutral in itself – an archetypal structure, in the language of analytical psychology (Freud 1933: 232–3). To say that the superego is an archetypal structure, even a complex, is to do more than score a Jungian point. What is involved is the realization that morality, conscience and so forth cannot even be conceived of, let alone discussed, outside of a context of morality and conscience.

As far as post-Jungian analytical psychology is concerned, there is Hillman's distinction between prohibition and inhibition (1975). The former is external, situational and mutable; the latter archetypal, internal and present in many human motivations where it may lead to a psychological deepening. In this conception of inhibition, we can further see why it is important not to write off original morality as primitive or as holding a person back.

A critic might argue that these depth psychologists have missed something. Man, as a part of nature, is red in tooth and claw. It is Freud's vision of *that* that ought to be stressed. Though morality is valuable, helping us to live together in peace for much of the time, it is secondary, a cultural product, even a fulfilled wish. Such a thinker might go on to talk about humans as animals, male dominance and authority, natural selection, the selfish gene, competition and even the archetypes (e.g. Stevens 1982). These arguments require replies.

To begin with, authority is not necessarily authoritarian. As Dieckmann suggests, authority may be seen as playing a necessary part in the unfolding and development of social co-operation. The exercise of authority, he says, is tantamount to an instinctual activity (Dieckmann 1977: 217–8). Extending Dieckmann's idea, we might remember that the genes themselves work together, they are interactive and interdependent.

Further, what ethologists tell us about animal behaviour depicts co-operation just as much as competition, sharing as commonly as ruthlessness, huddling together for warmth, hunting together, sometimes helping each other to build nests, uniting for defence (Bateson 1984). Co-operation has always co-existed with competition, both are 'archetypal'. Similarly, inhibitions upon aggression have as established a history as impulses to discharge it.

After all, what does 'animal' signify? The paradigmatic animal may be a wolf *or* a cow. Similarly, concentration camps speak to us of sadistic aggression *and* of passive compliance. The Oedipus complex is about competitive rivalry and father-murder *and* about intergenerational co-operation and lineage (see Kohut 1982). As Mary Shelley knew, man and monster are one.

But, as I have said, original morality seems to be insufficient for the leading of a moral life. In Hesse's words, 'a man may keep the commandments but be far from God'. It can be experienced as harsh, vengeful, primitive and cold; it grapples with the appetites – in Money-Kyrle's words, 'zonal bite will be reversed into moral beat' (quoted in Newton 1981: 190). In an adult, in adverse circumstances, this takes the form of a profound suspiciousness of others, a tendency to jump to the worst possible conclusions, to rejoice in the other's misery when it seems deserved, and, ultimately, to retreat into the wilderness to feed on locusts and honey. Occasionally, such a psychology may buttress social order but somewhere there will always be an inferior element in it, and occasionally, unhappily, the patient plays this part.

For the fatal flaw in original morality is its vertical perspective, its obsession with the superior–inferior dynamic. The need to maintain the vertical split (superior–inferior), which is central to original morality, fuels the horizontal split that threatens the world so pressingly just now (Russia–America). The vertical split (superior–inferior) is superimposed on the horizontal plane (self/other, them and us, Russia and America). If we ask ourselves what it is that enables such shadow projections to occur and be effective, we have to posit some hypothetical force such as original morality. *For something* enables me to take the superior position in relation to you, leaving you smelling of my shit. It's the judgemental flavour of shadow projections that gives them their power and this may be laid at the door of original morality. In its isolated, 'pure' form, original morality has helped to create our divided world, slouching towards apocalypse.

Nonetheless, it remains vital to see beyond the developmental aspects of original morality, to value it as a lifelong capacity, as well as concentrating on what has to be achieved to overcome it. Even if original morality may be seen to dominate a certain phase of development, it contributes a potential richness of texture and quality to all phases, not merely as a 'moral defence' or 'anti-libidinal ego' (Fairbairn 1952).

Original morality casts things in black and white, but black and white are genuine colours. In them, images of perfection and perfectibility are kept alive. It is true that they are body-less, humour-less, care-less – but, nevertheless, they are reassuringly perfect. It is true that original morality is essentially a morality of narcissism, of the uroboros, of once-and-for-all redemption. But it is precisely these problematic features that we often need. Original morality saturates behaviour, serving us as a well into which we can dip, regenerating ourselves, overcoming cynicism, recapturing enthusiasm, relieving pain. Original morality keeps alive our dreams of getting things done as planned. In pathological form, this may be an addiction to perfection but original morality also stands as a prefiguring of its partner, moral imagination, just as the self prefigures the ego, later to coexist with it.

Original morality has a function, then. As Jung noted, striving after moral perfection is 'not only legitimate but is inborn in man as a peculiarity which provides civilisation with one of its strongest roots' (Jung, 1954: para. 123). Original morality is a broad-horizon reality for all its oversimplification and certainty. 'Insight [exists] along with obtuseness, loving-kindness along with cruelty, creative power with destructiveness' (Jung, 1952: para. 560). Original morality is present in the experience of being in love, when the loved one can do no wrong, and in the experience of hate, when the hated one can do nothing right. Even when original morality leads to experiences of persecution and guilt, this may be seen as providing an emotional foundation for thought and, hence, for maturation. A picture emerges in which the task of the one confronted with original morality – parent, friend, or analyst – is to defuse, moderate, mediate such morality, tenderize it, round it out, render it fruitful, de-idealize it, shake it up a bit – *but not to do away with it altogether.*

The point can be illustrated further by reference to primary and secondary process. Though secondary process is undoubtedly more developed, primary process continues throughout life and, without it, there is no *prima materia* for secondary process. Similarly, primitive forms of consciousness continue alongside more developed forms (Plaut 1959; Samuels 1985: 69–83; Zinkin 1979). Moral words are among the first to be learned.

From this perspective, an *equation* of moral imagination with the so-called 'mature' superego or the depressive position, or an *equation* of original morality with the paranoid-schizoid position would be too hasty. Both moralities interact with each other and in both positions – and we know from Bion how it is that the positions themselves enjoy an interdependence and interplay (1965). So there are two different axes to consider:

paranoid-schizoid ⟷ depressive position
and
original morality ⟷ moral imagination

Moral imagination

So, by now the reader is probably asking, what is this thing called 'moral imagination'? Broadly speaking, as the moral aspect of imagination, it is moral imagination that we use when confronted with a pressing, problematic and, especially, conflict-laden situation. Moral imagination is one means by which we apply our imagination to complex social and political issues. *Moral* because a choice may have to be made; *imagination* because that choice may have to be ingenious, less than clear-cut, a compromise or a creatively improved adaptation. Let's now look in detail at what is involved; at first, my approach is going to be an oblique one.

Right at the start of the Jewish Day of Atonement service (Yom Kippur), there is a short prayer that is of fundamental importance. So central is this prayer that in some congregations it is not recited by the reader alone but together with two members of the congregation. In all versions of the ritual, the prayer is recited *three times* and therefore may be assumed to be of supreme significance. This is the prayer:

> All vows, bonds, oaths, devotions, promises, penalties and obligations: wherewith we have vowed, sworn, devoted and bound ourselves: from this Day of Atonement unto the next Day of Atonement, may it come unto us for good: lo, all these, we repent us in them. They shall be absolved, released, annulled, made void and of none effect: they shall not be binding nor shall they have any power. Our vows shall not be vows: our bonds shall not be bonds: and our oaths shall not be oaths.

Our vows shall not be vows. What are we to make of this extraordinary pronouncement, the equivalent of cancelling all resolutions at the very moment of making them? Remember, this is *the* high, holy day. There are three possible understandings of the prayer. First, we must be careful not to aim too high, making promises for the future that we cannot keep because of our human limitations. Given the massive sanctions laid down in the Old Testament against those who break their vows, it is crucial to state, right at the start of the process of repentance and atonement, the possibility that it will not work out as intended in the future. Thus, reference is made to the period between this Day of Atonement and the one next year. The second interpretation of this Kol Nidrei prayer is exactly the opposite: that the vows, bonds, promises that are being annulled refer to those made last year, which experience has shown to be unfulfilled or unfulfillable. It is urgently necessary to cancel these promises for we are even now in breach of them. Finally, a third reading: by cancelling all human moral contracts, we are free to contract with God. The compulsions of original morality are anticipated and, hopefully, purged.

I have introduced these reflections on the Yom Kippur ritual to show that a recognition of the unlivable nature of original morality on its own lies at the heart of Judaism, and perhaps of all religions. Jung unfairly castigated Judaism as a source of repressive and legalistic moralism, overlooking the more generous side. What Jung failed to recognize, before the war in his *Zentralblatt* papers on racial psychology (1934) and after it in *Answer to Job* (1952), is that Judaism enjoys and suffers the tension between original morality (certainly not lacking therein) and moral imagination.

It is not a case of contrasting absolute moral principle with relative quasi-moral behaviour. Both original morality and moral imagination have principles. What follows is an attempt to outline some of the principles of moral imagination.

Moral imagination contains an intuitive and psychological understanding of what a moral principle really is. As the philosopher Philippa Foot points out, morality differs from etiquette or good manners in that:

> Moral rules are not taught as rigid rules that it is sometimes right to ignore (as in the case of etiquette); rather we teach that it is sometimes *morally permissible* to tell lies (social lies), break promises (as e.g. when ill on the day of an appointment) and refuse help (when the cost of giving it would be as we say disproportionate). So we tend, in our teaching, to accommodate the exceptions *within* morality, and with this flexibility it is not surprising that morality can seem 'unconditional' and 'absolute'.
>
> (Foot 1978: 186–7)

Accommodating the exceptions within morality is a good enough summary of moral imagination. With this perspective on moral principle, we lessen the intimidation that is attached to obligation, hence enlarging the area of choice.

If original morality is about manifestos, moral imagination is about that Mediterranean shrug of the shoulders when faced with inconvenience or even disaster. Sometimes accompanied with an exclamation, 'Boh!', the gesture signifies an acceptance of imperfection, a worldly and wise reluctance to hope for too much, and sometimes it signals a creative improvisation to try to deal with things.

Steiner, a British psychoanalyst, makes a helpful contribution here. Discussing the question of Oedipus's knowledge or lack of knowledge of his plight, Steiner argues that 'we are meant to accept the idea that *both* can be simultaneously true, that he knew and at the same time did not know' (Steiner 1985: 165). Nothing could be further from the all-knowingness, maintaining narcissistic equilibrium, that we encounter in original morality. But if we are to avoid turning a blind eye to the plight of Oedipus, we also need that *certainty* that is the benchmark of original morality.

Continuing to search for the principles of moral imagination, let us focus on two specific themes: forgiveness and moral pluralism.

Forgiveness, and not blame, characterizes moral imagination. Forgiveness of one part of the self by another part, forgiveness of another person, or by another person, forgiveness of one group by another. Forgiveness is important because it can bring a new element into a situation; it is therefore creative (hence imaginative) and, to a degree, an autonomous force in psyche and culture. Forgiveness has much to do with suffering. For the sinner to *feel* a sinner, he or she experiences suffering. At the same time, the one who is to forgive will also have to suffer – for there can hardly be any forgiveness where there is no price to pay. Looked at in this way, the process of forgiveness rests on the ubiquity of suffering.

Forgiveness, as an image and as an experience, makes us question the operation of linear time. When forgiveness is coupled with repentance, then the present may be regarded as shaping the past. Associated promises of good behaviour in the future may be regarded as shaping the present. Forgiveness frees the imagination from the shackles of linear time. The value of forgiveness can be seen in analysis when the patient explores the possibility of forgiving his or her parents for the damage he or she feels they have inflicted. The patient leaves off his or her armour and displays hospitality towards images of the past; this process is the justification of reductive analysis.

In addition, we might query the conventional forgiveness–blame dichotomy. There is a middle position in which I partly blame the malefactor (or bad side of myself) and partly forgive him or it. We can then speak of part-punishment and part-redemption. Whatever the standing of these terms theologically or philosophically, we often encounter what is involved in an emotional form in the consulting room.

On the other hand, the patient gripped by original morality will know the moral score and will strive to become wholly virtuous before he or she forgives him/herself. As far as forgiving sinful others is concerned, the originally moral patient is unlikely to entertain the idea or, if he or she does, it will be in a form that reduces the other to nothing but a blob of contemptible and penitential stuff – hence easily pardonable from on high.

The next theme I want to pursue concerns moral pluralism. Though I intend to develop a different set of ideas here, I am thinking also of a morality of transition, liminal morality, differing moralities attached to the erotogenic zones, to specific images, to the various gods or to the stages of life.

If one looks at the multifarious moral commandments and prohibitions that exist, it is very difficult to state the one general principle, or even a few general principles, that connect all of them. They are unavoidably plural; it is their essence to discriminate numberless kinds of approved and disapproved behaviour. This can be seen in the Day of Atonement ritual, in which enormous lists of specific sins are confessed out loud; general confession seems inadequate even though it is general absolution that is sought. The specific, the nitty-gritty, the plural images of sin are thrust forward. This is so because human beings do not have a single dominating concern or goal, no one supreme interest – and the concerns, goals and interests that may be observed are, again innumerable. It is not a question of moral perception but of moral perceptions. There is a need to reconcile, or to downplay, or to privilege and accentuate very different concerns, and this is true for individuals and society alike. What we admire and value in ourselves and others need not follow any logical format: warmth and openness together with careful attention to detail, driving ambition with pervasive self-doubt. Such illogical combinations occur in the external world as well: societal conflicts and political pluralism are mirror and model for the moral conflicts of the personality.

It follows that moral imagination typically requires a weighing up of conflicting claims: for example, should I support a friend whom I know to be in the wrong? My response to this kind of question, coupled with my responses to myriad others of equal difficulty, informs the dynamics of social *communitas* and of moral imagination. Here, in the weighing of claims in conflict, original morality comes into its own, vital for the workings of moral imagination. We must endeavour to *use* the moral knowledge we have always had.

Thus far, I have been pitting moral imagination against the adoption of single-criterion ethics. Here I would like to recall Jung's admonition to follow the inner voice even when this risks being shunned as a deviant (Jung 1964: paras. 825–57). I find myself undecided as to whether this constitutes a single-criterion ethic. Sometimes in his constant preference for a subjective, intuitive and emotionalist morality, Jung can be seen as an exemplar of original morality; knowing and biased. Does sharing Jung's morality mean opening the inner ear and closing the outer one? On the other hand, the inner voice may itself be plural in its nature, expressing more than one point of view.

I have been arguing that there is a psychological value in facing a conflict of claims, something more than a mere acceptance of practical realities, which would be moral relativism or situation ethics. It is important not to see moral imagination as just the daily version of original morality, or as the relative outcome of absolute principle. *Pluralism is not the same as relativism.* Perceiving a conflict of moral principles is not the same as claiming that, in life, principle has to be watered down. Moral *relativism* implies a hierarchy in which principle is placed above and distinct from praxis. Moral *pluralism* sees no value in unlivable principle, nor does it take such a pat-on-the-head, there-there attitude to moral failure, based on concessions to human appetites. There's a name for that: casuistry. The principles involved in moral pluralism embrace their own tricksterish failure in the world; we accommodate the exceptions within morality; *the exceptions make the rules.*

After all, as the philosopher Anthony Kenny points out, what we mean by 'goodness' is itself plural and may vary when discussing either a thing or a state of affairs:

> The criteria for the goodness of a thing depend on the nature of the thing in question: an earthworm who does well the things that earthworms do is a good earthworm, no matter whether anybody wants an earthworm or not. The criteria for the goodness of a state of affairs depend on what people want: good weather is not weather which is good of its kind, or which does well the things which weather does, but weather which enables you to do well whatever it is you want to do.
>
> (Kenny 1963: 221n)

Of course, moral imagination itself could be represented as a single-criterion ethic, with *its* value wedded to pluralism and conflict. I don't see any defence against that save to recall that one leitmotif of this chapter has been to point out the co-presence of original morality, the acme of single-criterion ethics, with moral imagination. The absolute has its place. Indeed, sometimes it is necessary to make a one-sided commitment, based on one moral criterion or a small set of criteria. Then moral imagination must cope with a tension within itself between the variety of pluralism and the intense strength of the moral absolute. This may be seen when a person makes a massive investment in a god, a profession, an art, a relationship. It is a part of human experience to be torn in this way and the rack is stretched between more than mere models of behaviour; variant self-images are at odds. Nowhere is this more marked than in the ways in which nation states present themselves to others or see themselves from within. The difficulty an individual might have in reconciling the competing claims of his inner units is multiplied when the problem is faced by the state.

The question of moral pluralism is also addressed in Diderot's brilliant dialogue entitled *Rameau's Nephew,* written *circa* 1761. The amoral, tricky, corrupt, wastrel musician challenges the validity of the moral principles by which his philosopher interlocutor is judging him. True, he says, there may be some kind of general conscience, just as there is a general grammar but, as in grammar, there are exceptions. In fact, as the Diderot scholar Peter France points out, Rameau is doing more than defending the exception against the rule; he, too, is arguing that the exception *is* the rule. It follows that 'so-called virtue is cold and unlovable, so-called vice is what makes the world go round' (France 1983: 79). In the end, like so many tricksters, Rameau 'turns the tables by casting doubts on the sanity of those who patronise him' (France 1983: 81).

In this clash of original morality and moral imagination, we should not assume that each protagonist represents one side in a clear-cut way. Both parties speak for both moralities at different times. Of course, Diderot is present in both of his creations. The point is that in original morality there is either no dialogue or, if there is a dialogue, it is one with overclear and unequivocal positions in it. In moral imagination, not only is there dialogue but it is difficult to say with certainty who speaks for what. The clinical parallel is with the dialogues of active imagination that become suspect when cut and dried. In *Rameau's Nephew,* we see how the relationship between the two men changes during and because of their communication.

Now, as promised at the outset, it is time to consider how depression drives a wedge between original morality and moral imagination, frustrating their dialogue and their mutual fertilization. In particular, when we reflect upon moral imagination, as an experience and in emotional terms, aggression cannot be avoided. Without aggression, 'conflict' remains a word and not a living and coruscating process. *Aggression fuels moral imagination.*

Depression

I want to present depression as a philosophy of our day, dedicated to the condemnation and suppression of aggression. As such, depression may be seen as a moral disorder and injurious to moral imagination. Depressed patients tell us of being overwhelmed by feelings of badness, destructiveness and, above all, self-blame. Psychodynamically, the connection with aggression lies in the fantasy of having destroyed the loved object or person who was necessary for emotional survival; ambivalence was not a possibility. Alternatively, depression may be a means of guaranteeing parental love and acceptance by gainsaying the aggression that is felt not to be permitted by the parents. The reader will note that I couple these opposing viewpoints, for I believe that the real value of theoretical disagreements among analysts is that they point to the nub of the matter, whatever it is, and suggest a starting point for the tyro theoretician.

This also applies to background speculation concerning the aetiology of depression, particularly where the debate polarizes along developmental/archetypal lines. From the personal historical perspective, we have to think of the vulnerable mother, in fact or fantasy, meaning her vulnerability in psychopathological and environmental terms. The depressed mother, the unmothered mother, the too-young mother – and then the poor, ill-housed, badly educated, unsupported mother (see Brown and Harris 1978). The mother's vulnerability performs a phenomenological work upon aggression. In plain language, the child's aggression seems to the child to be worse than it really is. From an archetypal perspective, we have to think tentatively of an adverse and inborn imbalance between love and hate in an individual. This is a very hard thing to stomach: some people are born constitutionally more aggressive than others. Given an unfavourable and unempathic response to the excess of aggression, and it is clear that depression in the adult may be the outcome. Here, it does not matter whether the archetypal view is expressed in terms of the gods or in the language of biochemistry, neurology and genetics.

One of the consequences of the moral certainty of depression is that the psychological value of aggressive fantasy is lost. Depression, functioning as a moral philosophy, promotes two well-known but seemingly intractable conflations: of aggressive fantasy and destructive fantasy, and then of fantasy and action. Let's consider these in turn.

Aggressive fantasy has its own *telos*. In saying this, I do not intend to minimize the damaging, negative, painful, perverted, controlling aspects of aggressive fantasy. However, the observation has often been made that aggressive *behaviour,* in the form of healthy self-assertion, is a necessity for survival in both an absolute and a social sense. My concern is more with aggressive images and images of aggression. Because the ground to be traversed is undoubtedly familiar, I would like to make a start by saying that the old debate about whether aggression is primary and innate, or a secondary reaction to frustration and fear, or both, has tended to mask a more significant question: what are the consequences for moral speculation if aggression *is* innate? It seems to me that there is no moral problem whatsoever with aggression as an innate factor, no need for shame or apologetics about that (but cf. Jung 1950: para. 504n, where he demurs at the death instinct). After all, sex is similarly innate and is not minimized on that ground nor are attempts made to eliminate it altogether.

Aggressive fantasy promotes a vital style of consciousness (images of tearing things up, dissecting them, controlling them, playing with them, making use of them). Aggressive fantasy has much to do with our desire to know; it is not, in itself, completely bloodstained and unreflective. (Bad science is not science *per se.*) Aggressive fantasy can bring into play that interpersonal separation without which the word 'relationship' would have no meaning. In this sense, aggressive fantasy may want to make contact, get in touch, relate. For some, mainly men perhaps, it may be the only way to relate. The same is true for internal units and processes; aggressive fantasy enables separate images of the parents to emerge, and other imagos, and inner discriminations – for example, what theory refers to as the ego–self axis. As Searles says, 'at one moment a violent urge may express a striving to be free and at the next a desire to relate' (Searles 1973: 325). Aggressive fantasy forces an individual to consider the conduct of personal relations. When one fantasizes an aggressive response to one's desires on the part of the other, one is learning something about that other as a being with a different but similar existence to one's own. Without aggressive fantasy, there would simply be no cause for concern about other people and so aggressive fantasy points beyond ruthlessness to discover the reality and mystery of persons. 'It is only when intense aggressiveness exists between two individuals that love can arise' (Storr 1970: 57). Finally, aggressive fantasy is playful at times, even humorous, a continuous cartoon of ejaculatory, exploratory enjoyment, a *jouissance* – for women, perhaps one way to be 'seminal', 'thrusting' and 'penetrative'.

Since it is composed of images as much as impulses, aggressive fantasy can be approached via its specifics. An example appears in Freud's 'A child is being beaten'

(1919). And Jung, writing about the treatment of depression, suggested that getting to the inherent fantasies leads to 'enrichment and clarification of the affect' (Jung 1960: para. 167). But it is clarification of the *image* that is needed in relation to aggressive imagery: biting is not tearing, nor smearing, nor cutting, nor punching, nor shooting, nor beating.

Aggressive fantasy, like incest fantasy, has a refuelling and regenerating function that is accentuated in more extreme fantasy. For aggressive fantasy returns us to basics, to evolutionary dangers just as much as to the mother's body or the father who bars our path.

When an instinctual impulse is blocked in terms of actual expression, the fantasies associated with it may be permitted space in which to take on more depth; it is not important whether we refer to this as sublimation or transformation. But if the fantasy is itself blocked, then this cannot happen. What Jung pioneered for fantasies of incestuous sexuality in *Symbols of Transformation* (1950) should be attempted for aggressive fantasy. This would mean, for example, that aggression between persons, or the aggressive fantasy of one about the other, may not only be about those two persons; its symbolic meaning as *coniunctio* as well as its literal potential engages our interest. The perversity and horror of aggressive fantasy may give it a creative capacity to nourish the soul. Just as with sexuality and spirituality, the transformation of aggressive fantasy tends to be in the *general* direction of its opposite: creativity and moral imagination – towards forgiveness and the new departure that that can bring; towards moral pluralism; and towards an acceptance of the body's irreducibly aggressive motions. We should not forget the thrill and excitement of aggressive fantasy, its action in and upon sexuality and feeding. Then there is the bliss of the calm after the storm. Aggressive fantasy, breaking taboos as it does, proposes an image of human moral creativity shorn of idealizations and full of eros; Jacob wrestling with his angel. Transformation is never easy, sometimes destructive, and impossible to order up. Renewal and aggression are twins.

Finally, in this survey, there is the part played by aggressive fantasy in a gut response – that free play of imagination that permits one to react outside of the 'rules', leading eventually to an aesthetic sense. (The reader might recall the discussion in Chapter 5 [of *The Plural Psyche*] of the father's role in the transformation of aggression.)

In myth, when Kronos turns on Uranus, one of the imaginal birth moments of Western culture, he cuts off his father's genitals with a sickle, casting them into the sea. From them, Aphrodite is born, the goddess of love. Out of the despairing, murdered, foamy ejaculate steps the epitome of beauty. Here, too, the imago of child as phallus has its archaic roots. It seems to be no accident that contemporary depth psychologists have needed to make the aggression–depression dynamic a central part of their theorizing. Nor is it coincidence that Hermann Hesse's counterpart to Narcissus, the one who leads a life of mind and spirit, is Goldmund, as often killer as fornicator. In its confusion of aggressive and destructive fantasy, a depressed ego stops the dialogue between the aggressive mind and the world.

I mentioned that depression promotes two conflations and we have just been looking at one of them, between aggressive fantasy and destructive fantasy. The other mix-up was between fantasy and action. Here the designation of depression as a moral philosophy makes sense. In depression we can see a distorted application of what, in philosophy, is referred to as intentionality. Any emotion (and that includes fantasy) will construct an object towards which it is directed, towards which it has intention. I cannot be aggressive save in relation to an object of aggression or believe without an object of belief. Such 'intentional objects' include ideas (objects of thoughts), individuals (objects of love and hate), or groups (objects of alliance and enmity).

In depression, the strength of aggressive fantasy, and the moral consequences ascribed to it by the ego, make for intentional objects of immense power. While the value of intentional objects is that they facilitate emotional expression, their coming to psychic dominance – as they do in the omnipotent, destructive fantasies of the depressed person – has absolutely the opposite effect: a paralysis of the imagination and a judgemental, landslide victory for original morality. The depressed person – or culture – is confronted with an utterly literal portrayal of the outcome of fantasy. In the language of philosophy, in depression 'intentional objects' become 'material objects'.

I am not saying that inner and outer are absolutely different or that fantasy and action are unconnected. But in depression the ego adopts an exclusively external perspective, forgetting, in Winnicott's phrase, that moral guilt belongs to inner reality (Winnicott 1958: 15). Therefore a depressed person cannot join in the dance of original morality and moral imagination.

I have been working up these ideas about depression at some length because they have particular relevance to our reactions and responses to the nuclear threat. (This is my case illustration, so to speak.) Consider: in almost every respect, the emotional dynamics of our confrontation with the nuclear situation replicate and stimulate those of depression. There is a confusion between inner and outer; inner fantasies of world destruction that have always existed are now literal fact. There is an enormous fear attached to the expression of aggression today; total war might result. Moral imagination is overwhelmed and the ego, dominated by original morality, searches for something to blame: history, the system, patriarchy, the enemy, the scientific ego itself.

The pressing issue is our powerlessness in the face of the nuclear problem. We need to distinguish between the psychological dynamics of the world political situation and the specific psychological dynamics of our inertia and impotence. Not what is felt about the Russians, nor why it is felt, but how we feel about a world in which Russians, Americans and others are locked into a certain kind of combination. If we look at things from this standpoint, the critically disabling anxiety from which we suffer is not paranoid anxiety, hence not characterized primarily by splitting, projective identification, projection of the shadow, and so forth. In the nuclear age such concepts, often quoted by depth psychologists, do not illuminate our paralysis when what used to be regarded as an overliteral apperception of aggressive fantasy has become the plain fact. *We can destroy our adversaries* – and, from that, depression will follow, silencing the articulation between original morality and moral imagination. We back away from the creative edge of our aggressive fantasies when, in reality, it is through their free play that we can begin to realize their opposites – forgiveness and compassion (J. Kirsch, personal communication 1986).

Like depression with its delusions of self-blame, the nuclear situation forces us to stay locked into original morality. For whether we anticipate with certainty total nuclear destruction or, with equal certainty, a peaceful balance based on the fear of retaliation, it is *such certainty itself* that keys us into original morality. When depression and original morality collude, one's sense of responsibility becomes the victim; 'integration of the shadow' becomes a pious nonsense. If nuclear weapons have injured our capacity for moral imagination, they certainly show our need for it. But cultural depression will prevent the need from being met. Hopelessness has become global and there is no space for good thoughts about ourselves.

In our culture, the depressive fear of our own destructiveness, and the corresponding paucity of moral imagination in relation to that, have reached epidemic proportions. The traditional institutions for its containment have become eroded. Our culture suffers from a collective, depressive delusion that it is all-bad, all-destructive. We are therefore alienated from the possibility of forgiveness. Moreover, the process is circular; depression and original morality feed into one another so that we cannot extract the value from our aggressive fantasies. When we talk of the positive side of the shadow or of healthy aggression, we should take care not to neglect the depressive block in us that prevents such gold from being mined. There is also the possibility that interruption of the flow between original morality and moral imagination may itself lead to (further) depression.

Women in our culture experience particular difficulties in expressing aggression; one result may be their statistically greater tendency to become depressed. For women have much to feel aggressive about; they have to be nice, adopt a passive social stance and worry about their appearance; they are said to be 'maternal' and their eroticism is limited by male preconceptions. Yet it is women who have led the way in protesting against the assumptions of nuclear proliferation. Perhaps their anger and aggression at what is required of them by society has freed their imaginations and enabled them to take action. However, for men and women, the depressive fear of losing parental love makes it hard to say 'no' to the political parent-figures; it is a problem that is not usually addressed by those who want 'the people' to act.

For some, global hopelessness is itself so intolerable that trust is placed in simplistic, single-strand solutions. Using the language of this chapter, this is original morality and not moral imagination at work.

Depth psychology and social analysis: A comment

It would concern me greatly if the question of the validity of applying concepts and intuitions from depth psychology to issues of a social and cultural nature was not addressed in this chapter. To begin with, psychological ideas are already part of culture. They are generated in a precise historical context even though their imagery may be recycled through the operation of the archetypes. We may find in our analyses of the internal world just what it is that is experienced in society. Conversely, how we perceive the world and what we perceive therein tells us about the psyche. The interpenetration is not an imposition; it already exists. However, it is important to carry out a necessary work of abstraction upon clinical material before applying it to social trends and issues. That is why I am interested in using theoretical *disputes* rather than single theories when discussing cultural and social matters: depression as personal-historical or as innate and endogenous; a consequence of aggressive fantasy or a learnt passivity. Focus on the debate permits a more flexible application of the psychology assuming, as it does, that psychological dialogue, discourse and dispute are cultural phenomena, reflecting cultural processes and preoccupations. We learn as much about clinical practice when we reflect upon culture as vice versa.

Another way for the analyst intent in communicating an analysis of culture to proceed is to stick close to the therapeutic method. Instead of a surreptitious identification of the culture (or an aspect of it) as the 'patient', such identification becomes open. According to Stein (1985: 22), this 'treatment' of a cultural phenomenon is demonstrated in Jung's approach to Christianity. Stein shows how Jung's method used three main planks of psychotherapeutic procedure.

These are: (a) historical reconstruction; (b) interpretation, both reductive and forward-looking; and (c) the transference–countertransference dynamic. Thus, when we examine a phenomenon (a case?) such as helplessness and hopelessness in the face of the nuclear threat, we are interested in how the problem has evolved, how we understand its origins, where it seems to be going and, finally, how we relate to it on an emotional level and how it (the problem) responds to our therapy. This last subject is important: even the social analyst writes out of a personal agenda; though this may be hidden, his or her countertransference has to be considered. Social problems, like patients, respond to treatment in differing ways. The hope is to avoid the self-deception of 'objective' analysis; this would be analogous with the inhuman application of the worst kind of 'high-tech' medical approach. Using psychotherapy as the model for cultural analysis makes use of the critic's affective engagement. Looked at like this, maybe all social and political enquiry is really therapy.

A further reason for including this 'comment' is that the nuclear threat is but one aspect of a general alienation of women and men from their social world: pollution, poverty, exploitation, sexism and racism are all part of the picture.

Coda

I had thought to stop the chapter here, with depression as 'the problem', so to speak. But, conscious that it is well known that there are many positive aspects to depression, I gradually became aware that depression, the problem, could also be visioned as a kind of solution, or at least as an ambience in which solutions could be worked upon (because there is no obvious solution).

Overcoming depression involves a reconstruction and reconstitution of the internal world so that losses are somehow made good or accommodated to; imagos of others (particularly parents) are allowed fruitful life; and personal responsibility for disaster is reassessed. All of these involve entering fantasy, owning the aggressive images and hence one's potential for aggressive, even warlike discharge. An alternative to discharge, though, is to be forgiven for one's aggression; by oneself or by its recipient whether friend, enemy or analyst.

Considered in this light, depression may be seen as lying at the *heart* of moral imagination and, especially, of forgiveness. Paradoxically, depression may then actually *constitute* a link between original morality and moral imagination. For depression forces us to take fantasy seriously, if not literally. This means facing the potential outer reality of aggressive fantasy alongside its inner creativity. When that happens, depression becomes the forum for an integration of the instinctual body and the imaginative soul and our aggressive dreams show us the meaning of our despair.

Finally, I want to introduce the metaphor of depression as a *search*. For the individual, such a search may be a search of collective memory – Memory, mother of the Muses and hence of creativity generally. The work of memory is the work of mourning. In the nuclear age, we have to search in our memory for the archaic fascination with death that spawned civilization and from which we have turned our faces. The search in depression reflects a need for continuity as a fundament of imagination. Depression enables imagination to be of service. Depression may be seen as a piecing together, over time, of a solution. That is partly why the writer has to get depressed when the book isn't going well, the mother when the baby won't feed, the worker when faced with unemployment, each of us when threatened by the bomb. All have to search for a solution. The depressive process, static on the surface, is a flow of information, intuitions and images leading to a reorganization of these. For that is all that is meant by 'solution'; it is not 'cure' or getting rid of depression. The misery of depression comes in part from the awful slowness of the search and its apparent futility.

References

Bateson, P. (1984) 'The biology of co-operation'. *New Society, 31*. May 1984.

Bion, W. (1965) *Transformations*. In *Seven Servants*. New York: Jason Aronson.

Brown, G. & Harris, T. (1978) *Social Origins of Depression*. London: Tavistock.

Davis, M. and Wallbridge, D. (1981) *Boundary and Space: An Introduction to the Work of D. W. Winnicott*. London: Karnac.

Dieckmann, H. (1977) 'Some aspects of the development of authority'. In A. Samuels (ed.), *The Father in Analytical Psychology*. London: Free Association Books (1985); New York: New York University Press (1986).

Fairbairn, W. (1952) *Psychoanalytic Studies of the Personality*. London: Tavistock.

Foot. P. (1978) *Virtues and Vices*. Oxford & New York: Oxford University Press.

France, P. (1983) *Diderot*. Oxford & New York: Oxford University Press.

Freud, S. (1905) *Three Essays on the Theory of Sexuality*. Std Edn 7. London: Hogarth.

Freud, S. (1916–17) *Introductory Lectures on Psychoanalysis*. Std Edn 15–16. London: Hogarth.

Freud, S. (1919) 'A child is being beaten'. Std Edn 17. London: Hogarth.

Freud, S. (1933) *New Introductory Lectures on Psycho-Analysis*. Standard Edition 22. London: Hogarth.

Gilligan, C. (1982) *In a Different Voice: Psychological Theory and Women's Development*. Cambridge, MA: Harvard University Press.

Hillman, J. (1975) *Loose Ends*. Dallas, TX: Spring Publications.

Jacoby, M. (1985) *Longing for Paradise: Psychological Reflections on an Archetype*. Boston, MA: Sigo.

Jung, C. G. (1934) 'Zur Gegenwartigen Lage der Psychotherapie'. *Zentrallblatt fur Psychotherapie* 7: 1&2.

Jung, C.G. (1950) *Symbols of Transformation*. CW 5.

Jung, C.G. (1952) *Answer to Job*. CW 11.

Jung, C. G. (1953) *Two Essays on Analytical Psychology*. CW 7.

Jung, C.G. (1954) *Archetypes of the Collective Unconscious*. CW 9i.

Jung, C. G. (1960) *The Structure and Dynamics of the Psyche*. CW 8.

Jung, C. G. (1964) *Civilization in Transition*. CW 10.

Kenny, A. (1963) *Action, Emotion and Will*. London: Routledge and Kegan Paul.

Kohlberg, I. (1968) 'Moral development'. In *International Encyclopaedia of Social Science*. New York: Macmillan Free Press.

Kohut, H. (1982) 'Introspection, empathy and the semi-circle of mental health'. *International Journal of Psycho-Analysis, 63*: 4.

Milner, M. (1977) *On Not Being Able to Paint*. London: Heinemann.

Newton, K. (1981) 'Comment on the Emergence of Child Analysis by M. Fordham'. *Journal of Analytical Psychology, 20*: 2.

Plaut, A. (1959) 'Hungry patients: Reflections on ego structure'. *Journal of Analytical Psychology*, 4: 2.

Samuels, A. (1985) *Jung and the Post-Jungians*. London & Boston: Routledge and Kegan Paul.

Sayers, J. (1986) *Biological Politics: Feminist and Anti-Feminist Perspectives*. London: Tavistock.

Searles, H. (1973) 'Violence in schizophrenia'. In *Countertransference and Related Subjects: Selected Papers*. London: Hogarth.

Stein, M. (1985) *Jung's Treatment of Christianity: The Psychotherapy of a Religious Tradition*. Wilmington, IL: Chiron Publications.

Steiner, J. (1985) 'Turning a blind eye: The cover up for Oedipus. *International Review of Psycho-Analysis, 12*: 2.

Stevens, A. (1982) *Archetype: A Natural History of the Self*. London: Routledge and Kegan Paul.
Storr, A. (1970) *Human Aggression*. Harmondsworth: Penguin.
Winnicott, D. W. (1958) 'Psycho-analysis and the sense of guilt'. In *The Maturational Processes and the Facilitating Environment*. London: Hogarth (1965).
Zinkin, L. (1979) 'The collective and the personal'. *Journal of Analytical Psychology*, *24*: 3.

CHAPTER 5

A NEW DEAL FOR WOMEN AND MEN

Retrospective introduction

This chapter comes from *Politics on the Couch* of 2001. I was interested in probing the balance between gender wars (a phrase of the time) and a new co-operative political and psychological partnership between the sexes. In particular, I was interested in whether men could change, whether they hated women, and whether they really were powerful. It might be interesting to look at what I wrote in a letter to the Guardian in August 2013 to see how these themes remain on my mind. A serious female journalist had written a piece on the importance of feminism not ignoring the role (negative and positive) of men. I responded:

> Therapists who work with and study men will applaud Yvonne Roberts' spot-on analysis (Don't forget men in the shifts that are reshaping society, 04.08.13). Among the many things we have learned is that there is a kind of 'male deal' that men sign up to from an early age. Provided men renounce softness and relatedness to others, provided they agree to compete with each other, then society will reward them with many goodies including power over women and children. But we've also learned that, for many men (and this is increasing under austerity), those goodies are not for them. In other words, we need to break up the monolith of 'men'. Some are powerful for sure; others are manifestly powerless and oppressed: black men, disabled men, imprisoned men.
>
> We also need to identify and celebrate intergenerational co-operation between men, something gay people have pioneered. Here, therapy theory has to be revised as the legacy from Freud is that men are psychologically bound to fight another: sons against the father, brothers against each other, every man against women. This is not how it always has to be, not even how it always is.

I found it interesting to relate this letter to the chapter below.

The 'New Deal' was the name given to the wide range of programmes, agencies and economic laws and institutions introduced by President Franklin Delano Roosevelt in the United States between 1933 and 1938. The term was also picked up by the Labour government in Britain in the 1990s. The new deal referred to in this chapter is a psychological as well as political new deal between the sexes . . . Roosevelt's economic and social reforms were responses to the trauma of the Great Depression. Who would disagree with the proposition that a traumatic situation has existed for women and men and the relations between them in most Western countries ever since the end of the Second World War?

'Gender' has come to mean the arrangements by which the supposedly biological raw material of sex and procreation is shaped by human and social intervention. Gender and the passionate politics it spawns have given rise to traumatic divisiveness in our world – West, East, South and North. But the very idea of gender also has a hidden bridge-building function: it sits on a threshold half way between the inner and outer worlds, and thus is already half way out into the world of politics. On the one hand, gender is a private, secret, sacred, mysterious story that we tell ourselves and are told by others about who we are. But it is also a set of experiences deeply implicated in and irradiated by the political and socio-economic realities of the outer world. The notion of gender, therefore, not only marries the inner and outer worlds, but actually calls into dispute the validity of the division. It is no wonder, then, that gender issues get so politicized as well as continuing to turn us on, that contemporary political discussions focus so often on gender issues such as the proportions of men and women in the various arms of government, paternity (as opposed to maternity) leave and the perennial issue of equality of pay.

Men and politics

Ironically, men have become the object of much political and psychological scrutiny in the West these days and are often seen as 'the problem' – 'ironically' because for millennia men were the ones to scrutinize other groups and make them problematic: women, children, Blacks, the fauna and flora of the natural world. Men were a sort of papal balcony from which to survey the universe. But in our age, a huge shift in cultural consciousness has taken place and new questions about men have arisen: men as (errant) fathers, men as (violent) criminals, men as (uninvolved) citizens.

The three underlying questions seem to be: Can men change? Are men powerful? Do men hate women? Today's men and women would probably want to answer 'Yes and No' to all three of those questions. Saying 'Yes and No' is not a high-octane or passionate position, but it may be the only reasonable, viable, pragmatically effective and imaginative position to take.

Can men change? Men *can* change, of course, and yet the statistics about who typically takes care of children or does the washing-up show that they have not altered their behaviour very much. Why not? In the past few years, far too much time has been spent on irresolvable philosophical, metaphysical and quasi-scientific discussions about the relative importance of nature and nurture in the formation of gender identity and performance. Yet it may still be politically useful to consider the limitations on men's capacity to change – not because of putative biological hard-wiring but because of psychological factors, in psychotherapy language 'internalization', a kind of psychological rather than biological 'inheritance' referring to the way men take in (internalize) images of manliness they see projected by the outside world and make them part of their inner world.

Are men powerful? They certainly have economic power. But Black men, homeless men, men in prisons, young men forced or tricked into armies, disabled men, gay men – these are often vulnerable figures. We have serious trouble contemplating male economic power and male economic vulnerability simultaneously. We know, too, that men are scared of women. Never mind their fear of 'the feminine', what scares men is *women*. How can a man be said to be powerful if he is scared of women? And men are also frightened of other men. When contemplating the question of male power, what each of us has internalized is crucial in determining our answer – which means that personal experience and circumstances are decisive.

At the same time, the undoubted economic power that males possess could be made to serve progressive ends. If men and their formal institutions put just a tiny proportion of their economic power to benevolent use, it would make an enormous difference. So whatever changes may be taking place in the world of men could have immense political and social effects.

Do men hate women? Here, the word 'ambivalence' comes to mind and, as we shall return to the concept later, its history will be useful. In 1910, when Jung's superior, Eugene Bleuler, coined the word ambivalence, he meant it as a very serious symptom of schizophrenia. By the 1930s and 1940s, it had become *the sign* of psychological maturity according to psychoanalysis. Ambivalence is the capacity to have simultaneously hating and loving feelings towards the same person. So it is *not* only a problem, but an extremely hard to achieve aspect of psychological and social maturity. (Similarly, F. Scott Fitzgerald said that the test of a first-rate intelligence is the ability to hold two opposed ideas in the mind at the same time and still retain the ability to function.) Therefore, later in this chapter, when considering the creation of temporary deals and alliances of a political nature between men and women on the basis of their ambivalent feelings towards each other, something elevated, difficult to achieve and worthwhile is being proposed, not something tawdry and short term.

In praise of gender confusion

Most people are wary now of any individuals who seem too settled and sure in their gender identity and gender role. Think of the tycoon – so capable and dynamic, such a marvellous self-starter. Do we not know that, secretly, he is a sobbing little boy, dependent on others, perhaps mostly females, for all his feelings of safety and security? Or the Don Juan, talking incessantly of the women he has seduced, who turns out to have fantasies of being female himself and yearns to be seduced by another man? Or the woman who seems so fulfilled as a mother, yet privately desires to express herself in ways other than maternity, to come into another kind of power, to protest her cultural 'castration'?

We have come to accept that behind excessive gender certainty lurk gender confusions like these. At the same time, even many people who are suspicious of too much gender certainty feel that it is basically a good thing to be pretty certain about one's gender, to know for sure that, in spite of all the problems one has with being a man or a woman, one is indeed a man or a woman.

Yet it may be that another ideal altogether is needed to make sense of what we are experiencing in the muddled and mysterious world of early twenty-first-century gender relations and gender politics. Many people who come for therapy are manifestly confused about their gender identity. They may know how a man or woman is *supposed* to behave; but they are not sure that, given what they know about their internal lives, a person who is really a man or a woman could possibly feel or fantasize what they are feeling and fantasizing.

For these profound feelings of gender confusion to exist, there has to be an equally profound feeling of gender certainty in operation at some level – certainty based on the images presented by society. You cannot know the details of your confusion without having an inkling of the certitude against which you are measuring it. The client sobbing his little boy heart out knows very well that 'real' 'manly' tycoons exist out there and evaluates himself negatively as a result. Indeed, we could even say: no gender certainty, no gender confusion. What this means is that, to a very great degree, people construct their gender confusion in relation to their gender certainty. If gender certainty is part of ordinary socialization, then gender confusion is equally constructed and not a deep personal wound or failure.

We need, therefore, to extend radically the by now conventional insight that gender confusion lies behind gender certainty to see that *gender certainty lies behind gender confusion.* To the extent that gender confusion is usually taken as a mental health problem or neurosis, we are making a colossal mistake and even playing a destructive con trick on those supposedly suffering from it. The problem, in fact, is gender certainty.

We can look at how this operates for men in Western societies. The clichéd idea that many men living in a feminism-affected culture feel confused about who they are *as men* takes on a rather different cast if we disown the idea of the desirability of gender certainty. From this angle, modern men are not so confused – or at least feeling confused is not their main problem. Their problem is being afflicted with a gender certainty that is of no emotional use to them in their lives, and may be actually harmful to their potential. (When men's movement leaders offer a certainty that seems to have been missing from the lives of men, they are unwittingly doing nothing more than bringing the unconscious gender certainty that was always there to the surface and reinforcing it. As that certainty came from the culture in the first place, there is nothing radical or scene-shifting about it at all.)

The really interesting question is what to do with the feelings of gender confusion from which everyone suffers these days. It all becomes easier to live with if we replace the word 'confusion' with something that sounds more positive, like 'fluidity' or 'flexibility' or even 'androgyny'. But the word 'confusion' has merits because it comes closer to capturing what contemporary people feel about their gender identity.

In fact, gender confusion can contribute something valuable to political and social reform and change. If gender is a story we tell about ourselves that is half private and half public, it is also something upon which most polities have erected a welter of oppressive practices and regulations, mostly favouring men. Unfortunately, many Western governments (such as Labour in Britain) may be turning back to a retrogressive form of gender politics fuelled by the certitudinous 'family values' of the past, a politics which has always tended to favour men.

But many men want to make a progressive contribution to gender politics and hence (as men) to the wider political scene. It is not necessary to refuse to be a man, or enter into spurious sociopolitical alliances with women that deny the existence of differing political agendas for the sexes. All that may be required in the first instance is a celebration of not knowing too well who we are in terms of gender, not knowing too well what we are supposed to know very well indeed.

In workshops I have conducted on male psychology, participants engage in an exercise using a rating scale that represents a continuum from 'old man' to 'new man'. Old man counts as zero; new man counts as 10. If the person is a man, he is asked to place himself on this scale; if a woman, she is asked to score the most significant man in her life, past or present.

One might imagine that this would be a straightforward business, and people would respond by saying 6, 1, 2, 8 and so on. But it never happens like that. Many people insist on giving multiple answers. A man will say that he sees himself as a 2 *and* a 9. Sometimes this gets expressed more precisely: 'When I'm with a woman

I'm more likely to be a 9, right at the new man end, but when I'm with men I find myself a 2 or 3.'

One man said: 'I would say I'm a 2. I consider myself traditional, but I'm trying to modify myself.' The number of participants of both sexes who mention words like *modify, change, improve* in connection with men is very high. Another man said: 'When I thought about it, I thought 5. This isn't out of not wanting to change, but out of confusion – the struggle, uncertainty and confusion of being a man.'

Many women mock the exercise, but what they say is quite revealing. One woman said: 'I think my husband is a 2 but *he* thinks he's an 8.' Another woman said: 'I've been married for 33 years. My husband started as a 3 and after bringing up the children together, which was terribly important to him, I think he's become a . . . 4!'

We need to access what is involved in gender confusion and gender certainty in a new language of fleshly images that speak more directly to people's experience. Children seem to grasp this instinctively. When my son was eight and my daughter seven, they taught me *their* theory of gender confusion, which has much more to do with self-image at depth than the more conventional, journalistic presentation of men as mixed up because of what women have managed to achieve. They identified four equal categories: boy-boy, boy-girl, girl-girl and girl-boy. Anatomy is important but not decisive in determining who belongs to which category. So my daughter could refer to herself as a girl-girl or a girl-boy while my son oscillated between being a boy-girl and a girl-boy. Context was important – it depended on whom they were with. This system gets beyond a simplistic heterosexual–homosexual or feminine–masculine divide. In the adult world, as many (or more) boy-girls are heterosexual as are homosexual. The certitudes upon which homophobia rests are subverted by this way of speaking.

In fact, the celebration of confusion embodied by such children's theories may be a more effective, interesting and radical way to enter gender politics than either the suspiciousness and judgementalism of the therapist or the nostalgia-fuelled return to certainty we see in some aspects of the men's movement or the advocacy of an ersatz merger of men's sociopolitical interests with those of women. Gender confusion unsettles all the main alternatives on offer.

What, then, does it mean that men are now increasingly seen as the problem? This new stance reverses the trend of centuries in which women – the other sex, the second sex, the dark sex, the sex which is not one – have been the problem men set themselves to solve. Nowadays, it is the men – sexually abusing, domestically violent, planet-despoiling creatures – who are depicted as the source of women's difficulties. There is little doubt that the accusation is valid. But a completely different set of images has also arisen, suggesting a breed of men who support the rights of women and children and are ecologically aware and non-violent. So we are faced with a split in our collective image of men. Conventionally, psychotherapists tell us that such splits come about when something (such as gender confusion) causes unbearable anxiety. It seems more likely that immense collective cultural anxiety is actually being caused by the false certitude of masculinity itself – what might be called 'the male deal'. It is the male deal that lies behind the deeply problematic gender certainty mentioned earlier. And it is the male deal that grounds our culture's assumptions about religion, science – and politics.

In the male deal, the little boy, at around the age of three or four, strikes a bargain with the social world in which he lives. If he will turn away from soft things, feminine things, maternal things, from the world of play wherein failure does not matter, then the world will reward his gender certainty by giving him all the goodies in its possession – all the women he can eat. In return for the gift of political power, he promises to be a good provider and to keep unruly and subversive women and children in their place. He also promises not to deviate from this function by loving other men too much (that is, becoming gay). Homophobia is a political defence of the family as capitalism has defined it.

The question is whether or not we can reframe the collective confusion about the male deal as an opportunity to rethink a number of things: the deal itself and its damaging as well as pleasurable effects on men; the nature of male authority and its roots in Western attitudes to work; the possibility of women and men facing the difficult economic times ahead as partners as well as (not instead of) adversaries.

Given that men control the sources of economic and political power, including the production of ideas and images of sexual difference, then if men are on the move at some level, adding male political power to the ideals of male change could be decisive. In other words, we could be confronted with a social movement as significant as feminism but with the crucial difference that men are fortified with possession of all the resources from which women have been excluded.

Nothing is more suspect than the complaint, fuelled by 'victim envy', that society now favours women over men. Nevertheless, as suggested earlier, it would be wrong to end by reasserting that males have all the power. Perhaps there isn't a monolith called 'men' after all. As a woman in one of the workshops said of her husband: 'Well, if you take 1–5 and put it on one side and if you take 6–10 and put it on the other side – *he's in the abyss!*'

CHAPTER 6

THE GOOD-ENOUGH FATHER OF WHATEVER SEX

L'être dont l'être est de n'être pas
(The being whose essence is in not having an essence)

Simone de Beauvoir

Retrospective introduction

Do we still lack accounts of what ordinary, devoted, good-enough fathering looks like, as I suggested here in *Politics on the Couch* in 2001? Maybe we now know more about why such accounts are lacking. In part, this is because the facts are not friendly towards the existence of a 'good-enough father'. But in addition, we are still so stunned by the realities of child sexual (and other) abuse by men, and by the realization that the culture supports such behaviour (for example in the BBC, which is currently embroiled in investigations into child abuse by BBC staff dating back to the 1970s). It could seem to be in very poor taste and be lousy politics to consider the positive erotics of the father's body or how he acts as a locus for the transformation of aggression. But, at a recent conference in 2013 in South Africa (attended by Africans as well as whites which is unusual for a therapy gathering in that land), where issues with 'the missing men' are at the heart of the violence that, alongside corruption, threatens to destroy the ANC's revolution, it became clear that people are recognizing that we do need inspiring accounts of what men can do. And that we also need compassionate accounts of the ways in which they suffer at the hands of other violent men.

The bits of this chapter that satisfy me the most are those in praise of lone-partner families and families headed by same-sex parents. What I wrote about the secret hardness of the female body has been understood (I think). I continue to query whether heterosexual marriage is in any way special and lend my voice not only in (qualified) support of same-sex marriage, but also in support of other styles and modes of relationship including polyamory and promiscuity.

The father in contemporary politics

In Britain and the United States, the pivotal place of lone-parent families in public debates about families and family policies remains a feature of the political scene. In 1995, the then Conservative British government announced plans to cut the benefits payable to lone-parent families and the early days of the 1997 Labour government were also marked by an attempt to cut such payments. The American story has been very similar.

Not surprisingly, then, when there are meetings about lone-parent family issues, they often take place in a politicized and tense atmosphere, with media interest and demonstrations. In such a situation, it is not too far-fetched to say that developmental psychology and psychotherapeutic perspectives on family process move implicitly and secretly to the heart of political life. Hence the presence of a chapter on 'the father' in a book on politics.

This chapter is both a psychological response to the challenge of fatherhood and a critique of social policies based on received wisdoms about the father. It tries to break up the monolith called father by introducing two figures whom I call the 'good-enough father' and the 'father of whatever sex'.

The idea is to show that there is both more and less to fathers than the continuing political and moral panic about lone parenthood suggests. If we listen to the psychological subtext of the passionate debate about the social and political consequences of lone parenthood being conducted in most of the West, it becomes clear that we are witnessing a damaging and misleading idealization of fathers and the roles men play in families. It is folly to base policy on this idealization. But the fact that such idealization exists gives political debate in the 1990s about lone parenthood a marked psychological dimension. The politics revolve around psychological theory and the psychology has become part of political debate.

What drives the continuing stigmatization of women who bring up children alone in many Western countries is our world's total failure to come to terms with the imminent collapse of some of the things that used to support male dominance in society – a collective failure that, as we have seen in previous chapters, has left many men unsure of their personal roles. Generally speaking, men still have the power, but they lack a fixed identity. As the British suicide figures for the 1990s show, this unsettles them so much that they find living with it difficult or impossible. Male suicide almost doubled; female suicide declined by about the same amount. It cannot simply be unemployment, for there have been recessions before.

It often seems that the only thing that governments, various sections of the media, certain academics and many therapists are able to do is to yearn for the return of the father as a source of stability, discipline and order in the family and, by some kind of magic, in society as well. This yearning persists in spite of what we now know about the so-called 'traditional' family; it was a very short-lived phenomenon (if it ever existed at all). As several recent historical studies have shown, the family has always mutated in a duet with economic and industrial organization.[1] That is why it is so important not to fall for the temptations of underclass theory and pillory today's lone parents and their families – never mind the scarcely hidden racism in that tendency. It is pointless to yearn for yesterday's ideal family. That family, source of much misery, was a staging post on a long journey. In fact, in Britain today, only a minority of families (about 23 per cent) consist of the conventional mixture of a male breadwinner, a female homemaker and two children. As Helen Wilkinson put it, as far as families are concerned, 'diversity is king'.[2]

In the mode of yearning to which so many segments of society seem addicted, the father is presented as a sort of public school 'fagmaster', the older boy who is assigned younger boys as servants and in return helps to form their characters. A first leader in *The Times* in 1993 showed this up very well by bemoaning the absence of fathers as a 'moral presence' in the family. The trouble is that, when faced with thinking like this, there is a vacuum where new ideas should exist.

Even in progressive circles there is a denial of the possibility of other styles and models of fathering. Perhaps we can come up with a model here, based on views and values that will neither implicitly condemn lone-parent, fatherless families nor leave them in the lurch. Such a model of fatherhood would stress the father's active, direct emotional involvement with his children from the earliest age. It would support an egalitarian, co-operative, non-hierarchical family, rather than pointlessly seeking to restore father and his authority as the (flawed) source of rules and regulations – whereby, presumably, he would also be reinstated as the source of sexual and physical abuse of women and children.

While not denying that many clients from lone-parent family backgrounds have psychological problems, twenty-five years of clinical research into lone-parent families leads me to dispute that there are *inevitable* damaging psychological effects of living in a lone-parent family. Damage would be still less inevitable were lone-parent families to be given adequate resources, approval and support from the community. When we talk about resources, we should perhaps think of more than money, housing and so forth – although these are clearly important. We should also think of what it does to the evolving personality of a child in a lone-parent family to know that the set-up at home is attacked in the real, adult world as inferior, bad, mad and in need of government control. My own children certainly picked up quite specific social and political values and assumptions about family life from television before they were five years old.

Playing the father role

There are two separate questions involved in the psycho-cultural debate over fatherhood. The first has to do with the consequences (or lack of them) of lone parenthood for child development. For convenience, we could call this *the lone-mother question*. The second has to do with the question of what fathering *is* these days. We could call this *the crisis-in-fatherhood question*. It is important to recognize that these two apparently different questions lead us in a surprisingly similar direction. Addressing one question helps us to engage with the other. Both questions stimulate thinking about what fathers do, or can do, that is life-affirming and related to others, beyond being a 'moral presence'.

We can begin to create and assemble a psychological information pool, or resource, for women bringing up children on their own or women bringing up children together with other women. When the father is revisioned as being 'unpatriarchal', such women can also be revisioned, not only as mothers but also as 'fathers of whatever sex'. Immediately, we undermine everything that our society assigns or wishes to assign to men. Anatomy ceases to determine parental destiny and the lone-mother question is completely re-framed.

The questions we need to ask of women are: can you do the things that male fathers do? Do you *want* to do them? We invite women to assert their capacities to be fathers of whatever sex, which would often make them good-enough fathers, rather than setting them up to fail as phoney ideal fathers. Men fail to be ideal fathers, too. Women may well choose not to perform every item on any list of fatherly functions, nor will they necessarily perform these functions in *precisely* the same way that men might. But would that matter? Some might say it would be a pretty good thing. Difference does not always mean deficit. The issue is not that mothering and fathering are identical – though there will be disagreement about the differences – but whether or not a woman can do much of what fathers do (and a man much of what mothers do).

Gathering information about fathering today could enable women to decide how many of its functions they could perform themselves. That is why the usual formulation has been twisted so as to call women who raise children alone good-enough fathers. Many women who raise children alone, or together with other women, are certainly already doing a lot of being a good-enough father of whatever sex without naming it as such. This group of women represents an incalculably valuable resource. What they do as parents could herald a whole new approach to parenting that plugs into the fluidity in gender roles that has evolved since the Second World War and which is not going to be wished and/or legislated away by governments.

To those who have a negative reaction to the idea that women can be good-enough fathers and play the father's role, let us say: men, too, only *play* the father's role. Fathering does not come 'naturally' to men, along with penises and stubble – it has to be learned, and every new father discovers that society has rules about how to do it; there is a masquerade of manliness, a male masquerade, to adapt Joan Rivière's term.[3] Women who father as good-enough fathers of whatever sex may teach things to men who father. I remember my daughter setting up a game with me by saying, 'You be the daddy, Daddy' – and then, at some point in our family play, announcing, 'Now I'll be the daddy, Daddy.'

This is the bottom-line lived experience behind the academic work on power and on the cultural construction of gender and gender roles.[4] Men already play the role of father, just as women may come to play the role. And they play it differently at different times and in different places; parenting is inherently multicultural. It is surely significant how much we all use the word 'role' in relation to being a parent. So, for the sake of completeness, let us recall that women who look after very small children are *playing* at being mothers, playing the role of mother. Motherhood, too, is not as 'natural' as some people continue delusively to think it is. Maternity and paternity have evolving histories.

What of the second question, the question of the crisis in fatherhood, what fatherhood is and means for men? We certainly need to make the role of the male parent more interesting and meaningful for younger men who have started to reject a dictatorial, Jurassic style of fathering – even if their female partners would accept such behaviour, which, these days, is unlikely. Women's increasing refusal to accept male dominance, coupled with men's beginning search for inspiring ideas about manhood and fatherhood, are crucial social and psychological changes on which the debate about fathers should be focusing. 'Men' have become a category, one of many, rather than some sort of privileged vantage point. But, as noted earlier, this huge change in Western consciousness does not mean that men and women now have identical agendas. Men will not give up their power that easily, and there is a lot of making up to be done. But writing as a man, a father, a therapist, I have come to see that it is not the actual maleness of the person from whom the child obtains fathering that is important. What matters is whether or not the relationship between the father of whatever sex and her or his children is good enough.

This chapter works on two levels: as a resource for women who raise children alone, and as an agenda for contemporary men who want to be fathers in a new way that is psychologically realistic. To underscore the two levels and to explain the terms and words used, let me pose a series of questions. When a man takes care of a very small baby, what should we call what he does? *Fathering*, part of an enhanced and expanded definition of father? *Mothering*, because looking after the newborn is what mothers traditionally do? Or plain parenting? Similarly, if a woman lays down the law in a family, is she *mothering*, part of an enhanced and expanded definition of a mother? Or is she *fathering*, because laying down the law is what fathers traditionally do? Or plain parenting?

If we opt for straightforward answers or desex the words for parents, we deny any differences between mothers and fathers. The questions show that our language for parenting has collapsed; that is why some want so desperately to speak a language they need to believe once existed. But the breakdown is not a disaster. It is an opportunity, and ushers in a new kind of transformative politics, fuelled by what people actually experience in their emotional and personal lives.

The politics of paternal warmth

In Chapters 4 and 5 [of *Politics on the Couch*], I argued that, in all the justified concern about child sexual abuse, we have perhaps forgotten to say enough about the positive aspects of a father's physical warmth. Many conventional families have lacked this kind of experience, a lack that can generate its own particularly pernicious brand of psychic pain. Any woman bringing up children alone or together with another woman is bound to give some thought to what it means that there is no father present. Here, she will think about the positive outcomes of providing fatherly warmth. She will want to decide whether or not to attempt to become the father of whatever sex, whether or not to try to provide similar experiences leading to similar outcomes, and how to do this.

Fatherly warmth leads to a recognition of daughters as people in their own right, not simply as little mothers, not only as creatures tied into the image and role of mother. As we saw, this has sociopolitical implications. Many feminist writers have shown convincingly that the 'reproduction of mothering' is terribly limiting for women. It ties them into the role of the one who looks after others, who responds and reacts to their needs, who puts her own needs last and who dares not risk disfavour and disapproval by expressing her assertiveness and demands. Fatherly recognition of the daughter as other than a mother can enable women to break out of the cycle of the reproduction of motherhood. Those other pathways that I mentioned earlier then emerge: the spiritual path, the work path, the path that integrates her assertive side, the path of sexual expression (not necessarily heterosexual), maybe the path of celibacy. It is crucial that there be pathways that are not man-oriented and that involve movement away from the father – for example, the path of solidarity and community with other women.

Women bringing up children alone can send similar messages to their daughters. They can understand and recognize their daughters' evolving sexual potential – and everyone has a sexual potential from birth – as taking those daughters away from a mix-up or overlap with the mother. The stress on the sexual daughter is deliberate here; mothers, too, can be sexual. A recognition of a daughter's evolving sexuality by either a female or a male parent plays a part in turning that daughter away from a path in life that is completely circumscribed by the maternal role. To function as the father of whatever sex may mean a woman who parents alone will actually seek out and accentuate the competition that goes on in families between parents and children of the same sex. The mother can communicate to her daughter that the daughter is a potential rival (in many diverse respects, not just Oedipal rivalry over a father). She can go on to communicate that this is not a bad thing and, if she does, she will make possible the kind of differentiation from the mother that a male father's recognition provides.

Paternal warmth challenges our cultural habit of splitting perceptions of the male body into something horribly abusive and violent (which it can be) or something meekly pretty, hairless and nice (which it usually is not). Nevertheless, male bodies have potential to do good as well as harm, and discussion about *both* possibilities will take us far beyond the idealized images of advertising.

Communicating positive physical warmth is pleasant and moving for both participants. The father as well as the daughter receives something out of this 'erotic playback'. Once the initial 'woman equals mother' equation is broken up, the outcome for a girl is unpredictable. She may want and need to grow away from as well as towards her father, away from the world of men in general as well as towards it, to seek out, work with, fall in love with and raise children with other women.

Fathers do not simply liberate or permit daughters to take up different psychosocial roles from that of maternity, but foster a *plurality* of psychosocial roles, meaning the ways in which they do or do not shake down for women into a workable blend of oneness and manyness. This is a key social issue for women – how to be more than one person while at the same time still managing to stay psychologically whole? The many mainstream books about superwoman and her balancing act with her time indicate that these ideas about the father–daughter connection are not just of professional psychological interest.

What about the father's physical warmth and erotic playback in relation to the son? For sons, a good-enough physical connection to the father helps lead to the growth of homo-sociality. The political implications of this are immense. Intimate father–son relating, prompted by positive physical warmth that is frankly expressed between them, could inspire the new forms of social and political organization that Western societies urgently need just now – emphasizing co-operation and non-hierarchical organization as modes of masculinity that are just as valid as the pecking order and the rat race. They are also modes of being that women will find more congenial than aping all the worst features of the male drive for success.

In these new forms of social organization, men learn from other men just as they love them. As far as fathering is concerned, we saw in Chapter 5 [of *Politics on the Couch*] that the most difficult hurdle to overcome is the fear that ordinary, devoted, good-enough fathers will somehow be effeminate, the code for 'homosexual'. Our culture has employed a fear and loathing of homosexuality as a weapon to keep men tied into the role of provider in the family, the ones who must therefore remain emotionally distant. The pay-off for men has been access to economic and political power. The cost has been the loss of the opportunity for intimacy and the expression of paternal warmth.

This is territory where the female father of whatever sex comes into *her* own and can function as a resource for male fathers. Women tend to know more about community and non hierarchical organization from the inside. Women who parent alone will probably already be considering how to make co-operation more attractive to their sons, rather than having them regard it as bland or, worse, non-manly. They may use what power they have to reinforce and support an *absence* of hierarchy and unbendable rules, asking, even challenging their sons to use their imaginations as much as their biceps. And many sons will respond to the challenge. They know at some level that being an old-style, oppositional man, testing the limits of authority, is only one way to be male. (Not that boundary-testing behaviour is going to vanish overnight; it even has some positive aspects, in that rules should be challenged, and gathering new knowledge may involve breaking rules.)

The father of whatever sex knows quite a lot already about working co-operatively – remember, in the old language, which has collapsed, she is a woman.

The politics of paternal aggression

So far, the argument has been about the more erotic side of parenting – physical warmth and recognition of the daughter as other than mother, father–son togetherness as leading to reforms in how we conceive of society itself. What about aggression, an altogether more problematic theme? Surely, some will say, only men can handle their sons' aggression?

Much depends on what we mean by 'handling' aggression. If we mean eliminating it from the picture altogether, either with discipline or by teaching stoicism in the face of frustration or adversity, we seem doomed to fail. But the question is not really how to handle, manage, discipline or eliminate aggression; it is part of life, and it is not all bad. Rather, the task is to see how aggression might be kept moving and prevented from degenerating into destructiveness. Aggression is part of communicating. It is a valid way of securing attention. But who is to say whether an act of aggression is horribly destructive or constructively self-assertive?

As I suggested in Chapter 4 [of *Politics on the Couch*], the human body can become a sort of index for aggression. Fathers rather often make use of chest aggression, exemplified by the ambivalence of the bear hug. Then there is male genital aggression exemplified by pornography. Men also go in for arm aggression, suggesting a range of images and acts from pressing a nuclear button to striking a blow with a weapon to strangling someone with bare hands. Leg aggression is often practised by fathers when they walk away and duck confrontation. Anal aggression, coming out of the bottom, involves enviously smearing the achievements of others, perhaps by snide comments – what was referred to in encounter groups as 'coming out sideways'.

The relationship between the child and the father of whatever sex is the arena in which movement between these different styles of aggression is worked on and developed. The main aim is to keep aggression fluid and moving through the various styles so as to avoid the predominance of one style over the others. When one style predominates, there is more likely to be movement from benevolent aggression to pure destructiveness. But there is more to communicating aggression between father and child than keeping several styles going at once. There is also the possibility of an element in fathering that can help to *transform* antisocial, sadistic, unrelated aggression into socially committed, self-assertive, related aggression. This transformation takes place on the social level as well as in families.

Fathers work on these issues without knowing it. For some the goal is to allow aggression its place in open and emotionally mobile relationships. For daughters, the goal is to validate and reinforce their capacity to challenge and fight with men. A woman's capacity to confront the patriarchy stems, to a certain extent, from the way her father played back her aggressive response to him.

As far as women who bring up daughters alone are concerned, the main thing is the need not to retreat into some spurious all-female, nicey-nicey, sisterly alliance. Lone parents usually are aware of how tempting it is for anyone who is isolated or fears rejection to do this. Equally, men and women who parent alone have simply had to come to terms with an unacceptable degree of physical aggression in the family already. Perhaps lone fathers of whatever sex need to know that it may even be a good thing if they and their daughters fight. (They are going to fight at some point anyway.) This would change the terms of debate about lone-parent families and pose a few challenges for two-parents families. Fathers of whatever sex need to encourage their daughters to challenge male authority; it is often intelligent and not always disloyal, for mothers to approve of this.

There is always going to be tension and frustration in the family, and thus the possibility of aggression. But it can be reframed from the beginning as part of a relationship, not something to be eliminated. In terms of actual parenting behaviour, women who parent alone need to be reassured of what many know already: it cannot be wrong to engage in rough-and-tumble play with boys, even though such play is bound to become a bit too real from time to time. It is not always a bad thing when events get a bit out of hand – just look at the psychological damage done to people who grow up in emotionally over-controlled families, where father was certainly and perhaps simply a moral presence. What kind of training in 'handling' aggression is that?

Can fathers change?

If some readers disagree that a father of whatever sex can be good-enough, they might note that it is not proven that only a male can do these things. Such readers should not forget how many men do not or cannot do them before concluding that it is impossible for a woman to do them.

Moreover, we have not yet mentioned the fact that many children living in families headed by one parent have regular contact with the other parent, or the ways in which women who parent alone can encourage contact between their children and adult males, or the part male mentors might play in some families. These issues have often been discussed.

Some readers may have less of a problem with women doing the fathering but do not like the idea that fathers, or men in general, can change. In fact, both the idea and the practice of fatherhood have shown incredible cross-cultural variation and changes over time; they are not written in stone. Consider the research on how fathers play with their children. Captured on video, fathers are seen to be much more active and physical, while mothers videoed playing with their children are quieter, more reflective and more protective. This result seems both logical and fixed. But if the play of fathers who, for whatever reason, have sole or primary care of their children is videoed, *it resembles that of mothers.* Fathers can change. Maybe men can change.[5]

One way in which men are changing is that they are becoming more sceptical of the male deal. Increasingly, and especially in mid-life, men are becoming aware that repudiating everything in themselves that was soft, vulnerable, 'feminine' in exchange for receiving the desire-fulfilling goodies of Western capitalism was not altogether a good deal after all. Among many experiences which it denied them is the experience of being a hands-on, actively involved father.

Parallels drawn between changes in the world of men and the women's movement are fallacious because of the reality that men already possess power and resources. Nor has there yet been a radical shift in the role of the father in many households. Empirical social scientists tell us about the unchanging picture in the majority of families: most do not look after children, do not do their share of the chores and are responsible for whatever is sexually and physically perpetrated.

But the aspirational atmosphere is changing. This is very hard to measure empirically, and the intuition of a depth psychologist sometimes does not pass muster when compared to 'real' social science. I was in the United States at the time of the Anita Hill–Clarence Thomas Congressional hearings (on the accusation of his sexual harassment of her and its impact on his nomination to the Supreme Court) and many commentators noted that the effect of these events on public consciousness was considerable. The general attack on lone-parent families and resistance attack may have a similar effect in many places. As political leaders have found, there are profound electoral spin-offs from paying heed to identity politics.[6] If men are changing and we are about to see good-enough fathers in larger numbers in Western societies, then the very existence of male power takes on a new significance. If changes are taking place in the world of men and fathers, they will have political and social effects now and in the future. Throughout *Politics on the Couch*, we have seen that gender issues are especially important for politics, just as they are for therapy, because of the unique position of gender midway between the outer and inner worlds. Both our public *and* our private lives are riddled with gender issues. Indeed, one way of understanding the unending wave of sex scandals in British and American politics is to see them as highlighting the shakiness and shifting nature of our present images of masculinity, and the problems we are having trying to work out what are and are not acceptable modes of behaviour for men.[7]

People living in lone-parent families have become experts at living with the changes in gender role that are sweeping over the Western world. Could we reframe lone parents and their children as today's experts at coping with changes that threaten to drive everyone crazy by their depth and rapidity? The attack on lone parents in many Western countries has presented us with an opportunity to inject psychological realism and sensitivity into our politics, acknowledging that the old politics, which sought to leave out personal experience, are falling to pieces. People living in lone-parent families may be the expert practitioners of this new kind of psychological politics. Can we learn from them?

Psychotherapy and the father

Although Winnicott coined the phrase 'the good-enough mother' in 1949, the good-enough *father* has not been written about very much.[8, 9] Yet retheorizing the father is necessary if psychoanalysis is to progress beyond a politically biased image of the father that reflects a specific historical and social period in Western culture. When Winnicott disputes the seriousness for a small baby of having a psychotic *father* (as opposed to a psychotic mother) or when he speaks of the father showing his gun to his children as a way of explaining what the outer world is like, his work reeks of cultural and historical contingency.[10] Yet psychoanalysis worldwide continues to offer what I call the 'insertion metaphor' as the root image of the father's penetrative, unwavering psychological role in a child's early life. The father of early childhood is supposed to insert himself, like a giant depriving and separating penis, between mother and baby, who would otherwise stay locked in a psychosis-inducing and phase-inappropriate symbiosis. In Margaret Mahler's psychoanalytic account, the father awakens a two-year-old from sleep and turns that child towards the (or is it his?) world.[11]

This comforting but reactionary story about fathers – father holding mother who holds baby (with its avoidance of the detail of a more direct relationship with children) – is one that urgently requires critique, not least because of the insult to mothers and babies contained in the notion that they have no commitment and capacities in themselves to becoming separate. Do mothers and babies really want to be psychotic? Moreover, what is so wonderful about the rupture of the mother–child relationship depicted by psychoanalysis, together with rapture over the strong ego that is supposed to result, a question well-posed by feminist theorists on both sides of the Atlantic?[12]

Jacques Lacan's work does focus on the father and in it we find a dematerialization of the father so complete that he crops up in accounts of development solely as a metaphor. Father is a name or Name in a complicated psychoanalytic theorem; a third term in relation to the mother–infant dyad. We should note that, even in Lacan's work, father and child are never really regarded as in immediate relationship. This approach fails to recognize the interplay between the father's concrete, literal presence and his metaphorical function.[13] For Lacan, as John Forrester says, 'the father's function is *strictly metaphorical* – he functions neither as real father (flesh and blood) nor as imaginary father (though he later figures in fantasy as an ideal or punitive agency).'[14] Is it really possible to divorce the literal and the metaphorical as Lacan does, either for purposes of description or as a mode of understanding? All of Lacan's abstractions about the phallus cannot do away with the fleshy actuality of the father's penis as the raw material from which the metaphor has fashioned itself.

Lacan was as culture-bound as anyone else. Could a conscious recognition of the positive, direct, physical, affirming father–infant relationship, dating from the earliest moment, have been possible either in the bourgeois France of Lacan's childhood (he was born in 1901) or during his adult life of psychoanalytic theory-making?

What of C. G. Jung and the post-Jungians? As he sought to identify the essential and invariant features of father–child relationships – the so called father archetype or archetypal father – Jung overlooked the way in which such relationships are built in culture. But if we do explore the father–child relation, we see that, in most cultures, it is dependent on the intersection of two other relationships: that between mother and child, and that between woman and man. A man does not become a father in either a formal or an emotional sense unless something happens simultaneously within the space created by these other two relationships. What that 'something' is, and what the father does, varies from culture to culture and across time. (Actually, the way that the father–child relationship is constructed is no different from the mother–child relationship, which, as many writers have argued, is not as natural, biological, innate, ahistorical, universal and 'given' as we used to think.)[15]

Fathers in the future

Realizing that the father is a culturally constructed creature leads to all kinds of possibilities. The father relation cannot be approached via absolute definition; it is a situational and relative matter. So a new judgement is required on what may seem like hopelessly idealistic and Utopian attempts to change the norms of the father's role. The father's role can change, because written into it is the refusal of absolute definition. This refusal is made possible by male political power and freedom and by the historical and cultural mutability of the father relation. Hence, the only 'archetypal' aspect of the father is that there is no archetypal aspect.

If there is no father archetype of the kind that would hold us back, what can *we* do to help the process of change along? It is still hard to find accounts of the father that depict his benevolent aspects as opposed to his undeniably malevolent ones.

Very little has been said about the father's potential to contribute to the political and psychological mobility, enfranchisement and emancipation of others.

Here are some areas in which psychotherapists might contribute to new social and political thinking about the father:

- changing the social expectation that only women will look after small babies
- fostering a culture in which parenthood and work may coexist
- working towards more co-operative and less hierarchical forms of political and social organization
- getting a clearer understanding of male sexuality in general and paternal sexuality in particular (partly to be able to do more effective work with problems such as child sexual abuse)
- changing how we define and what we expect from good-enough families to include lone-parent families and other transgressive modes of family life.

Traditionally, the father is not only the locus and source of power in the family (and, hence, in society) but also the parent who radiates and deals in spirituality. This is, of course, another kind of power. The spiritual realm, like that of gender, is a liminal one, straddling the divide between 'higher' and 'lower' or between 'transcendent' and 'earth-bound'. Like gender, spirituality generates its own special politics, and these form the spine of the next chapter [of *Politics on the Couch*].

Notes

1 Walter Seccombe, *Weathering the Storm: The History of Working Class Families* (London: Verso, 1993). Helen Wilkinson, 'Celebrate the new family', *New Statesman*, 9 August 1999.
2 Charles Murray, 'Underclass'. In Digby Anderson (ed.), *Family Portraits* (London: Social Affairs Unit, 1990). Helen Wilkinson, 'Celebrate the new family', *New Statesman*, 9 August 1999.
3 Joan Rivière, 'Womanliness as masquerade', *International Journal of Psycho-Analysis*, *10*: 35–44.
4 Michel Foucault, *The History of Sexuality* (London: Allen Lane, 1979–88). Jeffrey Weeks, *Sexuality and its Discontents* (London & New York: Routledge, 1985).
5 Joan Raphael-Leff, *Psychological Processes of Childbearing* (London & New York: Chapman & Hall, 1991: 372, 533).
6 Judith Butler, *Gender Trouble: Feminism and the Subversion of Identity* (London & New York: Routledge).
7 Jonathan Dollimore, *Sexual Dissidence: Augustine to Wilde* (Oxford: Oxford University Press, 1991).
8 Donald Winnicott, 'Mind and its relation to the psyche-soma'. In *Through Paediatrics to Psychoanalysis* (London: Hogarth, 1958). Written in 1949. Also, Winnicott, 'The effect of psychotic parents on the emotional development of the child'. In *The Family and Individual Development* (London: Tavistock, 1968).
9 See also the 'Bowlby complex' in the 1960s where some mothers were said not to leave their children alone because of what the psychoanalyst John Bowlby had said about 'separation'.
10 Donald Winnicott, 'What about father?' In *Getting to Know Your Baby* (London: Heinemann, 1944).
11 Margaret Mahler, 'A study of the separation-individuation process', *The Psychoanalytic Study of the Child*, 1971: 401–27.

12 Judith Jordan, Ann Kaplan, Jean Baker Miller, Irene Stiver, Janet Surry. *Women's Growth in Connection: Writings from the Stone Center* (New York: Guilford Press, 1991).
13 Jacques Lacan, *Ecrits* (trans. Alan Sheridan) (London: Tavistock, 1977).
14 John Forrester, *The Seductions of Psychoanalysis: Freud, Lacan and Derrida* (Cambridge: Cambridge University Press, 1990: 110–1.
15 Elizabeth Badinger, *The Myth of Motherhood: An Historical View of the Maternal Instinct* (London: Souvenir Press, 1981).

CHAPTER 7

BEYOND THE FEMININE PRINCIPLE

Retrospective introduction

I hope this chapter from *The Plural Psyche* of 1989 will still be of interest. It is, on one level, a critique of gender essentialism in the Jungian community and in its theorizing. As such, students of analytical psychology and Jungian Studies could well be interested. They should note that the chapter was very controversial in its time and led to attempts to claim that I was not a real Jungian because I had abandoned the interior perspective in which 'masculine' and 'feminine' were exclusively metaphorical matters.

In addition, the chapter was my first attempt to sketch out a contemporary variant of animus-anima theory that led to a subsequent suggestion that the theory was useful in underpinning an approach to gendered behaviour that greatly extends what we understand as male/masculine or female/feminine behaviour for men and women. In this sense, Jung's antiquated gender theory gets given new legs.

In this chapter, I look at developments in analytical psychology concerning gender identity, gender characteristics and gender role. This is set against the background of a general debate about the psychology of sex and gender and the question of sex-based psychology. As in [all my work], the linkage between gender certainty and gender confusion is a central concern, as is the tracking of fluidity, flexibility and a pluralistic ethos in connection with gender.

The gender debate

Some questions: are men innately more aggressive than women? Does that explain their social and political dominance? Is there such a thing as innately 'masculine' or innately 'feminine' psychology?

In his book *Archetype: A Natural History of the Self,* Anthony Stevens drew on the work of the sociobiologists Wilson and Goldberg to reach the conclusion that 'male dominance is a manifestation of the "psychophysiological reality" of our species. In addition [there is] genetic and neurophysiological evidence relating to the biology of sexual differentiation . . . Patriarchy, it seems is the natural condition of mankind' (Stevens 1982: 188–92).

In *Jung and the Post-Jungians,* I drew on the work of Janet Sayers to critique Stevens's position (Samuels 1985: 220–2). Sayers felt that those opposed to changes in women's role had appropriated biology to their cause and she demolished the sociobiological case in a witty and learned way. For instance, Wilson quoted studies that showed that boys were consistently more able than girls at mathematics but that girls have a higher degree of verbal ability. And boys are, in Wilson's view, more aggressive in social play. From these bases, Wilson concluded that 'even with identical education and equal access to all professions men are likely to continue to play a disproportionate role in political life, business and science' (quoted in Sayers 1982: 77). Sayers wryly remarks that it is hard to see how males' lesser verbal ability leads to their being better fitted for political life. Surely, if biology really does determine social role, it should be the other way round?

Recently I came across the work of another academic psychologist, Gerda Siann (1985). She comprehensively surveyed the various research findings that purport to link aggression to the male hormones. She concluded that 'no specific areas in the brain or nervous system have been pinpointed as controlling aggression' and that an overview of the repeated studies shows that androgenized girls do not seem more aggressive than their peers, siblings or mothers. Overandrogenized males do not display noteworthy dominance, assertion or aggression in spite of the fact that their greater size would guarantee victory (they seem to be rather gentle people). What is more, Siann's careful reading of the research findings shows that castration has no effect on the overall aggressive behaviour of sex offenders, save in relation to actual sexual behaviour. Finally, plasma testosterone levels do not seem to relate directly to aggressive behaviour. Siann's overall conclusion was that

> the evidence does not show any clear and unambiguous relationship between male hormones and the propensity to display violent behaviour or feel aggressive emotion. Indeed the likelihood of such a simple unidirectional relationship has been thrown into doubt by two additional lines of investigation. The first shows that the secretion of male hormones is itself directly affected by environmental and social variables, and the second is concerned with the speculation that female hormones may also be implicated in violent behaviour and aggressive emotion.
>
> (Siann 1985: 37)

Siann also investigated the published research linking genetic inheritance and aggression. Her findings, which make interesting reading when read in conjunction with the discussion in the next chapter [of *The Plural Psyche*] on the hereditary factor in borderline disorder, was that there is no evidence for the genetic transmission of aggression or violence (Siann 1985: 39). *In sum, there is no corporeal innate factor in aggression.* The possibility remains that there is a noncorporeal innate factor – that aggression is linked to sex by invisible, psychological factors. We shall consider that possibility in a moment.

To sustain Stevens's sociobiological viewpoint, female aggression has to be overlooked or minimized. What is more, there is a confusion between 'aggression' and 'dominance'. Not all human dominance depends on aggression. We have to explain phenomena such as altruistic or self-sacrificing behaviour, conscience, the checks placed on the power of a leader, the human capacity for collective decision-making, and so forth.

What follows is a discussion of the third question with which we started this section: are there such things as innate 'masculine' and, more pertinently perhaps, innate 'feminine' psychologies? If there are, then there could be a noncorporeal innate factor in aggression.

Beyond the feminine principle

It is hard to write flexibly and fluidly about what is flexible and fluid. The danger when trying to reflect on our current preoccupation with gender is that we might become too clear and too organized – a reaction formation to the inevitable anxiety (and guilt) we experience at finding that what we thought was solid and fixed is perforated and shifting. Humanity is not just divided into women and men but also into those who are certain about gender and those who are confused about gender. As we have seen, getting the balance between gender certainty and gender confusion is a hard task. Clinically, we see the negative effects of an excess of either position and working with individual patients in the area of gender identity is a kind of research work before moving on to the collective stage and a wider scale.

For gender confusions have as important a role to play as gender certainties. They contribute something imaginative to social and political reform and change. I refer to 'confusion' and not to something that sounds more laudable like 'flexibility' because, experientially, that is precisely what it is, no bones about it. Not for the first time in psychology, we can fashion the strengths out of an apparent weakness. To do this, I have found that I have had to learn from women about what they have been through.

Does use of the word confusion not imply the possibility of definition and clarity concerning gender? The way I use the word 'certainty' in relation to gender is intended to suggest that, while clear definition is theoretically possible, it is, for the most part, illusory and/or problematic.

In order to discuss the subject at all, the distinction between sex and gender should be noted, allowing for some overlap as well. *Sex* (male and female) refers to anatomy and the biological substrate to behaviour, to the extent that there is one. *Gender* (masculine and feminine) is a cultural or psychological term, arising in part from observations and identifications within the family, hence relative and flexible, and capable of sustaining change. Now, in some approaches, particularly in analytical psychology, what can happen is that a form of determinism creeps in and the invariant nature of gender is assumed, just as if gender characteristics and qualities were as fixed as sexual ones. The history of women shows that change is possible just because the social meaning of womanhood is malleable. But when this is ignored, as by Stevens, the possibilities of change, other than as part of ordinary maturation and individuation, are lost.

Is there such a thing as a 'feminine psychology'? I'll begin with a general discussion, then consider whether there is a feminine psychology that applies to women. In a moment, I'll look at the 'feminine' in relation to men, and, after that, at femininity and masculinity as metaphors.

Males and females do have experiences that vary markedly. But it is a huge step from that to a claim that they actually *function* sufficiently discrepantly psychologically for us to speak of two distinct psychologies. The evidence concerning this is muddled and hard to assess. For instance, the discovery that boys build towers and girls build enclosures when they are given bricks can be taken to show a *similarity* of functioning rather than difference (which is what is usually claimed). Both sexes are interested in their bodies and, possibly, in the differences between male and female bodies. Both sexes express that interest in the same way – *symbolically*, in play with bricks. Or, put in another form, *both sexes approach the difference between the sexes in the same way.* The differences that we see in gender role and gender identity can then be looked at as having arisen in the same manner. The psychological *processes* by which a male becomes an aggressive businessman and a female a nurturing and submissive housewife are the *same* and one should not be deceived by the dissimilarity in the end product.

What I have been describing is not a woman's relation to an *innate* femininity or to an *innate* masculinity. Rather I am talking of her *relation to the phenomenon of difference*. Then we can consider the social or cultural structures erected on the basis of that difference. Each woman lives her life in interplay with such difference. This leads at once to questions of gender role (for example, how a woman can best express her aggression in our culture) but these questions need not be couched in terms of innate femininity or innate masculinity, nor in terms of a feminine–masculine spectrum. Rather, they might be expressed in terms of *difference*. In the example, the difference between aggression and submission needs to be seen as different from the difference between men and women! Or, put another way, whatever differences there might be between women and men are not illuminated or signified by the difference between submission and aggression. In the previous two chapters [of *The Plural Psyche*], we have been exploring how gender difference is formed in relations between parents and children and by cultural and social organization.

I am aware that *men* are said to have access to the 'feminine', or to the 'feminine principle', and I used to think that such an unremittingly interior view was the jewel in the Jungian crown. Now I am not so sure. If we're attempting to describe psychological performance, we have to be sure *why* terms with gendered associations and appellations are being used at all. Otherwise we end up with statements such as that 'masculine' aggression is available to women via their relation to the animus, or 'feminine' reflection in the man via his anima. But aggression is part of woman and reflection is part of man. What is more, there are so many kinds of aggression open to women that even current attempts to speak of a woman's aggression as 'feminine' rather than 'masculine' still bind her as tightly as ever. Let us begin to speak merely of aggression. Gender engenders confusion – and this is made worse when gender terms are used exclusively in an inner way. When we speak of 'inner' femininity in a man, we bring in all the unnecessary problems of reification and substantive abstraction that I have been describing. We still cannot assume that psychological *functioning* is different in men and women, *though we know that the creatures 'man' and 'woman' are different*.

The question of 'difference' brings us to a point where we can play back these ideas into analytical psychology. From Jung's overall theory of opposites, which hamstrings us by its insistence on contrasexuality ('masculine' assertion via the animus, etc.), we can extract the theme of *difference*. The notion of difference, I suggest, can help us in the discussion about gender. Not innate 'opposites', which lead us to create an unjustified psychological division expressed in lists of antithetical qualities, each list yearning for the other list so as to become 'whole'. A marriage made on paper. No, I am referring to the fact, image, and social reality of difference *itself*. Not what differences between women and men there are, or have always been; if we pursue that, we end up captured by our captivation and obsession with myth and with the eternal, part of the legacy from Jung. I am interested in *what difference is like*, what the experience of difference is like (and how that experience is distorted in the borderline disorders). Not what a woman *is*, but what being a woman is *like*. Not the archetypal structuring of woman's world but woman's personal experience in today's world. Not the *meaning* of a woman's life but her *experience* of her life. Each person remains a 'man' or a 'woman', but what that means to each becomes immediate and relative, and hence capable of generational expansion and cultural challenge.

My suggestion has been that *paternal deficits constrict the expansion and truncate the challenge.*

In both the collective, external debate about gender characteristics and the personal, internal debate about gender identity, the question of 'masculine' and 'feminine' is best left in suspension – even, and the word is used advisedly, in some confusion. *'Gender confusion' is a necessary antidote to gender certainty* and has its own creative contribution to make. This is particularly true in the treatment of borderline disorders, as we shall see in the next chapter [of *The Plural Psyche*]. For, when we consider gender and the borderline we will see how gender confusion and gender certainty can operate in isolation from each other. *Inadvertently, those who propound a 'feminine principle' play into and replicate the dynamics of unconscious gender certainty,* denying gender confusion.

It is probably fair to say that post-Jungian analytical psychology has become preoccupied with gender certainty and gender confusion in its concern with the 'feminine principle'. Here, I am not referring to the writings on women and 'feminine psychology' by Jung and his early circle of followers. The problems with that body of work are well known and often repeated. But in the 1970s and 1980s, mainly in the United States, women writers in analytical psychology have set out to revise, or revolutionize, the early work. Such writers are struggling to be 'post-Jungian' in their attempt to critique those of Jung's ideas that seem unsatisfactory or just plain wrong without dismissing Jung altogether.

The reason why there has been a concentration on the 'feminine principle' in recent Jungian writing is that it has provided a means to celebrate the specificity of women's identity, life and experience. In addition, having the notion of a 'feminine principle' in mind helps to make a critique of culture out of personal confrontations with it. The basic desire of feminists who are involved in Jungian psychology has been to refuse and refute the denigration of women that is perceived in analytical psychology, to bring the feminine gender in from the condescending margins, and to promote an alternative philosophy of life to that expressed in the power institutions of a male-dominated society.

Taken as a whole, and I realize I am generalizing, feminism which draws on Jung's ideas stands out from other varieties, with which I feel more in sympathy, in two main ways. Both of these stem from Jung's approach, resist eradication and cause great difficulties. It is assumed that there is something eternal about *femininity* and, hence, about *women*; that women, therefore, display certain essential transcultural and ahistorical characteristics; and that these can be described in psychological terms. What is omitted is the ongoing role of the prevailing culture in the construction of the 'feminine' and a confusion develops between what is claimed to be eternal and what is currently observed to be the case. It is here that the deadweight of the heritage of archetypal theory is felt, but as the mirror image of Jung's problem. He assumed that there is something eternal about *women* and, hence, about *femininity.* As Young-Eisendrath (1987: 47) writes, 'certain beliefs about difference – for example, about gender and racial differences – have influenced our thinking about the meaning of symbolic representations, behaviours, style, and manner of people who are alien to the roots of our psychology in Switzerland.' She goes on to say that we need 'something more than maps and charts of our own design.'

I would like to say what I find problematic in the many attempts to locate eternal models or maps for the psychological activity of women in mythology and goddess imagery. When such imagery is used as a kind of role model or resource for a woman in her here-and-now pain and struggle, that is one thing. But when it is claimed that such endeavour is a reclamation of qualities and characteristics that once prevailed in human society only to be smashed by the patriarchy, then that is altogether more suspect. For it is a highly disputed point, to put it mildly, that such an era ever existed. Could this be a case of taking myth too literally? And isn't there a hidden danger here? For if men were to claim that they are in the direct line of psychic inheritance of the characteristics and qualities of gods and heroes, then we'd end up with the status quo, with things just as they are, for they couldn't be any other way. As far as role-modelling and resource provision goes, surely any woman, even or especially an analyst, can perform this task for another woman.

It could be argued that referring to a goddess as a role model or resource is to miss the point about what is special in a divine figure – the numinosity that attaches to such a figure and hence provides a special form of authority. I am not convinced by this argument, for any figure can constellate the kind of venerating transference that is exemplified in the mortal–divine relation. This is something well known to any and every analyst who has experienced an idealizing transference. If the numinosity is not what is specific to the goddess, then, as I suggested, it is her a-temporality, that which is claimed as eternal and absolute in her.

The search for hidden sources of authority is a project constellated by what is seen as a flawed cultural tradition. But there may also be a 'flaw' in the project itself, for such a search demonstrates the very sense of weakness and lack of authority which it seeks to overcome. Engaging in a rivalrous search for female archetypes could lead to a new set of restrictions on female experience, as several writers have observed (Lauter and Rupprecht 1985: 9 discuss this point in detail).

Could we try to play the feminine principle in a pragmatic and not an eternal or absolute key? If so, then its truth would be measured, in William James's words, 'by the extent to which it brings us into satisfactory relations with other parts of our experience' (1911: 157). We would have to start assembling material on the experience of difference as well as on the experience of womanhood and manhood. Sociologists and academic psychologists may have done this but depth psychologists have not – or not yet. Then, in Shorter's words, we would become less concerned with the 'image' of woman and more with 'likeness' to that image. She says: 'Likeness is consciousness of image and its embodiment . . . It is not a question of imitation; each person becomes in part and to the measure that he (sic) is able "like to" the image' (Shorter 1987: 40). Or in Caroline Stevens's words: 'as a woman, anything I do is feminine' (personal communication, 1987).

The second point of disagreement between feminism in analytical psychology and feminism generally has to do with the impression that much Jungian discourse on the 'feminine' seems directed away from political and social action. Dwelling upon interiority and feeling becomes an end in itself. So, just as middle-class Victorian women were believed to be the repository of sensibility and confined to hearth and home, in the Jungian manner of it, women in the nuclear age are meant to be mainly private creatures.

My concern is that much thinking and writing around the 'feminine principle' has opened a secret door into analytical psychology for the return of what is, paradoxically and ironically, an overstructured approach to psyche, heavily dependent upon abstraction and decidedly moralistic. What I'm suggesting is that much contemporary Jungian work on feminine psychology may be seen as far more of an 'imitation of Jung' than was consciously intended. The intention of rectifying Jung's mistakes and prejudices has been perverted.

Trawling the recent literature, I have been struck by the massiveness of the feminine problematic, signified in numerous phrases such as: feminine elements of being, feminine modality of being, femininity of self, feminine ways of knowing, feminine authority, feminine assertion, feminine reflection, feminine dimensions of the soul, primal feminine energy pattern, feminine power, feminine response, feminine creativity, feminine mysteries, feminine body, feminine subjectivity, feminine transformation. I could have quadrupled the list; for ease of reference, I have subsumed all these terms under the general heading of the 'feminine principle'.

Something oppressive has come into being – not, repeat not, because what is claimed as the *content* of the 'feminine principle' is oppressive but because celebrating the feminine has raised it to the status of an ego-ideal, leading to a simple and pointless reversal of power positions. Further, perhaps it is the shadow of feminism generally to make women feel inadequate when they don't come up to its mark – or cannot emulate notable feminist figures.

Gender, metaphor and the body

I would like to say a few words now about the literal and metaphoric relationships between anatomy and psychology to draw together the psychological and scientific aspects of the gender debate, and because I will be talking again about this towards the end of the chapter. A literal determinism has seduced those who seek to make a simple equation between body and psyche. We do not really know what the relationship between them is but it is probably *indirect*. The fact that a penis penetrates and a womb contains tells us absolutely nothing about the psychological qualities of those who actually possess such organs. One does not have to be a clinician to recognize penetrative women and receptive men – nor to conclude that psychology has projected its fantasies onto the body.

A claim is often made that a female's body contains in it certain qualities and characteristics that lead to there being a quite specific and innate female psychology, based on the female body and quite divorced from male psychology, based on the male body. Now, as I just mentioned, there seems to be no problem with the idea that males and females have experiences of their bodies as different from the other sex's body. But the argument that innate psychological differences between the sexes are based on the body has serious and insidious difficulties in it. It *sounds* so grounded, so reasonable, so common-sensical, so different from social or ideological styles of exploring gender issues. However, if psychological activity is body-based then, as body is more or less a constant over the entire history of humanity, body-based psychological theory can only *support* the horrendous gender situation with which we are faced just now. For, if it is body-based, how can it be altered? It must be an inevitability and we would have to agree with Stevens when he argues that 'patriarchy is the natural condition of mankind' (Stevens 1982: 188).

Of course, psychology cannot be split off from the body. But the link is on a deeper level even than that of anatomical or endocrinological distinctiveness. The link between psyche and body surely refers to the body *as a whole* – its moods and movements, its pride and shame, its rigour and its messiness. On this level, the body in question is already a psychological body, a psychesoma, an imaginal body even – providing a whole range of experiences. Sometimes, this imaginal body provides crossover experiences, 'masculine' for women and 'feminine' for men. When the link between psyche and body is envisioned in terms of the body as a whole, then whether that body is anatomically male or anatomically female is less significant. But I am not attempting to deny anyone's experience of their body, nor to dispute the value of paying attention to the body. Indeed, the descriptions in this book [*The Plural Psyche*] of the father's relations with his children are markedly oriented towards physical experience and activity.

Even on a literal, bodily level, recent advances in anatomical research show that things are not what they seem to be. This renders attempts to link bodily and psychological characteristics, even of a subtle and metaphorical kind, highly relative, mutable, and conditioned by the state of knowledge and belief at any one time. In her book *Eve's Secrets* (1987), Lowndes engages in a comparative study of women's and men's sex organs. It turns out that the results of such studies depend completely upon what is compared. For instance, we usually compare penis and vagina, or penis and clitoris. But what if we compare the penis to the sum of clitoris, urethra and vagina (the so called CUV)? Then, according to Lowndes, the fact that the clitoris does have a much longer and deeper structure under the skin that merely culminates in the visible crown means that the female possesses an organ equal in size to the penis and composed of the same erectile material. What is more, a woman has a glans – this is not to be found on her clitoris but close by the opening of her urethra, a raised area as yet possessing no consensual medical name. Looking at the man, Lowndes points out how little is known about the inside of the penis and suggests that in the *corpora cavernosa* there is an area, or spot, that is as sensitive as the clitoris and performs the same functions: a male clitoris.

Lowndes has also found that men and women both have erections, though the charging with blood is visible more markedly in the male. She has also established, by means of careful test measurement, that there is a female ejaculation, composed of fluid that is neither urine nor vaginal secretion.

Anatomical differences between sex organs of men and women are, on the basis of Lowndes's work, quite literally skin-deep. *However, the point is not whether she is right or wrong about it but rather to underline the problems with regarding the body as a fixed element in a body–psyche linkage.* Again, this is not to deny such a link, merely to point out the impossibility of dismissing fantasy and/or changing knowledge from our eventual conclusions.

A further instance of the psychological significance of such work is that it is not at all new. In 400 BC Hippocrates said that men and women both ejaculate. In AD 150 Galen said that the vagina and ovaries are penis and testicles 'inside out'. In 1561 Fallopio discovered, as well as his tubes, that the clitoris has deep structures. In 1672 Regnier de Graaf looked for and found evidence of female ejaculation. It seems that what we say is the case about the body is already psychological (e.g. Freud or, indeed, Kinsey).

Why is this issue of the body as a possible base for sex-specific psychology so critical? I can give two suggestions about this. First, the whole cultural versus innate gender debate is, or has become, numinous. If I have taken one side rather than advancing a multifactorial theory, this is partly because it is what *I* think, partly because that's my personal style, and partly because a clash of doctrines is where the life in psychology is to be found. Again, though I think I'm right, it does not matter so much whether I am right or wrong, but whether what I am talking about can be recognized.

The second reason why the gender debate stirs us has to do with our ambivalence about our constitution, the psychological make-up that we bring into the world. On the one hand, how secure and fulfilling to know that one is quite definitely a man or a woman! I certainly feel a need for certainty and at no time do I suggest that there are no such entities as men or women. On the other hand, I am sure that anatomy is not destiny and am trying to work my resentment at the idea that it might be into a critique of those who tell me it is. There are no *direct* messages from the body.

Which leads back to the great problem with an overdependence in theory-making on the body's impact on psychology. If anatomy is destiny, then nothing can be done to change the position of women. So women who base their quest for a new and positive meaning for femininity on the body inadvertently undermine their own cause. On the contrary, we know how definitions of women and men change over time. Up until the end of the eighteenth century, for instance, representations of men in literature and drama quite often had them as crying – so different from this century, in which big boys don't cry. The body is not an icon in a vacuum.

It follows that animus and anima images are not of men and women because animus and anima qualities are 'masculine' and 'feminine'. No – here, for the individual woman or man, anatomy is a metaphor for the richness and potential of the 'other'. A man will imagine what is 'other' to him in the symbolic form of a woman – a being with another anatomy. A woman will symbolize what is foreign to her in terms of the kind of body she does not herself have. The so-called contrasexuality is more something 'contra-psychological'; anatomy is a metaphor for that. But anatomy is absolutely *not* a metaphor for any particular emotional characteristic or set of characteristics. That depends on the individual and on whatever is presently outside her or his conscious grasp and hence in need of being represented by a personification of the opposite sex. *The difference between you and your animus or anima is very different from the difference between you and a man or woman.* (I do realize that I am discussing animus and anima in their personified forms but I am bringing them in as illustrative of the indirect nature of the relation between body and psyche.)

What I am saying is that *'metaphor' can be as seductively misleading and one-sided as 'literalism'*. Sometimes, it is claimed that 'masculine' and 'feminine' are metaphors (you know, 'just' metaphors) for two distinct *Weltanschauungen* or the typical styles of operating of the two cerebral hemispheres. Why can't we just talk of *Weltanschauungen* or just of hemispheres? When we bring in either masculinity and femininity *or* maleness and femaleness we are projecting a dichotomy that certainly exists in human ideation and functioning onto convenient receptors for the projections. Then the argument that masculinity and femininity should be understood nonliterally, as really having nothing to do with bodily men and bodily women in a social context, may be taken as a recognition that a projection has been made, but falling far short of a successful recollection of it, certainly as far as our culture is concerned. All the other divisions that we know about – rational/irrational, Apollonian/Dionysian, classical/romantic, digital/analogic, and so forth – all these exist in every human being. They cannot conveniently be assigned by gender (or sex), save by the kind of bifurcated projection I have depicted. Why do we make such a projection? Surely it is more than a question of language? It could be because we find difficulty in living with both sides of our murky human natures. In our borderline way, we import a degree of certainty and clarity, and hence reduce anxiety by making the projection. Summarizing my view: it is in this projection that we find the origins of dualist ambitions to construct distinct psychologies for the two sexes and of the attempt to use 'masculinity' and 'femininity' solely as metaphors.

The whole gender debate suggests that, as with the father's relations to his children, we need to question whether heterosexuality itself should be taken as innate and therefore as something fundamental and beyond discussion, or whether it, too, has a nonbiological dimension. Freud' s perception was of an innate *bisexuality* followed later by heterosexuality. Jung's view was that man and woman are each incomplete without the other: heterosexuality is therefore a given. In this sense he differs from Freud's emphasis on bisexuality as the natural state of mankind. In Freud's approach, sexual identity arises from the enforced twin demands of reproduction and society. What I have been arguing shifts the concept of bisexuality from something undifferentiated (polymorphous or polyvalent) into a vision of *there being available to all a variety of positions in relation to gender role – without recourse to the illusion of androgyny.*

Feminist art critics have faced up to many of these problems concerning the body. In a critique of the relation between the biologic and the cultural, Parker and Pollock state that 'acknowledging the importance of events of the body . . . is not reducible to biological essentialism, a facet of patriarchal ideology which supposes a primordial difference between the sexes determined by anatomical and specifically genital structures. How the body is lived and experienced is implicated at all levels in social or societally determined psychic processes' (Parker and Pollock 1987: 29). Parker and Pollock go on to describe an artwork entitled 'Menstruation II' by Cate Elwes. During her period, dressed in white and seated in a white, glass-fronted box, she could be watched bleeding. Questions and her answers could be written on the walls of the box. Elwes wrote, 'The work reconstitutes menstruation as a metaphorical framework in which it becomes the medium for the expression of ideas and experience by giving it the authority of cultural form and placing it within an art context' (quoted in Parker and Pollock 1987: 30).

If discriminations like these are not made, then those analytical psychologists who espouse the idea of innate, body-based, sex-specific psychologies find themselves lined up with those groupings often referred to as the 'New Right'. New Right assumptions about sex-specific psychology tend to be based on appeals to tradition and often have a romantic appeal but, as Di Statham has argued in her paper 'Women, the new right and social work' (1987), those working therapeutically need to be aware of the way in which the assumptions can be used to promote the notion of 'order' and of how women's activities, in particular, are decisively limited.

The same point is made, with a good deal of passion, by Anne McManus in the August 1987 issue of the British feminist journal *Spare Rib*. She wrote:

> Feminism is flowing with the rightward tide, its critical radical spirit diluted beyond recognition . . . A decisive shift came in the transformation of women's *liberation* from oppression, to today's *confirmation* of that oppression in a type of popular feminism which unashamedly embraces anything female. Never mind that this implies a conservative re-embracing of traditional women's roles that the original movement was all about denouncing. Now any old gullible gush practised by women is feminist, especially if it's emotive, and authentic (what isn't authentic anyway at this level?), and anti-male rationality. A false dichotomy between thinking men and feeling women evacuates reason to men while women's fates are sealed, trapped again in eternal emotionality which leaves male power safely intact. Thus women are immobilised and trivialised by their very softness and tenderness, voluntarily abdicating the dirty power struggle, and *thereby* the power, to those who have it.

References

James, W. (1911) *Pragmatism*. London: Longmans Green; Cambridge, MA: Harvard University Press.

Lauter, E. and Rupprecht, C. (1985) *Feminist Archetypal Theory: Interdisciplinary Re-Visions of Jungian Thought*. Knoxville, TN: University of Tennessee Press.
Lowndes, J. (1987) *Eve's Secrets*. London: Bloomsbury.
Parker, R. & Pollock, G. (1987) *Framing Feminism: Art and the Women's Movement 1970–1984*. London & New York: Pandora.
Samuels, A. (1985) *Jung and the Post-Jungians*. London & Boston, MA: Routledge and Kegan Paul.
Sayers, J. (1982) *Sexual Contradictions: Psychology, Psychoanalysis, and Feminism*. London: Tavistock.
Shorter, B. (1987) *An Image Darkly Forming: Women and Initiation*. London & New York: Routledge and Kegan Paul.
Siann, G. (1985) *Accounting for Aggression: Perspectives on Aggression and Violence*. London & Boston, MA: Allen & Unwin.
Statham, D. (1987) 'Women, the new right and social work'. *Journal of Social Work Practice, 2*: 4.
Stevens, A. (1982) *Archetype: A Natural History of the Self*. London: Routledge and Kegan Paul.
Young-Eisendrath, P. (1987) 'The absence of Black Americans as Jungian analysts'. *Quadrant, 20*: 2.

CHAPTER 8

COUNTERTRANSFERENCE AND THE IMAGINAL WORLD

Retrospective introduction

This is the first of three clinical chapters in this book. It was originally published in 1989 in *The Plural Psyche* but first appeared as a journal paper in 1987. It has been much cited and usually given a good deal of approval as prescient, innovative and so on. In the chapter, I give an account of what I felt was the single most important clinical development in the therapy field: the permission given to the therapist to regard his or her subjective reactions to the client as communications from the client. Hence the therapist could, subject to the usual cautionary notes, use him or herself as an active participant in the work.

But the chapter did more than praise 'the countertransference revolution'. It also challenged the psychoanalytic account of this turn in clinical technique, replacing the role in Kleinian theory of projective identification by a usage of the notion of 'the imaginal world'. I saw this as a connecting link between the participants in therapy that somehow pre-existed the coming into being of the therapy pair, and not, as Winnicott stated, as being created by them. Hence the imaginal world was, as I saw it, the foundation of the therapy relationship and clinical work generally.

After that, I began to consider if what really linked therapist and client was not a buried 'rhizome' or a pre-existent imaginal world or their unconscious to unconscious communication, but rather their joint immersion in the political and social order of whatever society in which they happened to live. So it would be citizenship that functioned as the in-depth link that underscores the therapy relationship, including differences in political position in society (for example, economic standing, country of origin and so on).

This chapter is primarily clinical in orientation with a focus on the experience of the analyst as he or she encounters the patient. However, the evolution of the idea of countertransference evokes the entire history of analysis itself. For I think it is true to say that there has been a move away from a biological, scientistic vision of the psyche to one that accentuates the human and also the imaginal factors. The enormous shifts in attitude to countertransference exemplify these moves.

In the chapter I explore some links between current understandings of countertransference and the *mundus imaginalis*, the imaginal world, a term deriving from a different discipline but useful and suggestive in a variety of ways. To effect the link between a clinical concept such as countertransference and the *mundus imaginalis,* I will be making use of a research project I have conducted in which the countertransference experiences of nearly thirty psychotherapists have been collected, collated and evaluated. I think this is one of the earliest projects of its kind and the empirical approach gives a firm base to my overall intent. This is to propose a theory that will, in a pluralistic vein, harness together the functional realities of the analyst's profession and its implicit value system or ideology – an interplay of technique and soul, data and emotion, questionnaire and rhetoric, process and content, relationship and image, left and right hemispheric activity. If I speak of the analyst's use of him/herself, I am concerned with his or her ethos, his or her altitude towards his or her behaviour, his or her self-conception.

Here is a brief illustration of the phenomena with which I am dealing. The words are those of one of the therapists who collaborated in the project:

> Veronica is twenty and single. She is depressed and lives at home with her parents; she works for a bank. At school she was a model pupil and head girl. She started drinking heavily in her late teens and turned down several offers of university places at the last moment. After my third session with her, as I was getting into my car, I experienced a sharp moment of anxiety, an image of a car crash came to me and I found myself thinking, 'What'll happen to Veronica if I have a car crash?'

The therapist knew she was not going mad and that what had happened related to her patient. She was an experienced worker and able to manage her shaken feelings. Her conclusion was that she was being affected by her patient's massive feelings of destructiveness towards her and that her worry about the patient's well-being was representative of the patient's own guilt. The therapist regarded her countertransference reactions as having been stimulated by communications from the patient. Though such reactions are by no means the only source of information about the patient, they play a special part because of the depth and intensity of their impact upon the therapist. My concern is with this type of countertransference experience, to try to understand it and explain how such things can happen at all.

Countertransference in psychoanalysis

In his discussions of psychoanalytic technique, Freud felt that countertransference obscured the analyst's capacity to function effectively, to use his mind as an 'instrument' (Freud 1913). By countertransference, Freud meant something more than the analyst's having feelings towards his patient of which he was aware. Freud was referring to the analyst's 'own complexes and internal resistances', hence to parts of the analyst's unconscious brought into active functioning by contact with a patient (Freud 1910). Freud scarcely revised this essentially negative view of countertransference (as he did with the concept of transference, also seen initially as a handicap).

Although I am focusing on an attitude much more positive than Freud's, it should not be forgotten that there *is* such a thing as neurotic countertransference. This needs to be considered in parallel with the general claim that *some countertransference reactions in the analyst are best seen as resulting from unconscious communications from the patient* and hence of use in the analysis, as in the opening illustration.

There seem to have been three strands in post-Freudian psychoanalytic thinking about countertransference. The first, associated with the names of Heimann and Little, stresses the analyst's emotionality, his or her total involvement in the analytical process. From this, it is then felt that the analyst's unconscious 'understands' that of the patient on a feeling level. Psychoanalysts who have developed this view stress that such countertransference feelings should not be discharged or expressed but rather lived with, reflected upon, used to help the work along (Heimann 1950; Little 1957). As far as the patient is concerned, it is his regression that is being facilitated and valued, an innovation in itself and best encapsulated in Kris's phrase, 'regression of ego in the service of ego' (Kris 1952). 'Token care' may be offered on occasion; for instance, small objects to which the patient has become attached may be taken home to bridge the gap between sessions, a glass of water or milk may be brought, cushions and blankets will be available. Such offerings may be seen as natural extensions of an emotionally based approach.

The second reconstruction of psychoanalytic thinking about countertransference is to be found in Langs's work on the therapeutic process, utilizing a form of communication theory (Langs 1978). Everything that happens in a session, whether originating in patient or analyst, may be regarded as a *symbolic communication,* and psychoanalysis is conceived as an interactional field. In this approach, the psychoanalyst's contribution becomes as analysable as that of the patient. Langs points out that each participant is attempting to place parts of his or her own inner mental state inside the other. The analyst is trying to reach into his or her patient with, perhaps, an understanding of what makes him or her tick. One reason why the patient places what is troublesome to him or her inside the analyst is so that it might, perhaps, be understood. This placement will have a profound and unsettling effect on the analyst. But, precisely because the analyst cannot ignore such an upheaval within him/herself, he or she gains an entrance to the difficult areas of his or her patient's psyche, the access route being through his or her own disturbance. In other words, an analyst *hopes* that he or she will have a countertransference reaction to his or her patient because, in that way, he or she can be an analyst. The logical outcome of this is that the patient must be regarded as the analyst's ally. Langs feels that, even now, many Freudian analysts do not see the patient in a positive light. He writes: 'The patient as enemy and as resisting dominates the analyst's unconscious images, while the patient as ally and as curative is far less appreciated' (Langs 1979: 100). This image of the patient as ally crops up in the more specifically Jungian contribution to countertransference developments that we shall discuss in a moment.

Searles, though by no means using the same conceptual vocabulary as Langs, strikes a similar chord when he suggests that an analyst should allow a more severely damaged or regressed patient to see how the work has affected him. Searles includes in this both the analyst's childlike feelings and his more adult emotions. For example, when the theme of the work is oedipal, Searles is most concerned not to repeat 'an unconscious denial of the child's importance to the parent' (Searles 1959: 302).

The third way in which contemporary psychoanalysts, such as Racker, have modified Freud's negativity about countertransference makes explicit use of projective and introjective processes (and, above all, of projective identification) to explain how it is that parts of the patient's psyche turn up in the analyst's emotions and behaviour (Racker 1968). Those ideas will be examined in a concluding section but, for now, it should be noted that the concept of projective identification refers to much more than an infantile defence or something pathological in an adult.

To summarize: post-Freudian evolution of the idea of countertransference as communication embraces the themes of involvement, emotion, containment, symbolism, self-revelation and projection. One outcome has been that a wider range of patients may be treated than previously (cf. Gorkin 1987: 85). This has been both caused and promoted by the acceptance of visible warmth as part of a psychoanalyst's professional behaviour. Though the psychoanalyst may at times behave *like* a mirror, he or she is not a mirror.

This general loosening in psychoanalysis has led to the emergence of one quality above all others as crucial to the practice of psychoanalysis. That quality is *empathy*.

Kohut has left us a mysterious definition of empathy (Kohut 1982). This, he says, may be defined as 'vicarious introspection'. The poetic phrase is quite stunning in the range of possibilities offered: examining the psyche of another in one's own psyche, examining one's own psyche in the psyche of another, using one's psyche to see what it is like to be another, letting another's psyche into one's own so as to look at it – and so forth. In the same way that there is a form of observation that is suited to the outer world, empathy is 'a mode of observation attuned to the inner life of man'. But empathy is more than a way of gathering emotional information; it also suggests an immensely powerful relationship between people. So Kohut has forged a stout connection between, first, understanding the inner life of a person and, then, an intense personal relationship between people. It is on that note that I want to end this review of what has happened in psychoanalysis: analysis as a relationship between people that helps in an inner exploration.

Countertransference in analytical psychology

The contribution of analytical psychology to the general area of countertransference is more that of an extension to the founder's work than an alteration of it, for, as in many other instances, Jung's sensings of what was central to psychological treatment have proved more prescient than Freud's. As early as 1929, Jung was saying that 'You can exert no influence if you are not susceptible to influence . . . The patient influences [the analyst] unconsciously . . . One of the best-known symptoms of this kind is *the countertransference evoked by the transference*' (Jung 1946: para. 163, my italics). And, in the same paper, Jung refers to countertransference as a 'highly important organ of information'.

It is against this sympathetic background that we should view Fordham's introduction in 1957 of the term 'syntonic countertransference'. The word 'syntonic' is used in radio communications to describe the accurate tuning of a receiver so that transmissions from one particular transmitter may be received. In Fordham's usage, the unconscious of the analyst is tuned into what emanates from the patient's transmitter. The analyst may find himself feeling something or behaving in a way that relates to, or is expressing, the patient's inner world, again as in my opening illustration.

It is through introjection that an analyst perceives a patient's unconscious processes in him/herself, and Fordham realized that it was necessary to *use* this syntonic countertransference to understand the patient better. But to reach this position Fordham had to move far beyond the orthodoxy of his time. Up to then, for the analyst to have a fantasy about his or her patient, or to experience impulses to behave strangely, had been regarded as cardinal sins, evidence of neurotic blind spots in the analyst – and nothing more. Of course, Fordham does not neglect the neurotic aspect of countertransference, referring to this as 'illusory countertransference'.

More recently, Fordham posed the following question: if the analyst's countertransference is a normal part of analysis, then why continue to refer to it as countertransference, with implications of pathological fantasy or delusion? Fordham suggested that we might talk simply of interaction (or dialectical interaction) and reserve countertransference for something neurotic. Though this amazing return to Freud's position is a logical outcrop of Fordham's whole approach to the analytical process, the idea has not been taken up (Fordham 1979; personal communication 1985).

It should not be thought that this psychoanalytically influenced approach of the Developmental School is the only relevant move in analytical psychology. There has also been an attempt by more classically inclined analytical psychologists to use the image of the Wounded Healer to further an understanding of countertransference (though the word 'countertransference' may not actually be used).

Meier (1949) drew parallels between the ancient healing practices of the temples of Asclepius and modern analysis. Though this was primarily an attempt to show historical continuity within the collective psyche, two points stand out for the clinician. The *temenos,* or temple precinct, in which healing took place, is the predecessor of the enclosed analytical setting. The teacher of the healing arts, Chiron the centaur, is depicted as suffering from an incurable wound – the modern analyst is also such a Wounded Healer.

Guggenbuhl-Craig (1971) continued to explore the image of the Wounded Healer. His idea was that we tend to split this archetypal image so that the analyst becomes all-powerful, strong, healthy and able. The patient remains nothing but a patient: passive, dependent and prone to compliance. Now, there is really a split *within* both patient and analyst. If it is the case that analysts have inner wounds, then to present oneself as totally healthy is to cut off from part of one's inner world. Likewise, if the patient is only seen as ill, then he or she is cut off from his or her own inner healer or capacity to heal him/herself.

When a person becomes sick, the 'healer-wounded' image comes into operation. The outer person is sick but there is also his or her inner healer to consider. Initially, and to get the treatment moving, this will be projected onto the analyst. But Guggenbuhl-Craig's point is that his projection must be taken back so that the patient can utilize his or her own healthy attributes. The analyst, too, must make an initial projection. This is of his or her wounded part onto the patient; thus he or she is helped to feel sympathetic, understanding and disposed to help. He or she, too, must withdraw this projection in due course so as to release his or her patient's capacity to be healthy. This implies the analyst staying in touch with his or her inner wounds. The process may be repeated over and over in an analysis.

Guggenbuhl-Craig's descriptions may be compared to Langs's catchphrase of the 'patient as ally'. Similarly, Money-Kyrle wrote that 'The aim of psychoanalysis is to help the patient understand, and so overcome, emotional impediments to his discovering what he innately already knows' (Money-Kyrle 1971: 104). And Sterba (1934) saw as fundamental to the analytical process that the patient must split his or her ego, identifying one part with the analyst, so observing and reflecting on the material he or she produces as patient. The patient's material constitutes the other part of his or her ego. The patient's reflecting ego may be regarded as an activation of his or her inner healer.

Continuing to look at what analytical psychology has to say about countertransference, a research project was carried out in Germany in the early 1970s. Four analytical psychologists met to study their various countertransferences and, in particular, to record their associations to the material of the patients at the same time as they recorded the patient's comments. Here is what the report of that project has to say about associations to dream imagery:

> The most astonishing result for us was the psychological connection between the analysts' chains of associations and the patients'. For the psychotherapist it is, of course, self-evident that the chain of associations should be connected together in a psychologically meaningful way. So it was to be expected that this connection would be found not only in the patient's chain of associations but in the analyst's as well; what we had not expected was that the two chains would again be connected with each other so that they again correspond meaningfully all along the line. Perhaps the situation may best be characterised by the spontaneous exclamation of one of our members: 'The patients continually say what I am thinking and feeling at the moment!'
>
> (Dieckmann 1974: 111)

The proposal of that research group was that such events are caused by the existence in man of a separate and more archaic perceptual system than the one of which he is aware.

To recapitulate: in analytical psychology, attention has been paid to the way projection and introjection combine to make an analyst function as if part of his or her patient's inner world. It has also been regarded as vital that excessive healer-wounded splits in both analyst and patient be brought together so that the patient's inner healer can be released. Finally, a wholly different perceptual system is proposed to explain how it is that analysts get so comprehensively in touch with their patients.

Putting the Jungian and Freudian ideas together, we may, dare I say it, even speak of an analytical consensus and one that may be used as an assumption: that some countertransference reactions in the analyst stem from, and may be regarded as communications from the patient, and that the analyst's inner world, as it appears to him or her, is the *via regia* into the inner world of the patient.

Research project: Hypothesis

Before introducing more of the research material, I want to state the hypothesis on which the project was based. My thinking is that there are two rather different sorts of usable countertransference – though both may be seen as communications from the patient. The difference between the two is shown in this simple example. Suppose, after a session with a particular patient, I feel depressed (this may be a single occurrence or part of a series). Now I may know from my own reading of myself that I am not actually depressed and certainly not seriously depressed. I may conclude that the depressed state I am in is a result of my close contact with this particular patient. It may be that the patient is feeling depressed right now and that neither of us is aware of that. In this instance, my depression is a reflection of his depression. So I would call this an example of *reflective countertransference*. In time, I may be able to make use of this knowledge, particularly if I had not realized the existence (or extent) of the patient's depression. But there is another possibility. My experience of becoming a depressed person may stem from the presence and operation of such a 'person' in the patient's psyche. The patient may have experienced a parent as depressed and my reaction precisely embodies the patient's emotionally experienced parent. I have also become a part of the patient's inner world. I stress 'inner world' rather than the patient's actual infancy or history to make the point that I am not attempting any kind of factual reconstruction. That 'person' will inevitably also be symbolic of a theme active in the patient's psyche or of a part of his personality. This entire state of affairs I have come to call *embodied countertransference* and it is to be distinguished from the former category of reflective countertransference. There is a considerable difference between, on the one hand, my reflecting of the here-and-now state of my patient, feeling just what he or she is unconscious of at the moment, and, on the other, my embodiment of an entity, theme, or person of a longstanding, intrapsychic, inner-world nature. One problem for the analyst is that, experientially, the two states may seem similar. Perhaps some countertransferences are both reflective and embodied.

'Embodied' is intended to suggest a physical, actual, material, sensual expression in the analyst of something in the patient's inner world, a drawing together and solidification of this, an incarnation by the analyst of a part of the patient's psyche and, as the *Shorter Oxford English Dictionary* defines it, a 'clothing' by the analyst of the patient's soul. If our psyche tends to personify, as Jung suggests, then embodiment speaks of the way the person/analyst plays his or her part in that.

I am grateful to Symington (personal communication 1986) for suggesting that it is important to distinguish between countertransference states in the analyst that refer to the patient's ego and countertransference states that refer more to the patient's objects. Reflective countertransferences would, I think, refer more to the patient's ego position whereas embodied countertransferences could refer to either the patient's ego or to his or her objects, according to the specific context. The main point is that the problem that the analyst and patient are working on can become embodied in the analyst.

Now any analyst who proposes new terms must explain why he or she does so in order not to be charged with word-mongering. This is particularly the case when, as in this instance, the new terms overlap with those already in use. Fordham's concept of syntonic countertransference is one for which I, in common with many analytical psychologists, am extremely grateful. His achievement was to drag analysts out of their ivory towers, help them truly to listen to what their patients were trying to tell them and make a reality out of pious commitments to 'the dialectical approach'. But gradually I began to feel that the term 'syntonic' was distant from my experience; often one does not feel in tune with the patient in these countertransferences and there may be dissonance inside oneself. Later, it may be clear that one was in tune. So 'syntonic' leans too much towards an Olympian standpoint, intellectual, even technical or technological, and, hence, radiates commitment to a mode of observation more suited to the outer world than to the empathic processes we are talking about. Embodiment, on the other hand, does imply a becoming, with its consequent involvements, and also a suggestion of a medium for countertransference communications from the patient; this, it will turn out, is often the analyst's body. Again, many of these countertransference states are nonverbal or pre-verbal – and embodiment speaks to that.

The unease with the notion of syntonic countertransference was a particular problem for me, as I was deliberately trying to keep my theorizing on the 'low road', 'experience-near', in Kohut's phrases, using the empirical stance and data collection together with an empathic attitude (Kohut 1982). So I chose the terms 'embodied' and 'reflective' quite deliberately, to be of help in the task of bracketing countertransference (specific to the practice of analysis) and the *mundus imaginalis,* a more general, cultural term employed in archetypal psychology. It may turn out that these ideas particularize and extend Fordham's theory – paradoxically by invoking an approach with which he is in total disagreement (numerous personal communications 1976–88).

The term 'incarnate', which was one of the associations to which embodiment led, has a history in analytical psychology. It was first used in 1956 by Plaut to describe how an analyst may have to let himself become what the patient's imagery dictates he be. However, Plaut's pioneering paper referred to the analyst's reactions to transference projections of which he was aware, and to his control (or lack of it) of his response. For example, what to do when a woman patient saw him as a remarkable teacher; should he contradict this, teach her about wise old men, or 'incarnate' the image so as to develop a knowledge of how to use it? Plaut's concern was not with states in the analyst that are apparently devoid of any causation outside of the analytic relationship.

It should be reiterated that not all countertransference reactions are usable communications from the patient. We need to bear neurotic countertransference in mind – identifying with the patient, idealizing the patient, the analyst's retaliation to the patient's aggression, his or her destruction of his or her own work, his or her attempt to satisfy his or her own infantile needs through the relationship with the patient. Nor is it always immediately clear what the patient's communications mean. As Jung said, the analyst may have to stay in a muddled, bewildered state for a period, allowing an understanding to germinate, if it will. An ability to rest with the anxiety and maintain an attitude of affective involvement becomes crucial.

Research project: Results

I will turn now to the material that I gathered through the research project in 1983. I embarked on it because I felt a need to check hypotheses like the reflective/embodied countertransference model and did not trust myself to use my own case material in isolation. Since 1976 I had been giving seminars to psychotherapy trainees in which I suggested that there were these two sorts of countertransference. I contacted thirty-two qualified psychotherapists who had been in supervision with me during this period and asked them for a few examples of countertransference reactions of theirs that they considered to result from the unconscious communications of their patients (see note at end of chapter). The hypothesis that there are two different kinds of countertransference was restated and the participants were reminded of the existence of neurotic countertransference. The countertransference reaction was to be reported in detail and I asked which kind of countertransference this was thought to be and how this experience had affected the work. The final question, which summarizes the intent of the whole project, was: 'Can you say how the patient may have provoked or evoked these feelings in you?'

Readers may wonder why the research hypothesis was made plain to the participants. This was no secret for they all knew of it anyway, having heard me expatiate on the subject. The transference to me could be managed by avoiding asking whether the hypothesis was 'true' and focusing enquiry on the way the participants were or were not using the concepts. The clinical validity of the hypothesis is expressed in its possession or lack of clinical usefulness.

Methodological justification came from Popper (1963). Using falsifiability as a yardstick, the classification of countertransference is offered as a predictive theory whose hypotheses may then be tested. There is a cumulative quality about this undertaking (and Popper regards such a quality as crucial to scientific enquiry). An attempt is made to preserve as much as possible of preceding theories. After all, we are dealing with nothing more than successive provisional approximations to the truth. There are further observations that might be made about this kind of theorizing, all deriving from Popper. It does not matter how I arrived at the hypothesis; this has no bearing on its standing. What is more, there is no value in having an open (in the sense of empty) mind; the inductive method, in which data is surveyed and generalizations about it formulated, is in no sense 'objective'. From that, we must affirm that it is perfectly in order that the research material is partially derived from the hypothesis it is intended to test; it always is.

As it turned out, the results of the project were of sufficiently manageable proportions for me also to be able to use the currently discredited but traditionally admired inductive approach. The results could be surveyed to see if a pattern emerged that might be generalizable into a theory. That is, if the theory had been in existence, the results obtained could have been explained by it. As we have seen, my interests and expectations meant that the survey was by no means a random one. Still, its outcome was that another, quite different, categorization of countertransference emerged to be set alongside the reflective/embodied distinction. I shall return to this later in the chapter.

It may also be necessary to justify such empiricism to those who see it as opposed to poetic, rhetorical, imaginal explorations. An empirical base does not necessarily lead to prosaic conclusions. The findings of the project are quite the opposite. Empiricism, as expressed in this research venture, supports a poetic, metaphorical, imaginal explanation for the mysterious workings of countertransference.

The 26 completed replies covered a total of 57 cases. Because some cases involved more than one example of a countertransference communication and because some countertransferences could be said to be both reflective and embodied, the total of such examples came to 76. Of these, 35 (46 per cent) were held by the respondents to be of embodied countertransference and 41 (54 per cent) of reflective countertransference.

It was abundantly clear that the participants could see how to use such a classification of countertransference. Here is an example said to be of embodied countertransference. The patient was a young, unmarried woman who had presented originally with a mixture of intolerable guilt accompanied by a sense of responsibility for the spiritual and moral welfare of others. She had also had a depressive breakdown. She had had several traumatic religious experiences in childhood. This is the therapist's account:

> This event happened after three years of work when we were thinking of adding a second session. She was always extremely controlled, with periods in every session which felt almost autistic. She said nothing which had not already been minutely examined 'inside'. She watched my face for the slightest move, flicker of an eye, for instance, and would interpret what she thought she saw there – to herself – as me laughing at her, getting fed up with her, getting irritated by her. I suggested that perhaps one day she might feel able to entrust a bit more of what was inside to me, with the feeling that I would not change it or take it away, that I could just hold it. As I was speaking I had a very strong

> impression or image of a large, black, open-mouthed pot which was strong yet open – like a big belly. The pot was huge and black and also like a witch's cauldron (I later realised). I said to her that it would be rather like having a pot which she could safely leave things in. Her immediate reaction was that it would be like a wall which something had been hurled at violently. My instantaneous image was of a violent expelling-type vomit, running down the wall, uncontained and wasted. We were both quite staggered by the strength and opposite nature of the two images we had had.

The therapist felt that the pot image demonstrated that the patient's mother had longed to be of use to her. But the witch's cauldron and the image of vomiting suggest something else besides. The cauldron was described as big enough to swallow up a human being – and hence a sinister and dangerous part-self or splinter psyche within the patient. Thus there were two aspects to this embodied countertransference: her mother's longing on the one hand and, on the other, an embodiment by the therapist of a split-off part of the patient's psyche.

The next illustration is an example of a reflective countertransference. This therapist found herself coming to supervision with me in clothes very like those worn by her patient at their most recent session. This was something she realized during the supervision, but, in fact, I had been struck by the clothes she was wearing the moment I met her at the door, a little-boy presentation, school sweater, crooked tie and collar, muddied, practical shoes. And, though I did not know it, she was wearing a coat of the same colour as her patient's, a coat she had not worn for years until that day. As we talked, it became clear that the patient had never felt able to relate closely to her mother. She was the middle of three daughters and had been 'assigned' to her father – memories of being placed, unwillingly, on his knee. She had never felt 'at one' with her mother. And she certainly could not let herself feel *like* her mother, like a woman. The way she had resolved this was to let herself be 'Daddy's girl' but in a way that ruled out incestuous involvement (the little-boy strategy).

The therapist's behaviour, in which she became merged with her patient, might have been considered neurotic. But the notion that it reflects her patient's desire to be at one with her therapist, and, indeed, her whole life struggle to obtain mothering, is equally plausible. For instance, the therapist writes: 'In some ways she had been treating me like a man although she had sought out a woman therapist. I found myself being more active and penetrating than my usual style and generally more assertive.' Mattinson (1975) has written of the way in which the dynamics of one situation (therapy) are reflected in those of an adjacent situation (supervision); this is also well illustrated in the workshop transcript that follows.

What I have been describing was, for me, a confirmation of a hypothesis. As I mentioned earlier, in addition to that, it was also possible to detect an overall pattern in the seventy-six countertransference responses and, moreover, one about which I had had no hypothesis. The countertransference responses described fell into distinct groups or categories, as follows.

First, *bodily and behavioural responses*. For example: wearing the same clothes as the patient, walking into a lamp-post, forgetting to discuss something important, a strange sensation in the solar plexus, a pain in a particular part of the body, sexual arousal, sleep.

Second, *feeling responses*. For example: anger, impatience, powerfulness, powerlessness, envy, irritation, depression, manipulation, redundancy, being flooded, being bored.

Finally, *fantasy responses*. For example: this is the wrong patient, there's something wrong with my feet, a large black pot, I killed her mother, I'm a prostitute, I feel reverence for her serious, private place, *he* has God on *his* side, all colour has gone out of the world, a car crash, he'll rummage through my desk and books if I leave the room, the patient is getting bigger and bigger and is filling the room.

Exposing myself to these accounts, this time without the protection of the reflective/embodied theory, made me aware that all these instances of countertransference may be said to be images, and this is true even of the bodily or feeling responses. They are images because they are active in the psyche in the absence of a direct stimulus that could be said to have caused them to exist. That is, nothing has been done to the analyst that would, in the usual way of things, explain the presence of such a reaction in him or her. A person may be conscious or unconscious of an image but, either way, the image may be regarded as promoting feelings and behaviour and not as secondary, a coded message about them (cf. Newton 1965; Kugler's [1982] use of a term such as 'acoustic image').

In the questionnaire, I also asked the participants what was the presenting problem of their patients. One finding is particularly interesting. It would seem that patients with instinctual (sex, aggression, food) problems are more likely to evoke reflective and embodied countertransference than other patients. What is highlighted, therefore, is the special part that may be played by the body in the patient's evocation of countertransference in the analyst. This bodily proposition will have to be looked at alongside the earlier idea that it is the image that is the decisive factor. Here, the *mundus imaginalis* turned out to be relevant.

In both the 'pot' example of embodied countertransference and the 'clothes' example of reflective countertransference, imagery and bodily perceptions played intermingled roles. In sum: the hope is that these findings justify a classification of usable countertransference responses into reflective and embodied, and that both terms accurately depict what happens. Further, the additional grouping of countertransferences under the headings of bodily and behavioural, feeling, and fantasy responses may also be justified.

Implications for technique

A central technical issue is constellated by a vision of countertransference as a possible communication from the patient: what is the analyst to do with the knowledge he or she may gain from an analysis of his or her countertransference experiences? Should he or she disclose them to the patient? If so, how? Should the analyst weld his or her understanding of the countertransference into his or her interpretations? If so, how? Should he or she do little more than stay in touch with what is being discovered?

When I first began to think about these matters, I expected to find a sharp divide between Freudians and Jungians, with the latter group being more willing, even eager, to disclose countertransference material. True, a few Jungian analysts (e.g. Stein 1987) are strong advocates of disclosure, particularly of feelings about the patient generated in the analyst. But even such an extreme viewpoint is also represented in psychoanalysis, for example by Winnicott in 'Hate in the countertransference' (1949). The comprehensive literature review in Gorkin (1987) suggests strongly that there are numerous psychoanalysts who can see occasions on which it is advisable and justifiable to disclose countertransference. In psychoanalysis much more has been written about the *kind* of patient with whom this is appropriate than in analytical psychology.

Perhaps because of the Freudian/Jungian consensus referred to above, most analysts seem to agree with Segal's position, summarized by Casement (1986a: 548):

> The analyst is in no position to interpret if the interpretation is based only upon what the analyst is feeling in the session. Unless it is possible to identify how the patient is contributing to what the analyst is feeling, and in such a way that the patient could recognise this, then it is better to remain silent.

Casement notes the twin dangers of gratifying patients who want a magician for an analyst and of persecuting others with omniscience. Precisely because of dangers like these, I felt it necessary to go on with my investigations of countertransference, so as to find an ideological basis for the careful use of the tacit knowledge of the patient that the countertransference can provide for the analyst. In other words, I think more is needed than an understanding of the dynamics of any one patient. What is required is an understanding of how these phenomena generally tend to function. I do not mean a tight theory or categorization, because that would defeat the purpose of utilizing countertransference, but I do mean something more than clinical pragmatics. My working out of the theme of the *mundus imaginalis* is intended to be that kind of ideological project.

Succinctly, an understanding of what it is that the analyst reflects or/and embodies can serve as a kind of resource out of which he or she fashions the actual words and images of the interpretation, rendering them fresh and, above all, related to the patient – hence not 'cliché interpretations' (Casement 1986b).

What I aim at is summarized thrillingly in this note sent by Bion to Meltzer (who quotes it in 1978: 126):

> Now I would use as a model: the diamond cutter's method of cutting a stone so that a ray of light entering the stone is reflected back *by the same path* in such a way that the light is augmented – the same 'free association' is reflected back by the same path, but with augmented 'brilliance'. So the patient is able to see his 'reflection', only more clearly than he can see his personality as expressed by himself alone (i.e. without an analyst).

At this point, I should like to introduce a transcription of an audio-tape recording of a workshop I conducted on countertransference. As with any such transcripts, the reader should be aware that group-associative and other processes and the natural focusing instigated by having a theme sometimes give a peculiar cast to the material.

Analyst A **(male):** This is a new person that I'm working with. About four sessions. My image is of her sitting on the couch in the office and she typically takes her shoes off and puts her feet up on the couch. She makes herself seem very comfortable though I don't think she is. She wears very dramatic clothes: white, attractive, striking. One of the issues in the therapy is that she has had or managed to have therapists abuse her, including sexually, as did her father. And now she has a desire to get vengeance on men. She also wants to protect other people from therapists' abuse so she is pursuing a legal action. I have this image of her as a *rather striking bird*. This complicates trying to sort out what is already a very difficult therapeutic interaction.

AS: My first reaction is to say don't try bioenergetics with this patient.
(Pause. Laughter.)

AS: I wonder why I said that disrespectful thing in relation to your patient – that's a countertransference on my part for sure. Have you thought of her as a sexual person; obviously, I was . . .

Analyst A: I have. But not of doing bioenergetics.

AS: This is the countertransference really because one doesn't make love to a bird draped in white. I expect you know about the self-protective aspects of the image for you?

Analyst A: Sure.

AS: But there's more to it. Here is a woman whose talk is all about sex but who produces an image in you of spirituality, virginity, something soaring, whiteness. The whole thing is the embodied countertransference, associations and image. What you are embodying is a conflict *in her* – a split if you like, between sexuality and spirituality. No doubt it's something that it might be possible to work on with her. It's a terrific incongruity. Jung had an idea about the relationship between sex and spirit. He was on about the conversion of sexual libido into spirituality. Being a boy, he did it from the perspective of a boy with mother! For the girl, it's probably what the father does with her. When the symbolic aspects of incest are swept away by its actuality, then the father has failed in helping with that conversion. Then your patient has to live superficially, sexually for sure, but without spiritual depth.

Analyst A: Yes, that's the problem, sex is something physical only, without much significance. I'm trying to follow, I'm not a Jungian, I'm a psychoanalyst. I did feel that this is an image she projects and it's also a defensive posture on my part. I can see now that it is perhaps a communication from her to me that I must help her with the transition you've been describing which has been impossible for her. Maybe then she could let herself be really sexual instead of projecting it into therapists.

AS: In simple language, she's never been taken seriously. That gives a prospective aspect to her sleeping with previous therapists because that certainly gets her taken seriously and as special and you end up in court.

***Participant* (female):** Could this image be the analyst's anima, or feminine side?
(Long pause.)

AS: I think the group dynamic is important here because he already said he isn't a Jungian and now you suddenly hit him with 'anima' and he doesn't know what to say! I think what's happening is this: you (as daughter) feel he (as father) said he didn't want to know you when he said he wasn't a Jungian. So you offer him your Jungian self once again, hoping for a better response. It's a father–daughter rejection/retaliation dynamic and it is dead relevant to this case.

Analyst A: I'm sitting on my hands here because I want to come in and say that anima is one Jungian concept I do know . . .
(Laughter.)

AS: So actually when she said 'anima' you were perfectly comfortable until I came lumbering in?

***Analyst A:* (male):** Well, no, I *was* uncomfortable when she said 'anima' but when you came in I started to feel protective towards her. Are you saying that this feeling of protectiveness is also one of these countertransferences?

AS: Probably. But I think still that what she said is the most important thing. She was saying (provocatively): 'I have a world view and depth that you as father are not taking seriously. I'm not being taken seriously.' What is tragic is that the father does want to take her seriously – he does know about anima but he couldn't say anything when she brought it up. He ends up 'sitting on his hands' in frustration. The whole episode is an embodiment of her problem. Going back to her own father: they couldn't meet because of the actualizing of the incest link and so the mutual understanding on a deep level got left out. What gets into people in a group is connected to the patient.

Participant I saw her more as a bird of prey, dangerous to therapists, so I understood your bioenergetics joke. But she chose another male therapist. Why?

AS: There's probably lots of reasons but I'm saying she needs to be noticed by the father in a very special way and she is in search of that. It's profound, not mere attention-seeking. She needs acknowledgement as a sexual being who can also have depths – that's the issue we're embodying. The incestuous father didn't give her that acknowledgement and she felt massively deprived as well as abused and attacked.

It is now the time to explore the underlying ideology, the idea of the *mundus imaginalis.*

The *mundus imaginalis*

The *mundus imaginalis,* the imaginal world, is a term employed by Henry Corbin, the French philosopher and scholar (Corbin 1972; 1978; 1983). To use this term in an analytic context is not in itself original. Hillman's suggestion that we practise 'Jung's technique with Corbin's vision' is a precursor (Hillman 1980). This enables us to include inside the *mundus imaginalis* those images that Corbin regarded as a 'secularisation of the imaginal': grotesque, painful, pathological – analytical material. The *mundus imaginalis* refers to a precise order or level of reality, located somewhere between primary sense impressions and more developed cognition or spirituality.

The *mundus imaginalis* (Hillman adds) enables us to speak of the location of the archetypal. So we begin to regard the psyche as structured by its images alone rather than by unknowable, irrepresentable, theoretical archetypes (see Samuels 1985: 31–2). Fordham also in a sense joined Hillman when he wondered whether the conventional archetypal structure/archetypal image split in analytical psychology has any meaning. Fordham's point was that the word 'image' in the term 'archetypal image' is redundant because no archetype can be discussed or have any being without an image; hence, 'archetype' includes and implies an image (Fordham 1970: 297). Hillman's version of the same argument was that, as we cannot even conceive of the so-called noumenal, hypothetical, archetype without an image, it is the image that is primary (Hillman 1980: 33n).

As Corbin sees it, the *mundus imaginalis* is an in-between state, an intermediate dimension, in his original French *entre-deux,* which may even have the meaning:

'neither one thing nor another' (Corbin 1983: 1). It is possible to see, therefore, how the *mundus imaginalis* acquired a relevance for the countertransference phenomena we have been discussing. They, too, are intermediate; in between patient and analyst, and also in between the analyst's conscious and unconscious. My use of Corbin's idea involves the suggestion that *two persons, in a certain kind of relationship, may constitute, or gain access to, or be linked by, that level of reality known as the mundus imaginalis.* For the patient, the analyst him/herself *is* an in-between, a real person and also a transference projection. For the analyst, the world he or she shares with the patient is also the patient's own imaginal world.

When the analyst experiences his or her countertransference on a personal level and yet knows its roots are in the patient, it is an in-between state. To be sure, it is *his or her* body, *his or her* imagery, *his or her* feelings or fantasies. But these things also belong to the patient, and have been squeezed into being and given substance by the analytical relationship. It would be a great mistake for the analyst to remain enmeshed in subjectivity (actually in possessiveness) or compulsive introspection or self-blame. What appeared to have happened to him or her and in him or her is truly in between the analyst and the patient, imaginally real not subjectively real.

My suggestion is that there is a two-person or shared *mundus imaginalis* that is constellated in analysis. To justify this, it is necessary to take the parallels further, and deeper, though bearing in mind what a further, literal translation of *entre-deux* as 'between two people' might suggest to us.

Corbin refers to the *mundus imaginalis* as having a 'central mediating function' so that all levels of reality may 'symbolise with each other' (Corbin 1972: 9). The parallel is with the way the analyst symbolizes something for the patient. The analyst's ego is a special kind of ego, highly permeable and flexible and having as its central mediating function the operation of the sluice gates between image and understanding. Again, Corbin writes of the way 'inner and hidden reality turns out to envelop, surround or contain that which at first was outer and visible' (Corbin 1972: 5). The analyst's countertransference response is outer and visible; what is inner and hidden is the patient's psychic reality that certainly envelops the analyst. For Corbin, the *mundus imaginalis* is a 'fully objective and real world with equivalents for everything existing in the sensible world without being perceptible by the senses' (Corbin 1972: 7). In the analyst's countertransference we see equivalents of the patient's internal reality, even though the sensory data for the analyst's experience is missing. Hence, the rationale for referring generally to these countertransferences as images.

Of all the suggestive possibilities for analysis to be found in Corbin's work, it is his equation of the *mundus imaginalis* with visionary states that I should like to develop (Corbin 1972: 4). The experiences of countertransference, as described in this chapter, may be regarded as visions. No direct sensory stimulus is involved in a vision and also the experience is not of an intellectual nature. Jung made the additional point that no deliberate act of imagination is involved either (Jung 1963: 327). All these facts are relevant to countertransference.

Many of the extraordinarily powerful experiences and images I have been discussing are also described by Jung when he refers to visions as 'disturbing spectacles of some tremendous process that in every way transcend our human feeling and understanding' (Jung 1930: para. 141). Jung goes on to ask: 'Is it a vision of other worlds, or of the darknesses of the spirit, or of the primal beginnings of the human psyche?' We may add to the list: visions of another's psyche, empathic visions, analytical visions. Corbin's reference (Corbin 1983: 1) is to 'the organ of visionary knowledge'; for an analyst, when he is doing analysis, that organ is his countertransference.

The argument so far is that the *mundus imaginalis* functions as a linking factor between patient and analyst and that some of the analyst's countertransference may be regarded as visions and hence part of this imaginal world. What I want to do now is to relate the proposed connection between countertransference and the *mundus imaginalis* to what emerged from the research project; in particular, to explore what the analyst's body and the *mundus imaginalis* have in common.

Using Corbin's metaphor, the analyst's body becomes less literal, a 'subtle body', a 'being in suspense', a link between soul and corporeality (Corbin 1972: 9). What I am trying to convey is that, in analysis, the analyst's body is not entirely his or her own and what it says to him or her is not a message for him or her alone. In pursuance of this healing of the body/soul dichotomy, I may add to the term 'analytical visions' another: bodily visions – 'not-me possessions' of the analyst.

It is not just Corbin who has explored this area; Jung, too, wrote of the in-between world, referring to it as *esse in anima.* And Jung also had something to say about these connections between body, sense-impressions, fantasy and the subjective/objective dynamic. He wrote:

> A third, mediating standpoint is needed. *Esse in intellectu* lacks tangible reality, *esse in re* lacks mind . . . Living reality is the product neither of the actual behaviour of things, nor of the formulated idea exclusively, but rather of the combination of both.
>
> (Jung 1921: para. 77)

Jung went on to refer to this combination as fantasy, adding that fantasy 'fashions the bridge between the *irreconcilable claims of subject and object*' (my italics).

Capturing what is meant by bodily visions takes me once more back to Corbin. He was interested in studying what he described as 'the organ which perceives', the *mundus imaginalis;* this he refers to as 'imaginative consciousness' (Corbin 1972: 2). The analyst's imaginative consciousness and his perception of his bodily visions, apparently so disparate, may more accurately be seen as two different ways of approaching the same goal. For bodily perception is quite different from other kinds of perception because there is no *specific* organ that comes to mind in connection with it. As the philosopher Armstrong puts it:

> When I feel the heat of my hand, the motion of my limbs, the beating of my heart or the distension of my stomach, and do not feel these things by exploring my body with another portion of my body, there is no natural answer to the question 'What do you feel these states of your body *with*?'
>
> (Armstrong 1962: 10)

It was this argument that led Armstrong to propose that notion of 'bodily perception' and, as I hinted just now, his use of it and Corbin's of 'imaginative consciousness' are rather similar. Whichever of these terms are used, the issue that then emerges concerns the fate of the *mundus imaginalis* in analysis. Corbin writes that the *mundus imaginalis* can be useful and productive in linking intellect and sense impressions (Corbin 1983: 1). Or it can remain subservient to sense impressions and not serve the intellect. If this occurs, there is a resemblance to the analyst's remaining unaware of the implications of his or her countertransference; his or her bodily vision will not have a use.

The link between body and image is waiting to be further verbalized. In *A Midsummer Night's Dream,* Shakespeare wrote that 'imagination bodies forth the forms of things unknown' (Act 5, Scene 1). If countertransference communications are both images and bodily visions, then body and image shimmer together almost to the point of fusion. Here we may find quite another message in the word 'incarnate', that outgrowth of 'embodied'. When Plaut explained in 1970 what he had meant in 1956, he was worried that the religious association to 'incarnate' (spirit made flesh) had been troublesome. It seems to me, however, that his intuition was reliable. In the countertransference experience, the image is being made flesh. Where that means that the Other (the patient's psyche) is becoming personal (in the analyst's body), I would conclude that an analyst's countertransference may be further understood by regarding it as a religious or mystical experience.

Before this is dismissed as fanciful, parallels might be drawn between countertransference and a well-known list of the characteristics of the mystical experience (Happold 1963: 45–7). First, mystical states are ineffable; that is, they cannot be fully described to one who has not experienced something similar. Second, mystical states lead to knowledge and insight, often delivered with a tremendous sense of authority. Third, mystical states are transient. Fourth, mystical states *happen* to a person; even if he or she prepared him/herself, he or she is gripped by a power that feels quite foreign. Fifth, there is a sense that everything is connected to everything else, an intimation of purpose. Sixth, the mystical experience is timeless. Finally, the familiar ego is sensed not to be the real 'I' (see Powell 1985).

These points can be compared to the countertransferences described in this chapter. It is difficult to explain them to one who has not experienced them. The analyst does gain insights from them, often in a shattering way. Countertransference states are momentary. Even analytical training cannot fully anticipate or prepare for the countertransference experience. One does feel connected to one's patient, in an intimacy at once beautiful and unbearable. Countertransference reactions have no sense of history; past and present are jumbled. Finally, the analyst knows his or her ego is not responsible for what is happening to him or her.

Koss (1986) also suggested that states of possession entered into by spirit healers may be compared to typical countertransference experiences. Similarly, in Chassidic mysticism, reference is made to a quality known as *Hitlahabut,* or ecstasy. Buber held that this quality transforms ordinary knowledge into a knowledge of the meaning of life. For the Chassids, *Hitlahabut* expresses itself bodily, in dance. As Buber says, in dance 'the whole body becomes subservient to the ecstatic soul' (Buber 1931: 35). Analysis, too, is a form of dance, and ecstasy is not an inappropriate word to describe some of the emotions generated (and reported in the research project).

Corbin regards the *mundus imaginalis* as 'indispensable for placing the visions of prophets and mystics, this is because it is there that they "take place" and deprived of the imaginal world they no longer "take place"' (Corbin 1978: 4). Both reflective and embodied countertransference have their location in the *mundus imaginalis,* which is also the medium for their transmission. These connections between mysticism and analysis need not seem surprising. Psychology and religion cannot simply let go of each other. It is not enough to say that one explores depths and the other heights, that one is about soul and the other about spirit, one about dreams and the other about miracles, that one is concerned with immanence and the other with transcendence. It is not the case that this analytical mysticism is a mysticism of the one true God. Far from it. Analysis is a mysticism of persons – and hence polyvalent, pluralistic, many-headed, many-bodied.

The idea of a mysticism of (or between) persons is one by which contemporary theology is captivated (and this in addition to Buber's work). For example, a theologian writes: 'There is no point at all in blinking at the fact that the raptures of the theistic mystic are closely akin to the transports of sexual union' (Zaehner 1957: 151). The erotic dimension is introduced purposefully: transference, incest, sexuality form one spine of analysis. This is how D. H. Lawrence describes love-making in *Sons and Lovers:* 'His hands were like creatures, living; his limbs, his body, were all life and consciousness, subject to no will of his, but living in themselves.'

Throwing out an idea for a future discussion, and leaning heavily on Bion (1970), may not the analyst also function as a mystic for the wider group of society as a whole, or some analysts so function within their own milieux? That is why it is so important to keep avenues of communication open to psychoanalysts and the psychodynamic mainstream to make sure that analytical mysticism has a context and does not expend itself onanistically and nihilistically.

So I will return to that mainstream for a while. In the way I have been writing about it, the *mundus imaginalis* has similar properties to what Winnicott called 'the third area', sometimes 'the area of experience', sometimes 'the area of illusion' (Winnicott 1974). This area of the psyche lies in between external life and internal reality but both contribute to it. Of course, there are differences between Winnicott and Corbin. Corbin writes of a pre-existing intermediate dimension, Winnicott of the intermediate as a joint creation of both poles. Corbin's metaphor struck me more forcibly than Winnicott's as far as countertransference is concerned. But Winnicott evolved his ideas out of his study of what two people experience in a very special relationship. This means he had interpersonal activity in mind as well as his concern for the internal world. This helps flesh out my suggestion that we can speak of a two-person *mundus imaginalis* or of a mysticism of persons. What Winnicott writes of the third area repays attention:

> It is an area that is not challenged, because no claims are made on its behalf except that it shall exist as a resting place for the individual engaged in the perpetual human task of keeping inner and outer reality separate yet interrelated.
>
> (Winnicott 1974: 3)

I will try to anticipate a few objections to what has been proposed. These could be on the traditional ground that anything to do with the archetypal must consist of the products of the collective unconscious. Mother, the analyst's anger, walking into a lamp-post – what have these to do with the objective psyche? I do not anticipate such an objection from those who have worked more deeply on what is to be understood as archetypal. Hillman, for instance, writes that 'archetypal psychology cannot separate the personal and the collective unconscious, for within every complex, fantasy, and image of the personal psyche is an archetypal power' (Hillman 1975: 179–80). Here, and in numerous other passages, Hillman has reached the same place as those who, from the developmental perspective, regard the personal and the collective as indivisible. The distinction is that whereas Hillman searches for an archetypal perspective on the personal, writers such as Williams are committed to a personal perspective on the archetypal (Williams 1963).

A further possible objection would be that the *mundus imaginalis* is too precise an explanation for reflective and embodied countertransference. These, it would be argued, are merely manifestations of the self in its transpersonal guise or the result of our common heritage. I would agree that it is our joint and mutual connection to these factors that permits us even to discuss countertransference as communication. But this is insufficient as either description or explanation and may rest upon an idealization of the self.

However, perhaps the *mundus imaginalis* hypothesis refers to the alternate, archetypal perceptual system posited by the German countertransference researchers? Although it *could* be said that archetypal images have a power that enables them to be experienced as shared, I would prefer to say that images that turn out to be shared generate an archetypal power.

For another group of objectors, the concept of projective identification may be sufficient to explain the aspects of countertransference phenomena I have been discussing. However, projective identification, while undoubtedly playing a part in the formation of transference and countertransference, lacks something as an explanatory theory. In fact, as Meltzer points out, 'we are still in the process of discovering what projective identification "means"'. Meltzer's suggestion is that projective identification is an 'empty' concept, the result of an intuition of Klein's, and requiring clinical substantiation which, in the nature of things, will in fact be based on the use of the concept itself, for analysts cannot ignore it (Meltzer 1978: 38–9). The *mundus imaginalis* hypothesis can be used alongside the concept of projective identification by postulating on what projective identification is based, and then what it is that enables its operation to take place. Using words from other disciplines, the search is, respectively, for the 'rhizome' that nurtures projective identification and for the 'ether' that facilitates its transmission. Such factors would, by definition, be 'objective' (that is, collective or nonpersonal) and also require distinguishing from projective identification as a defence mechanism for an individual, even with an extension of its meaning to include normal, lifelong mental functioning.

By bringing in the images of the ether and a rhizome, I am trying to challenge the notion of empty space. We don't need to ask why projections travel, because they don't travel – the individuals concerned are already linked. It seems that the *mundus imaginalis* hypothesis fits in well with theories of personality development that postulate an initial togetherness, with *fantasies* of oneness. The baby in a state of being and the baby's objects are one (cf. Winnicott 1974: 80).

Meltzer speaks to this last point when, discussing Bion's work, he makes a fundamental distinction between, on the one hand, an analyst's response to his patient's productions via an examination of the structure of his own mind and, on the other, his scrutiny of its emotive and fantasy content (Meltzer 1978: 23). Meltzer goes on to pose a question that was a spur to the writing of the present chapter. When Klein first introduced the concept of projective identification, she did so in terms of *external* rather than internal objects. Later writers, such as Meltzer himself, applied the idea to internal objects. In the latter case, there is less difficulty in understanding how the process operates. For, in the internal world, psychic processes such as substitution and symbolization play the major part. But, Meltzer goes on:

> If [projective identification] operated with external objects, serious questions arose regarding the means by which it was brought about, the actual impact on other people, including the analyst, and the ultimate fate of split-off and projected parts of the personality.
>
> (Meltzer 1978: 23)

The *mundus imaginalis* hypothesis is an attempt to answer these questions. For it is a pre-existing environment for images that are produced relevantly and spontaneously. Images pertaining to one person crop up in the experience of another person because, on the imaginal level of reality, all images pertain to both.

The need to establish the phylogenetic background to projective identification was also explored by Gordon when she suggested that its role in the construction of countertransference reactions was based on the psychoid unconscious in which distinctions between psyche and soma do not apply. The relevance of projective identification is that its main occurrence is at a time in early development before soma and psyche have been truly differentiated (Gordon 1965: 129).

In the same way that a relationship requires a facilitating environment, a psychological process (such as projective identification) requires its own 'environment'; that can be expressed by the postulation of a certain realm or level of experience in the background. The *mundus imaginalis* meets the particular need because, by implication, it is to be regarded as a pre-existent, ready, as it were, to facilitate psychological processes. I have already mentioned this as the main difference between Corbin's and Winnicott's ideas. A similar point was made by Hamilton in relation to projective identification when she criticized the concept for its lack of reference to any pre-existing 'primary mutuality' between mother and child (Hamilton 1982: 60). The *mundus imaginalis* is an attempt to express the psychological basis of that mutuality at least as it appears in analysis.

Winnicott's contribution to the discussion is found in the distinction he makes between talking about 'mental mechanisms' and an 'experience of communication'. Winnicott's view is that an analyst cannot explore the latter without 'peddling in the intermediate area' (Winnicott 1963: 184). Davis and Wallbridge expand the point as follows:

> Although a two-way exchange can be explained in terms of projection and introjection, and though these terms can cover the source of our feeling for other people, and how we are able to identify with them, something is still left unsaid about the vehicle of inter-communication.
>
> (Davis and Wallbridge 1981: 124)

Similarly, the *mundus imaginalis* idea places less stress on movement and interaction, whether ——>, or <——, or <——>. It is an attempt to describe a 'vehicle' that encompasses the whole analytic field – interpersonal, interactive, intrapsychic and intersubjective.

A further contrast between the *mundus imaginalis* hypothesis and projective identification is to be found in their relation to the idea of psychic reality. Meltzer points out that one of Klein's main contributions to psychoanalysis was her stress on 'the concreteness of psychic reality (Meltzer 1978: 69). Jung's reference was to the necessity for his critics to recognize that 'a psychic process is something that really exists, and a psychic content is as real as a plant or an animal' (Jung 1955–56: para. 651). A problem with projective identification, however, is that it is usually described in terms of fantasy, which is the exact opposite of what is required. Several attempts have been made to remedy this. For example, Gordon suggested that identification is the psychic equivalent of ingestion, projection of excretion, and projective identification of fusion fantasies at the breast or adult coitus (Gordon 1965: 129). The fact that such an attempt is undertaken at all, coupled with Meltzer's observation, led me to consider the *mundus imaginalis* as a place where the concrete and the imagistic are intermingled; 'subtle body' being the best term to describe this.

There is little doubt that projective identification forms a part of empathy (the putting of oneself in the shoes of another). But a logical problem arises when an attempt is made to apply the projective identification/empathy link to countertransference. For the analyst is making use of the patient's projective identification to fashion his or her own empathic response. It is not usually a case of the patient using his or her transference projection to empathize with the analyst. What may be seen in analysis is the conversion of the *patient's projection* into the *analyst's empathy.* The problem can be stated another way: projective identification refers to the blurring of boundaries to the point of fantasies of fusion. At the same time, as Gordon points out, projective identification also involves the clarification or disentanglement of an internal muddle by the engagement of an external object (Gordon 1965: 143). The apparent contradiction may be resolved by postulating an area in the psyche wherein 'blurring' leads to 'disentanglement'.

Projective identifications are composed of images or imagos (cf. Racker 1968: 57, 73, 96, 119–120). This sense of the centrality of image is reinforced by Jung's definition of it. We are not dealing with parts of the personality but with a 'condensed expression of the psychic situation as a whole' (Jung 1921: para. 745). Jung goes on to discuss images in terms strikingly similar to those used by Corbin in relation to the *mundus imaginalis*: as mediators between undifferentiated emotion and more developed ideas (Jung 1921: para. 749).

Recent developments in this field

Since first communicating these ideas in 1983, I have become aware of others working along similar lines. For instance, Goodheart writes of 'the marriage of *imaginatio* and interaction', the former term referring to the portrayal of inner facts in the form of images and the latter to the protection of this development within the analytical relationship (Goodheart 1984: 101). Similarly, Schwartz-Salant writes of a 'mutually and imaginally experienced *coniunctio*' underpinning 'a Self structure between two people'. The attempt is to capture 'experiences that happen in a realm that is felt to be outside normal time sense and in a space felt to have substance. This space, long known as the subtle body, exists because of imagination, yet it also has autonomy' (Schwartz-Salant 1984: 10–11).

Schwartz-Salant has also proposed that we conceive of a series of unconscious couples that are always present in analysis: within each participant and as a counterpart to the analysing pair. Becoming aware of the interaction within and between these unconscious couples calls for a form of 'imaginal sight' on the part of the analyst (Schwartz-Salant 1986). Although I am in agreement with the main tenor of his thought, on these two points I am not in agreement. Schwartz-Salant suggests that the analyst be active in a quest for imaginal sight (1986: 33–4) whereas, in my approach, the analyst does nothing but wait for the countertransference experience to happen. I am not sure that the conceptualization (or image) of the unconscious couple is helpful for I would prefer to envision such phenomena as a normal part of either couple or individual functioning. The realms or levels of experience through which the couple(s) move are indeed radically different (and one of them is the imaginal realm), but the couple is still just a couple. By introducing a plethora of couples, there is a risk that what couples do could become idealized to the point that only material connected to the *coniunctio oppositorum* will be adequately analysed.

The interpersonal and the intrapsychic: On persons and images

In this chapter I set out to act as matchmaker for two world views, one empirical and the other poetic, one in which countertransference becomes the root of the analyst's technique of interpretation and one in which such a clinical confine is anathema. Fordham's technique with Hillman's vision? Let me conclude by saying that the offspring of this particular marriage confronts us with a fascinating problem: do we gain anything from our habitual division between the interpersonal (that is, relationship) and the intrapsychic (that is, image)? What the project showed is that the interaction of patient and analyst and their relationship can be placed firmly *within* the imaginal realm without forgetting that there are two people present. An analyst can think, feel or behave as if he or she were the patient, and also he or she can function as a part of the patient's psyche so that the *mundus imaginalis* becomes a shared dimension of experience. When we consider or reconsider our attitude to the division between the interpersonal and the intrapsychic, there is no need to fear an abandonment of the human element. In fact, I would suggest that, in the same way that our notion of the intrapsychic, internal world includes the part played by relations with other persons, our definition of what is interpersonal may also be enriched and expanded. Then internal imagery becomes seen as linking two people, the patient and analyst, and as fostering their relationship. It follows that to divorce work on the apparently imaginal and work on the apparently interpersonal is conceptually in error and practically limiting.

For it is no longer a question of opposing an examination of interpersonal communication to an examination of the imaginal world. If the idea of a two-person *mundus imaginalis* is taken seriously, then we must regard the interpersonal in terms of psyche speaking, and the imaginal in terms of an avenue of communication between two people, a relationship. Persons may carry imagery; imagery may originate in persons. It is necessary to see our field of reference in analysis as seamless and continuous so that ostensible 'images' and ostensible 'interpersonal communications' do not get separated, nor one gain ascendancy over the other on the basis of a preconceived hierarchy of importance. The coin is three-sided: to body and image can be added relationship.

This overlay between an interpersonal relationship and the intrapsychic image is addressed by Jung when he writes of alchemy, particularly in *The Psychology of the Transference* (1946). Looking at the woodcuts of *the Rosarium* (in the next chapter [of *The Plural Psyche*]), one finds it quite impossible to say with conviction that this is solely about a two-person process. Equally, what is being depicted is not just one person's individuation. The focus of enquiry includes both – the seamless field of reference mentioned just now. This led Jung to say in a letter that 'the living mystery of life is *always* hidden between Two' (Jaffé 1979). Or, put another way, the soul (says Jung) 'is the very essence of relationship' (Jung 1946: para. 504).

Note

These were the questions I asked the participants in the research project:

1 Age of client.
2 Your age.
3 Marital status of client.
4 Your marital status.
5 Presenting problem(s).

6 Brief history of client.
7 Countertransference experience in detail.
8 Is this reflective or embodied?
9 How did this affect the future of the work?
10 How did this affect your understanding of the history?
11 Can you say how the client may have provoked or evoked these feelings in you? What did they say or do?
12 Any other comments?

References

Armstrong, D. (1962) *Bodily Sensations*. London: Routledge and Kegan Paul.
Bion, W. (1970) *Attention and Interpretation*. In *Seven Servants*. New York: Jason Aaronson, 1977.
Buber, M. (1931) *Jewish Mysticism*. London: Dent.
Casement, P. (1986a) 'Countertransference and interpretation'. *Contemporary Psychoanalysis, 22*: 4.
Casement, P. (1986b) 'Interpretation: Fresh insight or cliché?' *Free Associations, 5*.
Corbin, H. (1972) '*Mundus Imaginalis*, or the imaginary and the imaginal'. *Spring*, 1972.
Corbin, H. (1978) Preface to D. Miller, *The New Polytheism*. Dallas, TX: Spring Publications.
Corbin, H. (1983) 'Theophanies and mirrors: Idols or icons?' *Spring*, 1983.
Davis, M. & Wallbridge, D. (1981) *Boundary and Space: An Introduction to the Work of D. W. Winnicott*. London: Karnac.
Dieckmann, H. (1974) 'The constellation of the countertransference'. In G. Adler (ed.) *Success and Failure in Analysis*. New York: Putnam's Sons.
Fordham, M. (1957) *New Developments in Analytical Psychology*. London: Routledge and Kegan Paul.
Fordham, M. (1970) 'A reply to Plaut's "Comment"'. In M. Fordham, J. Hubback, R. Gordon and K. Lambert (eds.), *Technique in Jungian Analysis*. London: Heinemann, 1974.
Fordham, M. (1979) 'Analytical psychology and countertransference'. In L. Epstein and A. Finer (eds.), *Countertransference*. New York: Jason Aronson.
Freud, S. (1910) 'The future prospects of psycho-analytic therapy'. Std Edn 7.
Freud, S. (1913) 'The disposition to obsessional neurosis'. Std Edn 12.
Goodheart, W. (1984) 'Successful and unsuccessful interventions in Jungian analysis: The construction and destruction of the spellbinding circle. *Chiron*, 1984.
Gordon, R. (1965) 'The concept of projective identification: An evaluation'. *Journal of Analytical Psychology, 10*: 2.
Gorkin, M. (1987) *The Uses of Countertransference*. Northvale, NJ and London: Jason Aronson.
Guggenbuhl-Craig, A. (1971) *Power in the Helping Professions*. New York: Spring Publications.
Hamilton, V. (1982) Narcissus and Oedipus: The Children of Psychoanalysis. London: Routledge and Kegan Paul.
Happold, F. (1963) *Mysticism: A Study and an Anthology*. Harmondsworth: Penguin.
Heimann, P. (1950) 'On countertransference'. *International Journal of Psycho-Analysis, 31*.
Hillman, J. (1975) *Loose Ends*. Dallas, TX: Spring Publications.
Hillman, J. (1980) 'On the necessity of abnormal psychology: Ananke and Athene'. In J. Hillman (ed.), *Facing the Gods*. Dallas, TX: Spring Publications.
Jaffé, A. (1979) *C. G. Jung: Word and Image*. Princeton: Princeton University Press.
Jung, C. G. (1921) *Psychological Types*. *CW* 6.
Jung, C. G. (1930) 'Psychology and literature'. *CW* 15.
Jung, C. G. (1946) *The Psychology of the Transference*. *CW* 16.
Jung, C. G. (1955–56) *Mysterium Coniunctionis*. *CW* 14.
Jung, C. G. (1963) *Memories, Dreams, Reflections*. London: Collins; Routledge and Kegan Paul.

Kohut, H. (1982) 'Introspection, empathy and the semi-circle of mental health'. *International Journal of Psycho-Analysis, 63*: 4.

Koss, J. (1986) 'Symbolic transformations in traditional healing: Perspectives from analytical psychology'. *Journal of Analytical Psychology, 31*: 4.

Kris, E. (1952) *Explorations in Art.* New York: International Universities Press.

Kugler, P. (1982) *The Alchemy of Discourse: An Archetypal Approach to Language.* Lewisburg, PA: Bucknell University Press.

Langs, R. (1978) *The Listening Process.* New York: Jason Aronson.

Langs, R. (1979) 'The interactional dimensions of countertransference'. In L. Epstein and A. Feiner (eds.), *Countertransference.* New York: Jason Aronson.

Little, M. (1957) '"R" – the analyst's total response to his patient's needs'. *International Journal of Psycho-Analysis, 38.*

Mattinson, J. (1975) *The Reflection Process in Casework Supervision.* London: Institute of Marital Studies.

Money-Kyrle, R. (1971) 'The aims of psychoanalysis'. In D. Meltzer (ed.), *Collected Papers.* Strathtay, Perthshire: Clunie Press, 1978.

Meier, C. A. (1949) *Ancient Incubation and Modern Psychotherapy.* Evanston, IL: Northwestern University Press, 1967.

Meltzer, D. (1978) *The Clinical Significance of the Work of Bion.* Part 3 of *The Kleinian Development.* Strathtay, Perthshire: Clunie Press.

Newton, K. (1965) 'Mediation of the image of infant–mother togetherness'. In M. Fordham *et al* (eds) *Analytical Psychology: A Modern Science.* London: Heinemann.

Plaut, A. (1956) 'The transference in analytical psychology'. In M. Fordham, J. Hubback, R. Gordon and K. Lambert (eds.), *Technique in Jungian Analysis.* London: Heinemann, 1974.

Plaut, A. (1970) 'On not incarnating the archetype'. In M. Fordham, J. Hubback, R. Gordon and K. Lambert (eds.), *Technique in Jungian Analysis.* London: Heinemann, 1974.

Popper, K. (1959) *The Logic of Scientific Discovery.* London: Hutchinson.

Popper, K. (1963) *The Logic of Scientific Discovery.* London: Hutchison.

Powell, S. (1985) 'A bridge to understanding: The transcendent function in the analyst'. *Journal of Analytical Psychology, 30*: 1.

Racker, H. (1968) *Transference and Countertransference.* London: Hogarth.

Samuels, A. (1985) *Jung and the Post-Jungians.* London & Boston, MA: Routledge and Kegan Paul.

Schwartz-Salant, N. (1984) 'Archetypal factors underlying sexual acting-out in the transference/countertransference process'. *Chiron*, 1984.

Schwartz-Salant, N. (1986) 'On the subtle-body concept in clinical practice'. *Chiron*, 1986.

Searles, H. (1959) 'Oedipal love in the countertransference'. In *Collected Papers on Schizophrenia and Related Subjects.* London: Hogarth, 1968.

Stein, R. (1987) *Incest and Human Love.* Baltimore, MD: Penguin.

Sterba, R. (1934) 'The fate of the ego in psychoanalytic therapy'. *International Journal of Psycho-Analysis, 15.*

Williams, M. (1963) 'The indivisibility of the personal and collective unconscious'. In M. Fordham (ed.), *Analytical Psychology: A Modern Science.* London: Heinemann, 1973.

Winnicott, D. W (1949) 'Hate in the countertransference'. In *Collected Papers: From Paediatrics to Psychoanalysis.* London: Tavistock, 1958.

Winnicott, D. W. (1963) 'Communicating and not communicating leading to a study of certain opposites'. In *The Maturational Processes and the Facilitating Environment.* London: Hogarth, 1965.

Winnicott, D. W. (1974) *Playing and Reality.* Harmondsworth: Penguin.

Zaehner, R. (1957) *Mysticism: Sacred and Profane.* Oxford: Oxford University Press.

CHAPTER 9

THE IMAGE OF THE PARENTS IN BED: FROM PRIMAL SCENE TO PLURALISM

Retrospective introduction

I felt that post-Jungian work on the primal scene was lacking and the field had been left to the post-Kleinians such as Meltzer. This chapter, from 1989's *The Plural Psyche*, was intended to highlight the role of the parental couple in personal development and also in clinical understandings. It is, in addition, a reworking of Jung's coniunctio idea.

I saw the parents both as fleshy, real creatures and also as metaphors for psychic bits that could take up almost any combination.

The reader will see that my interest in Hermes remains unabated in connection with the parents! In particular, I was looking to create a non-normative, non-judgemental, non-pathologizing text about grotesque sexual fantasy (and, I suppose, behaviour). Then I wanted to link this to a 'higher discourse of divinity or at least fecundity and probity'. This approach to heteronormativity and onslaught on hypocrisy continues to be a concern of mine in my writings about sexuality and new, transgressive relational styles (see my 2009 'Carnal Critiques: Promiscuity, Politics, Imagination, Spirituality and Hypocrisy'. *Psychotherapy and Politics International, 7*: 1).

Images and experiences of parental intercourse and the parental marriage hover between and connect inner and outer, personal and archetypal, destructive and creative. Images are the operant element in fantasy; it is they who permit talk of subjective reality. Because the primal scene has to do with origins and the mystery of a beginning it exerts a fascination; because it has to do with outcome and a tangible result it has a compulsive attraction. We know this from our own analyses, from our work with patients and from the history of the early days of the psychoanalytic movement.

Why 'in bed'? Concepts (such as the primal scene) need and create contexts, thereby becoming images. Jung points out that 'the term "image" is intended to express not only the form of the activity taking place, but the typical situation in which the activity is released' (Jung 1954: para. 152). The image of the parents in bed is, quite literally, a matter of chicken and egg. The individual is created out of primal scene activity but the scene, *qua* scene, does not itself exist except as part of a combining of endowment with experience. As a colleague has said, it is hard to get the image of the parents in bed together. It is a creation and a symbol for life as it develops. Bringing things together is a précis of creativity.

The question of the role of parental images in the development of personality is an interesting one. Issues such as the balance between reality and fantasy in the formation of internal imagery, the degree of importance of sexuality, and the purposive uses to which inner conceptions and preconceptions may be put are as relevant now as they ever were. In this chapter I am concerned with imagery developing over a period of time, changing or not changing as the case may be. Imagery is seen as deriving from the synthesis of fantasy and fact, subjective with objective elements.

In this chapter I argue that imagery around the parents in bed can be seen as a conjunction of the divine and the grotesque. Not only are these linked, but what is divine is sometimes primitive and what is grotesque is sometimes sublime. In any event, there is a connection which, it is argued, is central to developing self-image, gender identity and personal relationships.

The conjunction of the grotesque and the divine suggests the presence of a god, and the god who fits the bill, who most aptly could be described as a grotesque divine, is Hermes. Hermes' positive, transforming, connecting aspect is considered together with his tricksterism, his dishonesty, and his sexual perversity and obscenity. Two strands of argument emerge from this. First, that the function of apparently criminal or immoral impulses and behaviour needs reviewing as a developmental factor. The second strand is that Hermes' pluralistic encapsulation of adaptability and flexibility signifies something central for the resolution of neurotic conflicts generated by the primal scene. Jung says that 'Mercurius consists of all conceivable opposites . . . is a unity in spite of the fact that his innumerable inner contradictions can dramatically fly apart into an equal number of disparate and apparently independent figures' (Jung 1967: para. 284). Hermes is 'many-sided' (ibid.: para. 267) and has 'a limitless number of names' (ibid.: para. 284). My interest in adaptability began first in relation to its opposite – uroboric omnipotence in which, for example, precise inner preconceptions as to the ideal partner controlled heterosexual activity (Samuels 1980).

The adaptation that is focused on is that which must occur between the world of two-person relationships and that of three-person relationships. As Jung puts it, Mercurius is 'called husband and wife, bridegroom and bride, or lover and beloved' (ibid.: para. 268). His hermaphroditism suggests not only early sexualized confusion, but also the possibility of psychic resolution. Jung connects Mercurius with the Trinity in particular and 'triune divinity in general' (ibid.: para. 271) and, while this chapter does not explore this, it can be said that threeness and triangles are of the essence of the Oedipus complex and, of course, the image of the parents in bed. Hermes is three-headed, but he is also a unity and therefore contains seeds of acceptance of the plurality of family and the emergence and integration of differentiated parental images.

The move from twoness to threeness takes place, on the one hand, in the outer world as the baby 'discovers' his father in reality and experiences differences from the mother. On the other hand, however, in the inner world of imagery, a move is also taking place in which images of twoness evolve into images of threeness as the father separates from the internal family matrix. There are two primary images of twoness – mother and baby, and then the baby's image of his parents – and in this chapter I attempt to describe the interactive processes between these images of twoness as the individual moves towards three-person operating. Similarities and differences in the style and tone of mother–infant imagery and parents-in-bed imagery are examined and it is hypothesized that a specific psychic activity is taking place in which these images of twoness create a climate in which images of threeness can exist and the paternal image emerge.

The antiquities of human development

Jung and Freud's argument over how literally to take analytical material concerning parental intercourse revolved around the question of whether an adult could produce what looked like actual memories but what were in fact subsequent fantasies. Jung's *ex post facto* explanations stimulated Freud to ask where the later fantasies came from. Freud's insistence that the fantasies must come from *somewhere* led him into man's prehistory. For example, in the *Introductory Lectures on Psychoanalysis* he writes:

> There can be no doubt that the sources [of primal scene phantasies] lie in the instincts; but it still has to be explained why the same phantasies with the same content are created on every occasion. I am prepared with an answer that I know will seem daring to you. I believe that these primal phantasies, and no doubt a few others as well, are a phylogenetic endowment. In them the individual reaches beyond his own experience into primeval experience at points where his own experience has been too rudimentary . . . I have repeatedly been led to suggest that the psychology of the neuroses may have more stored up in it of the antiquities of human development than any other source.
>
> (Freud 1916–17: 370–1)

Freud suggests the existence of pre-subjective schemata that might even be strong enough to predominate over the experience of the individual: 'Wherever experiences fail to fit in with the hereditary schema they become remodelled in the imagination' (Freud 1918: 119).

We may not agree with Freud's Lamarckian overtones – the suggestion that primal fantasies are a residue of specific memories of prehistoric experiences – but there is less problem with the position that, in general terms, mental structures have a phylogenetic base. In *The Language of Psychoanalysis,* Laplanche and Pontalis point out that all the so-called primal fantasies relate to the origins and that 'like collective myths they claim to provide a representation of and a "solution" to whatever constitutes an enigma for the child' (Laplanche and Pontalis 1980: 332). In many respects these views correspond to Jung's theory of archetypes (see Samuels 1985: 42–4).

In 'From the history of an infantile neurosis' (1918) Freud observed that, for the Wolf Man, the main determinants of the primal scene were that it constituted paternal aggression, that therefore the parental marriage was sadomasochistic, that by identifying with either partner in turn the child derived sadomasochistic sexual pleasure causing guilt and anxiety, and that the child fantasized what happened in intercourse as involving anal penetration with attendant imagery of dirt, mess and power struggle. A key problem for the Wolf Man was caused by his feminine side. He conceived of the sexual opposites in terms of active and passive rather than male and female (Freud 1918: 46). In Jungian terms, the Wolf Man's archetypal images remain unmediated by experiences in the outer world. Summarizing Freud's findings, we can say that the child both projects inner contents and misunderstands on a cognitive level what is happening – his experience is too 'rudimentary'.

The 'parents' are not the parents at all

As many readers will know, Jung disputed the solely sexual significance of incest fantasies, stressing, in addition, the role of incestuous sexuality in psychic growth. What does the image of the copulating parents represent? Remember, 'in reality the whole drama takes place in the individual's own psyche, where the "parents" are not the parents at all but only their images' (Jung 1952: para. 507). The image of the parents in bed is a metaphor for a *coniunctio oppositorum*. Though this Latin tag can be understood literally as a coming together of *opposites*, a more satisfactory reading would refer us to an *integration* of all manner of psychological phenomena and characteristics, many of which appear to us as so unlikely to belong together as to be 'opposites'. That is, the opposites *seem* to be opposites and therefore the emotional task feels like one of bringing them together. But there is no need to postulate a psyche entirely characterized by oppositional organization.

Thus the question of the image of the parents in bed as a coming together of opposites can be worked on in more detail, according to the degree and quality of differentiation a person makes between the images of mother and father. For a *coniunctio oppositorum* only becomes fertile when the elements are distinguishable. In plain language, it's not a *stuck* image of parental togetherness that we see in a fertile primal scene, but something divided and unstuck, hence vital – but also linked, hence imaginable. Image holds the linked division in momentary balance.

Differentiation of the parents facilitates looking beyond or through the real parents to membership of the human race and to issues of ontology, purpose and meaning. 'Mankind has always instinctively added the pre-existent divine pair to the personal parents – the "god" father and "god" mother of the newborn child – so that from sheer unconsciousness or short-sighted rationalism, he should never forget himself so far as to invest his own parents with divinity' (Jung 1954: para. 172). Differentiation within the image of the parents in bed connects directly with the numinous and with ideas regarding the purpose of life. This seems appropriate, for the primal scene is about genesis and you cannot split alpha from omega. Differentiation implies plurality and conflict; granted sufficient ego-strength, this can lead to conjunction.

However, just as 'the opposites' need to be understood nonliterally, so, too, does the notion of conjunction. One need not think of an annihilation of the initial separate entities, rather of a tripartite possibility: each of the two initial separate entities *and* whatever is implicated in their conjunction – a pluralistic formulation: unity and diversity.

The images of the two parents form the most appropriate raw material for what Jung termed the syzygy – meaning a pair of linked opposites but most often referring to masculine and feminine images (or a pairing of animus and anima). If the psyche 'wanted' to express its multifarious and variegated nature and the possibility of an integration of its plurality, then images of the parents in bed perform this job perfectly. Not because the parents are literally 'opposites'; not because all they do is 'conjoin'; but because they want to be together, have been together, in the individual's mind are still together – and want to be apart, have been apart, and are still apart.

The problem of differentiation remains – indeed, we have to differentiate different kinds of differentiation. For example, a patient referred to her parents' marriage as a 'great big circular jigsaw fuck-up'. She was referring to her incomprehension, her envy, and her feeling of exclusion. The word 'jigsaw' contains the seed of a puzzling experience of differentiation – but, for the moment, only an intellectual solution.

My view is that *personal experiences of primal scene imagery and their working through determine, to a considerable extent, a person's capacity to sustain conflict constructively.* This general point becomes more pertinent when applied to the field of depth psychology. Stuck parental imagery implies intolerance, fantasies of superiority and difficulties with hearing the views of others. Primal scene imagery in vigorous motion suggests other possibilities – pluralistic possibilities – and other, variegated archetypal states of mind.

Merger and differentiation

Neumann (1954) took up the point about discrimination and worked on the differentiation of an early, merged parental imago. My idea is that a process of separating an image of each parent out of an image in which they are merged goes on at the same time as (i.e. is synchronous with) attachment and separation processes with regard to the mother. The distinction between separation *of* the parents and separation *from* mother is not primarily a chronological one.

It can be argued that the image of merged parents arises from a relatively undifferentiated state of mother–infant relations. As Newton points out, there is a problem here of point of view, both with regard to mother–infant and parent-in-bed imagery, because the lack of twoness in both images is what is experienced psychically even if we, the observers, can see that twoness is 'objectively' the case (Newton 1981: 73). If the merged parental image persists beyond an age-appropriate point then it becomes psychopathological and hence an example of the 'stuckness' that is not, and cannot be, a true *coniunctio.* The transition on which we are focusing is from images of mergedness and stuckness towards images of true union of separate entities with attendant conflict.

For the 'unsticking' to take place, Neumann ascribed to the infant affect and behaviour of a vigorous, instinctual and hence guilt-inducing kind:

> This destruction [of the merged parents] is closely associated with the act of eating and assimilation . . . The formation of consciousness goes hand in hand with a fragmentation of the world continuum into separate objects, parts, figures, which can only then be assimilated, taken in, integrated, made conscious . . . in a word, eaten . . . Aggression, destruction, dismemberment and killing are intimately associated with the corresponding bodily functions of eating, chewing, biting and particularly with the symbolism of the teeth as instruments of these activities, all of which are essential for the formation of an independent ego.
>
> (Neumann 1954: 124)

Neumann is arguing that the act of biting and its accompanying fantasies constitute an attempt to differentiate the stuck parental image, to comprehend imaginatively a primal scene in which two distinct parents may have intercourse. 'Not only do . . . male and female grow out of this development of opposites . . . but opposites like "sacred" and "profane", "good" and "evil" are now assigned their place in the world' (Neumann 1954: 109).

Neumann goes on to make an interesting point. He refers to the image of the merged parents as a 'primal deity' in the inner life of the child. It follows that the differentiation of the merged parents into the opposites of mother and father clears the way for the emergence of a type of polytheism – 'God is now experienced and revealed under as many aspects as there are Gods. This means that the ego's powers of expression and understanding have increased enormously' (Neumann 1954: 325). I would add that one facet of this increase in range is the capacity to tolerate the presence of the father. Polytheism is a way of describing the move from paranoid-schizoid mechanisms of control towards variegated two-person exchange and the depressive position. It also stands for the positive aspects of polymorphousness, namely fertility and creative potency. Polytheism rejects idealized fantasies of unitary fusion states (monotheism, if you like). But pluralism, as an expression of psychic vitality, embraces both polytheism and monotheism. Its capacity to do this is a primal-scene capacity: parents joined (monotheism) and parents apart but related (polytheism) and a linkage of parents-joined and parents-apart (pluralism).

Projection, introjection and the image of the parents in bed

Klein approached the problem from a different direction. She stated that the infant conceives of his parents in an almost continuous state of intercourse and is thus able to project any bodily impulse whatsoever on to the image of the parental couple (or, to be more precise, the image of the parents coupling). As Segal says, 'The infant will phantasy his parents as exchanging gratifications, oral, urethral, anal or genital, according to the prevalence of his own impulses . . . This gives rise to feelings of the most acute deprivation, jealousy and envy, since the parents are perceived as giving each other precisely those gratifications which the infant wishes for himself' (Segal 1973: 103). The infant then internalizes this heavily coloured image of parental intercourse and the image is now ready for reprojecting, for example, when the individual contemplates a marriage of his own.

One interesting overlap between Klein and Jung and involving the figure of Hermes might be mentioned. Jung shows that Mercurius represents 'continuous cohabitation' and comments on the numerous obscene representations of the *coniunctio*. He adds to this 'pictures in old manuscripts of excretory acts including vomiting' (Jung 1967: para. 278).

It is noticeable that Klein's source of positive connotation within the infant concerning the parents in bed is confined to projections of the infant's own real or fantasized gratifications and wishes, leading to envy of the parents in coitus (Klein 1929: 111). Jung's stress on the images of the parents in bed symbolizing an innate potential for integration and individuation is foreign to Klein's theory. She argues that

> the Oedipus conflict begins under the complete dominance of sadism . . . the attack launched [upon the objects] with all the weapons of sadism rouses the subject's dread of an analogous attack upon himself from the external and the internalized objects . . . a special intensity is imparted by the fact that a union of the two parents is in question . . . these united parents are extremely cruel and much dreaded assailants.
>
> (Klein 1929: 212–13)

Earlier she noted with regard to case material that 'aggressive motor discharges' are provoked by the primal scene (Klein 1929: 122). Riviere demonstrated the extremity of the position in her remark that a patient's unconscious feeling that he has good parents inside him means that the parents are 'idealized . . . and he is filled with a sense of omnipotence, perfection, grandeur and so on' (Riviere 1952: 21). In essence, Klein is taking what is happening at the breast or anus and, as it were, 'applying' it to the primal scene. There is therefore some interplay between feeding fantasies and primal scene fantasies. One might speculate about the extent to which the interplay in the adult psyche is *two-way.* We can ask: What is the influence of primal scene fantasies on feeding fantasies?

For instance, a patient is deeply involved in the animal welfare movement. While making love, she fantasizes that she is a cow being experimented on by scientists, being cut open and so on. She also fantasizes that within her vagina are teeth-like syringes that emit fluids that 'neutralize' her husband's sperm. Her oral aggression is projected into her primal scene imagery, but she also reports her father as supercilious and sadistic towards a less well-educated mother. The two sets of imagery influence each other and follow a similar pattern in their movement from states of identity and subjective merging to the formation of positive and negative attachments involving some differentiation and finally to full differentiation and creative or destructive intercourse.

There is a sense in which it is only after the recognition of the primal scene as involving two people, and the emergence of the father, that a full two-person relationship between mother and infant may be said to be constellated. When the infant becomes aware of the existence of a third person, he or she is forced to give up any identification with the mother, or fantasies of being fused with her. We find that chronology is not always the most satisfactory perspective from which to view psychic events; threeness may precede twoness, psychologically speaking.

Emergence of the father image

At this point it might be useful to consider the emergence and development of the infant's image of his or her father and his or her relationship to him. There would seem to be three strands in this. First, the infant experiences his or her real father as different from the mother – for example, by discovering a different sort of chest, or smell, or voice. Second, the image of the father has always been there for the infant as potentiality requiring fleshing out through experience. Finally, there is a sense in which the image of the father can be looked at as constructed or synthesized out of the interaction of images of mother and infant with images of the parents in bed. The image of the father and the infant's relation to him is predicated in part on their common relation to the mother. This last factor is of great significance.

What we can see is image creating image, the transitivity of imagery. The separation of the infant out of an intense feeding dyad and his or her differentiation of his or her parents are interactive processes. In the case of the mother–infant relationship the sequence is togetherness-separation-rapprochement. The infant experiences and develops an image of a relationship *he or she is in.* In the case of the image of the parents the sequence for the infant is stuckness-differentiation-conjunction; the infant is confronted by a relationship and an image of a relationship *he or she is not in.* The image of mother and infant and the image of the parents are themselves linked. Their transitive interaction and mutual mediation lead to the image of the father.

Parthenogenetic delusion

Money-Kyrle's remarks concerning parental intercourse in his paper 'The aims of psychoanalysis' are helpful in bringing out the subtle interweave between the developing relationship of mother and infant and the infant's perception and experience of the parental marriage. He says, 'All you can do is to allow your internal parents to come together and they will beget and conceive the child' and 'remember that, in the inner world, parthenogenetic creativity is a megalomanic delusion' (Money-Kyrle 1971: 103). Money-Kyrle's bringing in of parthenogenesis is significant for two reasons. First, because accepting that one has been created is the foundation of a religious attitude and second, because a teleological factor is implied in parental intercourse from the point of view of the child. Differentiating the parents gives the individual a chance to create something. But, as the following example shows, this does not always happen.

A successful entrepreneur felt his parents always closed ranks against him in family arguments. He could not see their togetherness as anything other than a ploy used against him, a fake trick. His image was of the parents arm-in-arm like an overposed early photograph – static and unreal. A feeling of togetherness with a woman was beyond him because it felt like the nothingness he fantasized in his parents' marriage. Mutuality had to be eliminated and was replaced by hypercriticism of his partner and competitiveness.

The grotesque and the divine

To conclude this section of the chapter I want to note Redfearn's comment that experiences of the primal scene antedate the emergence of the human self-image. Thus, one gets 'bizarre and monstrous forms on the one hand or god-like forms on the other' (Redfearn 1978: 235). I think that the bizarre and the monstrous, and the divine and the sublime, may be involved in another important *coniunctio oppositorum*. The linking of grotesque and divine would then take its place alongside the linked human and divine parents of Jung's theory. As we shall see, grotesque, divine and human dance a figure round the image of the parents in bed.

Recapitulation

I should like to recapitulate the themes that I shall develop further. From Freud, the need to look at man's prehistory and also to learn how grotesque fantasy about sexuality fills the gaps in rudimentary knowledge. From Jung, valuing of the image of parental intercourse as containing seeds of psychic integration for the individual and also the paramount need for conscious discrimination. Neumann, taking the problem of differentiation further, allocating to the baby's bite the function of separating the merged parental image and also pointing out the increase in experiential variety and flexibility that follows the emergence of masculine and feminine – polytheism. Klein, showing how mother–infant fantasy and primal scene fantasy interact. Money-Kyrle, stating how vital it is to allow the parents their creativity and warning against parthenogenetic inflation. Finally, Redfearn, underlining the enormous range of imagery involved in the primal scene from the most sublime to the most horrendous.

In many people there is a movement between an undifferentiated image of the parents and an image of union involving conflict as well as harmony. Psychopathologically there are two main possibilities: either a failure of the image of merged parents to differentiate or the creation of extreme images representing only one of the opposites. Each of these would lead to a negative and destructive archetypal state of mind.

It might be useful to list some of the conjunctions:

conjunction of human and divine;
conjunction of masculine and feminine;
conjunction of grotesque and divine;

and some of the undifferentiated images:

image of the parents in bed 'stuck' together;
image of the parents in bed fused with mother–infant imagery;

and some of the extremities:

grotesque sexual fantasy (Wolf Man);
idealization – confusion with divine parents.

In the next section of the chapter I go more deeply into some of the connecting factors between these ideas.

Hermes and his family

As I have been trying to demonstrate, thoughts about and reactions to the image of the parents in bed tend to polarize around the divine and the grotesque ends of a spectrum. Freud, Klein, Neumann and others, while not regarding the process as unhealthy, tend to see and to stress images of a violent, perverted, animal kind. Jung and Money-Kyrle, on the other hand, tend to see harmony and conjunction first and then the darker side. It occurs to me that this swinging, which is apparent in the theoreticians when perceived as a group, may tell us something about the way in which a child (and later the child in the adult) develops and experiences primal scene imagery. Psychological theory reflects psyche itself.

The individual needs some sort of thematic organizer around the polarities of grotesque and divine – which is where Hermes comes in. The god is used as a way of describing the ego's attempts to come to terms with what is involved in the primal scene. I am saying that it is all very well for Money-Kyrle to identify a 'direct line' connecting 'favourable development', 'the first good object', the recognition of parental coitus as a 'supremely creative act', and a good subsequent sexual and marital relationship (Money-Kyrle 1971: 105). This is a healthy sounding description of a healthy process and of course Money-Kyrle in no way avoids issues of psychopathology; but his unfolding seems more redolent of a hierarchy of (ideal) goals than of journey or process. Although what I detect in the figure of Hermes may ultimately move towards such goals, there is much twisting and turning through which the individual must live. Hermes' multi-faceted nature permits him to link what sometimes seems unlinkable even to the theorist – and how much more difficult to bring together for the infant. My contention is that although the hermetic strand in the working through of primal-scene emotions may appear to leave us stranded on the darker side of things, in reality this is not the case.

Meltzer, writing of metapsychology, states that 'every person has to have what you might describe as a religion in which his internal objects perform the functions of gods' (Meltzer 1981: 179). He argues that this religion derives its power not from belief, but because these gods do actually perform functions in the mind. Meltzer stresses the godlike functions of internal objects such as parental figures, but does not rule out the idea that part-selves ('the child parts of the personality') with archetypal potentials have a similar divine role. Hermes would then stand as a representation of a part-self.

In the literature, Hermes is seen as an agent and as a principle of transformation and connection; he is also a psychopomp or soul guide. As such he is much involved with change and development. Called Mercurius (quicksilver) he is elusive, always on the move, which is why he has to be contained in the alchemical vessel or consulting room. In alchemy Mercurius acts as a catalytic or linking element. As well as linking 'masculine' and 'feminine' he also links highest and lowest: Holy Ghost and Devil, wisdom and matter. Like any god he is two-faced – for Hermes the other side is his trickster nature. He is inventive in both senses of the word.

This two-facedness causes problems for commentators. In informal discussions with colleagues the introduction of the word 'Hermes' produced two radically different responses. Either all the 'good' aspects were listed (transformation, psychopomp, etc.) or all the 'bad' ones (trickster, thief, liar). It is hard to hold both sides together and of course there is overlap between Hermes/Mercury the classical god and the alchemical Mercurius. Hermes is part of what Jung calls 'the psychology . . . of the Mercurius duplex who on the one hand is Hermes the mystagogue and psychopomp and on the other hand is the poisonous dragon, the evil spirit and "trickster"' (Jung 1954: para. 689, Jung's quotation marks). Jung says this in connection with an artistically gifted patient who produced a 'typical tetradic mandala' and stuck it on a sheet of thick paper. On the other side there was a matching circle packed with drawings of sexual perversions. Jung connects that with the 'chaos' (again, for some reason, the quotation marks) that hides behind the self.

Elsewhere, Jung insists that the trickster myth is actively sustained and promoted by consciousness as a sort of reference point for human origins and indicates that, in the cycle, the trickster does become more civilized and even 'useful and sensible' (Jung 1954: para. 474). I hope to expand these points in connection with Hermes and primal scene imagery.

Let us now look at the myth in more detail. In the Hermes story he is the son of Zeus and the nymph Maia, who is the daughter of Atlas. On the day of his birth he sees a tortoise near the cave and is overcome by delight. He kills the tortoise and discovers that he can make a musical instrument from the shell, a lyre. He returns to the cave and sings a song to his mother and father referring to their love affair and telling, in the words of *The Homeric Hymn to Hermes,* 'all the glorious tale of his own begetting'. The next thing Hermes experiences is hunger and he wants very much to eat meat. He steals a herd of cattle from his brother Apollo and drives the cattle backwards to the cave, thus cleverly creating confusing tracks. He makes a sacrifice. He manages to fool Apollo and Zeus for a while about what he has done but eventually Apollo finds out and tries to bind Hermes but cannot. A peace deal is made in which each brother imparts or donates certain of his skills to his brother-god. Hermes teaches Apollo music and Apollo becomes the god of music. Apollo hands the role of psychopomp to Hermes. The crowning event of Hermes' first day is his audience with Zeus where he is made one of the Olympiads, the messenger of the gods.

Hermes is portrayed as a highly social god, interested in trade and commerce and exchange, befriending men on numerous occasions – for example, he gives

Odysseus a magic plant to help him resist Circe and also accompanies Herakles on his descent into Hades. He befriends the gods too – most notably when he rescues his father, Zeus, in a war with the giants. Interestingly, in the myth Hera consents to suckle Hermes, though she is usually represented as being extremely jealous of Zeus' affairs and the results of them. Apart from being helpful, Hermes plays numerous practical jokes on mortals and immortals alike. He contributes deceit and lies to the contents of Pandora's box. He is intelligent, flexible and creative; he can make fires for cooking and heating, for example. On the other hand, he can take the form of a sudden silence. His altars seem to have been phallic as were many of his representations. His role as the guide of souls to Hades overlaps with his functions as the god of travellers and of the crossroads.

Hermes is often depicted as chasing and/or raping some nymph or other – he is sexually rampant. Two of his offspring express this graphically. Priapus, who is sometimes stated to be Hermes' father as well as his son, is highly promiscuous, doubly phallic, front and rear, grotesque, obscene, pornographic, transsexual, transvestite, horrendous. The other son, Pan, is, *inter alia,* the god of masturbation and of nightmares.

Discussion of the myth

Let us look more closely at this archetypal metaphor for a developmental phase. Lopez-Pedraza points out that Hermes does not seem to have a complex about the primal scene, though his genogram would make interesting reading (Lopez-Pedraza 1977: 28). His father, Zeus, is a well-known tyrant, highly insecure and moody. His mother's father feels he carries the world on his shoulders, and so on. In fact Hermes *celebrates* his begetting in a song. One thinks here of Money-Kyrle's word 'allow' in connection with creative parental intercourse. Hermes does not indulge in parthenogenetic inflated fantasy; he sings of the act that brought him into being, specifically acknowledging the participation of both parents. Music-making connects with the idea that differentiating the parents is a creative act. Does Hermes deny primal scene envy here? Apparently not, but there is a humorous or even mocking tone to some of his song. And his later actions concerning the cattle theft need to be considered. He takes the meat he craves from the one who has it – his brother Apollo. That is, he makes an envious onslaught on Apollo's wealth. The *envy* can be twinned with the *celebration* mentioned earlier – is not this what we often feel at someone else's good fortune? Then Hermes is deceitful about his theft . . .

What does his thieving or taking mean? Why is a god a thief? Jung, following Schopenhauer and Buddhism, points out that it is individuation that lies behind such evils as stealing. In Christianity, similarly, human nature has to be tainted by original sin in order to be redeemed by Christ's self-sacrifice. This is because man in a completely natural state would be like an animal, neither good nor pure. Instinctuality and total unconsciousness would prevail if a distinction between good and evil was not drawn. Jung puts it like this:

> Since without guilt there is no moral consciousness and without awareness of differences no consciousness at all, we must concede that the strange intervention [of God introducing the distinction between good and evil to the world] was absolutely necessary for the development of any kind of consciousness and in this sense was for the good.
>
> (Jung 1967: para. 244)

Hermes' many good acts and his 'good' development (for example the way in which he and Apollo sort things out) come out of and after the evil act of stealing.

Perhaps the words 'stealing' and 'thieving' have connotations that make them invariably negative. Do they rule out the possibility of the freely offered gift, for instance, the mother's devoted offer of her breast? Hermes does get this from Hera, who is able to control any impulse to transfer her hostility towards Zeus onto the baby. So that *is* present in the story; the thieving is something else. I think that taking or stealing are words for what we call today introjection and internalization. Following Laplanche and Pontalis (1980: 229), introjection means that 'in phantasy the subject transposes objects and their inherent qualities from the "outside" to the "inside" of himself.' Internalization can be said to mean much the same but with one important difference. In the case of internalization what is transposed is the image of a *relationship* or interpersonal process (ibid.: 226). Hermes' thieving has much in common with this transposition, which is central to the idea of internalization.

This throws a different light on Hermes' mendacity and stealing. These features would then be part of a developmental process that would make considerations of morality and approval or disapproval irrelevant. Pre-morality (and even immorality) is fundamental to being human. The anthropologist Edmund Leach was reported in *The Times* of 3 September 1981 as saying, 'Nature cannot tell lies, but human beings can and do . . . Human beings engage in wilful deception on a massive scale. The ability to tell lies is perhaps our most striking human characteristic.'

Hermes and sexuality

Hermes is not a conventionally heroic figure; he is basic, down to earth, vital. Nowhere does this vitality show more than in his sexuality. Hermes and his sons, Priapus and Pan, bring together rape, sadomasochism, posterior intercourse and all manner of obscenities. These are not completely divorced from genital sexuality – Hermes does have intercourse with his nymphs. But, remembering our search for the god of the primal scene, consider the following. Freud saw paternal aggression, sadomasochism and posterior intercourse as the main grotesque fantasies occasioned by the primal scene. He wondered where they 'came from'. This archetypal metaphor is a partial answer to Freud's archetypal question.

Pan is the god of masturbation and masturbation fantasies and hence closely connected with the signs and symbols of infantile sexuality. He is also the god of nightmares from which we awake or are awoken sweating and frightened. If the primal scene, as a real event, has impact on a child then it will be mainly in the middle of the night. Parents report how often the baby cries or the child intrudes during lovemaking. The other son, Priapus, is both homo- and heteroerotic, truly polymorphous in both Freud's and Meltzer's (1981) sense.

Hermes is more than pervert or trickster; like any god he is something less than individuated. In his lack of a settled relationship with a female partner his is not an image of maturity either. His naughtiness is babylike and appealing, it is part of his eternal youth. Part, too, of youth and of growing up is, as Lopez-Pedraza says, 'to be initiated into sexual fantasies . . . Hermes is the god of sexuality, including cheap sexuality and love by chance' (Lopez-Pedraza 1977: 99). My feeling about Hermes' trickster side is that it is enacted in mocking the parents, denying and envying their separateness and creativeness, and in grandiose, parthenogenetic fantasy – sometimes he is described as his own parents and sometimes as parentless.

Case illustration

A patient of mine, aged forty, is a social worker (all details have been disguised). He is a large, bulky, hunched man with a gruff, abrupt manner, superficially masculine. In his inner world he sees himself as a teenage girl. His background involved a home dominated by women, a classic description of a weak father, and a fantasy of parental intercourse in which mother initiated, was on top, and brought about father's early death by sexual voraciousness. A major theme of the therapy has been a work conflict with his dynamic, quick-thinking and tricky boss who belittles him and interferes with his areas of responsibility. However, in his dreams the boss, far from being an enemy, is seen as a helpful figure – for instance giving him a rifle in a war and saving him because of knowing a foreign language. The boss appears as a tour guide and as an emissary from the Pope. The Hermetic overtones of all this are clear. To complete the picture, on the shady side, my patient and his boss have to hide some stolen goods and when the boss gives my patient some money there is some missing.

It has become clear to me that I, too, adopted a Hermetic stance. I felt tempted to become my patient's discussant and devise plans or even tricks with which to fight back. Gradually, the work situation improved as my patient won the respect of his boss and in dreams a more male self-image slowly appeared. Two dreams (nearly three years apart) concerning the death of his father show this. In the first there is to be a lawsuit against him, concerning a society lady, which he must be educated to contest. In the second, the dream emphasizes that he is not to blame for his father's death. A further dream on this theme involves him berating an uncle for backing out of a border crossing somewhere in Europe. The uncle *always* backs out. My patient advances into no man's land (!) alone and crosses into the new country (in his association, Poland – this was dreamt at the time of a Soviet-Polish crisis).

The emergent masculinity produced changes in primal scene imagery. The following two dreams are also separated by approximately three years:

> I am in the river floating downstream. There are sleeping people in all the houses. I don't have keys so I smash a hole in the window to get in. I am afraid. I come across a rat and a space monster copulating. They are lying on a ramp like a crucifix. Small monkeylike creatures dance around and in a box there is a sort of insect that reproduces by splitting itself. I know it has no sex life.

The second, later, dream:

> I am watching a man diving under the water. I tell my wife's brother that *this* is how to dive. On the seabed the diver meets his wife who is an animal of some sort but also human. She gives the man an oxygen tube and they have beautiful intercourse buoyed up by the water. As they continue their lovemaking, a glass dome fills with beads of many colours in regular and soothing patterns. Then the couple sit in armchairs like we had at home.

Recently his wife dreamt that they were getting married again.

This example naturally leaves out much analytic interaction, interpretation of homosexual transference and aggression towards me. The adoption of a Hermetic criminality did lead to the psychic developments outlined above. I cannot say that I remained uninvolved or in control of what was happening.

The patient produced a blending of images of the relation to his mother with images of his parents in bed. By tolerating considerable acting-out on his part in the form of flirtations with other types of therapy and growth activity, I fostered a mother–son differentiation and that, in turn, permitted the emergence of differentiated parental imagery. Our Hermetic activity also contributed to producing an impetus that put the primal scene into motion as an act that unites two separate entities.

References

Freud, S. (1916–17) *Introductory Lectures on Psychoanalysis*. Std Edn. 15–16. London: Hogarth.
Freud, S. (1918) 'From the history of an infantile neurosis'. Std Edn 17. London: Hogarth.
Jung, C. G. (1952) *Symbols of Transformation*. CW 5.
Jung, C. G. (1954) *The Archetypes and the Collective Unconscious*. CW 9i.
Jung, C. G. (1967) *Alchemical Studies*. CW 13.
Klein, M. (1929) 'Infantile anxiety situations reflected in a work of art and in the creative impulse'. In *The Writings of Melanie Klein*, Vol. 1. London: Hogarth, 1975.
Laplanche, J. and Pontalis, J.-B. (1980) *The Language of Psychoanalysis*. London: Hogarth.
Lopez-Pedraza, R. (1977) *Hermes and His Children*. Zurich: Spring Publications.
Meltzer, D. (1981) *Sexual States of Mind*. Strath Tay, Perthshire: Clunie Press.
Money-Kyrle, R. (1971) 'The aims of psychoanalysis'. In D. Meltzer (ed.), *Collected Papers*. Strath Tay, Perthshire: Clunie Press.
Neumann, E. (1954) *The Origins and History of Consciousness*. London: Routledge and Kegan Paul.
Newton, K. (1981) 'Comment on the emergence of child analysis' by M. Fordham. *Journal of Analytical Psychology*, 26: 1.
Redfearn, J. (1978) 'The energy of warring and combining opposites: Problems for the psychotic patient and the therapist in achieving the symbolic situation'. *Journal of Analytical Psychology*, 23: 3.
Riviere, J. (1952) 'General Introduction' to M. Klein, *Developments in Psychoanalysis*. London: Hogarth.
Samuels, A. (1980) 'Incest and omnipotence in the internal family'. *Journal of Analytical Psychology*, 25: 1.
Samuels, A. (1985) *Jung and the Post-Jungians*. London & Boston, MA: Routledge and Kegan Paul.
Segal, H. (1973) *Introduction to the Work of Melanie Klein*. London: Hogarth.

CHAPTER 10

JUNG, ANTI-SEMITISM AND THE NAZIS

Retrospective introduction

The next two chapters constitute my work on the question of Jung and anti-semitism. They were published in 1993 in *The Political Psyche* but were first conceived and started in 1987. I still believe that tackling this issue in a historically informed and psychologically sensitive manner is vital for the future of Jungian and post-Jungian analysis and studies. For it is the allegation of anti-semitism, and the linked allegation of indifference or mendacity on the part of the Jungian professional and scholarly communities, that are the major obstacles to the expansion and acceptance of Jungian approaches in both clinic and academy.

Some Jungians felt it was a betrayal for me to write these chapters. Some non-Jungians (incredibly) felt that I had whitewashed Jung.

I wish that similar reparative work would now be done on Jung's ideas about race and ethnicity.

I would like to take the opportunity to record that the attitude of the Jung heirs and their somewhat complacent advisers to a full and frank discussion of these issues has not been helpful. After this material was published, the heirs withdrew their consent for an introduction I had written to Jung's book on the events of the 1930s in Europe. The introduction had been in print for eleven years when the permission was retrospectively withdraw and the edition had to be pulped.

Introduction

In this chapter and the next one, I try to show that it was Jung's attempt to establish a psychology of nations that brought him into the same frame as Nazi anti-semitic ideology. In addition, Jung was absorbed by the question of leadership. Exploring these ideas as thoroughly as possible leads to a re-evaluation in more positive terms of what Jung was trying to do. Moreover, such an exploration is itself a necessary act of reparation.

In 1988 the London Library, a private institution much favoured in intellectual and literary circles, set up an appeal to mark the centenary of the birth of their onetime president, T. S. Eliot. The appeal was to benefit young writers. Instead, a storm of controversy broke out because of the great poet's alleged anti-semitism. Examples were not hard to find. In poems such as 'Burbank with a Baedeker: Bleistein with a Cigar' or 'Gerontian', Eliot compressed a whole range of anti-semitic stereotypes, from the small and avaricious businessman to the

Rothschild-like aristocrat. The poems were written in the 1920s, but their sting persisted. In 1948, a young Jewish poet, Emanuel Litvinoff, gave a reading of a poem he had written in the same year. Eliot was present at the reading of the poem, which included the lines:

> I am not accepted in your parish.
> Bleistein was my relative.[1]

By the time the furore over Eliot had entered the columns of popular newspapers, similar revelations concerning the philosophers Martin Heidegger and Paul de Man were the subject of scrutiny. Questions were also raised, by no means for the first time, about C. G. Jung's alleged anti-semitism and pro-Nazi stance. At least five letters, either attacking or defending Jung, appeared on the correspondence page of the *New York Times* during 1988. A lengthy piece written by a popular American psychiatrist-columnist, critical of Jung, appeared in the *Psychiatric Times* of September 1988. Peter Gay, Freud's most recent biographer, devoted a third of a review published in *The Guardian,* also in 1988, of a recent Jung biography to the subject.

My own experience, as an analytical psychologist interested in relating Jung's work and legacy to that of psychoanalytic thinkers, is that relations between Freudians and Jungians are increasingly hampered by the repeated claims that Jung was a Nazi sympathizer and anti-semite. In 1987, I presented a clinical paper to a study group of the New York Psychoanalytic Institute. The first question concerned Jung's supposed 'admiration of Hitler' (in the questioner's words). I had already noted that the entire audience on that occasion was, or seemed to be, Jewish, a fact which had produced in me a feeling of at-homeness up to the moment of that question.

To accomplish my task, I need to ask the reader to join me in due course in exploring two burning issues that were central to the ideology of fascism in the 1930s. The two themes are (1) the idea of *nation* and (2) the principle of *leadership*.

On not analyzing Jung

Readers of what follows may be disappointed that I scarcely mention Jung's personal psychology or psychopathology – his father-complex, the scars of the break with Freud, his shadow problems, his Swiss bourgeois mentality, and so forth. Nor do I give much space to the abundant personal testimonies that exist, intended to show that Jung cannot be regarded as anti-semitic, or to those accounts which prove the contrary, that he had a positive attitude to Jews and helped many Jews to achieve a relationship with their Jewishness for the first time. I must say here that I do not feel any sense of disappointment in Jung, that he has, in some personal way, let me down. Clichés about Jung's shadow problems concerning Jews strike me as rather shallow. I never saw him as 'a perfect leader, a saint, someone who guides us, a guru', so I do not have a reaction when he turns out to be a 'very average collective human being' (to use the dichotomy set out by Adolf Guggenbühl-Craig).[2]

For a while I worried that these omissions added up to a failure of feeling on my part. Obviously, I do not think that we should totally ignore Jung's experiences and experiences of Jung, forgetting the usefulness of a simple answer. Indeed, in the next chapter, I consider Jung the man as an example of a leader or potential leader.

But gradually I have come to see that *the true failure of feeling is found when the personal dimension is given too much weight or used to close an awkward issue once and for all.* A similar point was made by the editor of the *Journal of Psychology and Judaism* when introducing an issue composed of two major papers on the subject of Jung, anti-semitism and the Nazis.[3] I am sure I am not the only one to have mixed feelings about an analysis-at-a-distance of Jung's internal life (his dreams, for example) that does not observe the rule of 'confidentiality' even to the slightest degree. I simply do not feel that this level of data is a fruitful one. One difficulty with any psychological analysis of Jung the man is that a conclusion that the whole thing is very complicated can almost always be known in advance: Jung, by his own admission (regarding Number One and Number Two personalities), was an extremely complex person who excited equally complex reactions. So, for me, analyzing Jung is not the best way to proceed. Instead, I would like to cast as actors in this drama not individuals, but *groups,* and suggest that the play is about to-ing and fro-ing between groups: Nazis, Jews, Jungians, Freudians. I was amazed, and sometimes shocked, to discover the extent to which the groups, apparently so different, share a common process.[4]

Was Jung anti-semitic?

I have chosen to locate my inquiry on an intergroup level, which is where the drama about Jung has been played out, a drama involving Christians as well as Jews, Freudians, Jungians and Nazis. This does not in itself constitute a magic solution to the difficulties inherent in our themes. But it does go some way to rectifying a serious problem with what has been written about Jung to date. We have history.[5] We have attack.[6] We have defence.[7] We have at least half a dozen biographies of Jung. We have the *New York Times* letters. We have pleas for an imaginal approach.[8] But we have virtually no political analysis of this drama. There is very little critical work on the relationship of what is politically dubious in Jung's writings to the general cultural problems of Nazism and anti-semitism.

So, rather than attempt a new analysis of Jung the man (for which, not having met him, I feel I have not the slightest evidential basis), I sought a new use of what I had read. In these chapters, I ask whether there is something in the fundamental structure of Jung's thinking about the Jews, in its heart or essence, that made anti-semitism inevitable. When Jung writes about the Jews and Jewish psychology, is there something in his whole attitude that brings him into the same frame as the Nazis, even if he were shown not to have been an active Nazi collaborator? Is there something to worry about?

My brief answer, in distinction to that of many well-known Jungians, is 'yes' and, as I said, my hope is that by exploring the matter as deeply as I can a kind of reparation will ensue. Then there will be the base from which to explore the full potential of what Jung was trying to do with his psychological thinking about culture in the 1930s.

Many of those who have heard me lecture on this topic have commented that the particular blend of intellect and emotion, logic and image, makes mine a post-modern contribution. Perhaps this is a consequence of exposure to modernism's shadow, the events, language and imagery of the Nazi era. As a Jewish man, I found that writing about Jung and anti-semitism turned into a personal odyssey. Travelling this road has enabled me to stay an analytical psychologist. But I know that, if the source of a thoughtless remark about Jewish people is the *Collected Works* of C. G. Jung, the possible outcome of the idea set loose in the political arena is the concentration camp and the gas chamber. The Jew of whom Jung writes is my relative and sometimes we do not feel accepted in Jung's parish. But this is not a parochial matter and others than Jews are involved. In 1946 the Foreign Office in London received a document entitled 'The case of Dr Carl G. Jung – pseudo-scientist Nazi auxiliary' suggesting a possible trial as a war criminal. I have seen this document, which did not excite the interest of the civil servants concerned; its significance does not lie in its content, which is familiar, but rather in the degree of political outrage Jung managed to elicit.[9]

Finally, I believe that the manifold strengths and subtleties of analytical psychology are being lost. Such loss results not only from the alleged Nazi collaboration and anti-semitism (both of which Jung denied), but also from what can sometimes seem like an inability on the part of many Jungians to react to such charges in an intelligent, humane and honest way. Thus, psychoanalysis and other intellectual disciplines are permitted to continue to ignore the pioneering nature of Jung's contributions and, hence, the work of post-Jungian analytical psychologists. As Eli Weisstub puts it:

> There is much to be done in answering some of these criticisms ... Only in so doing can we (that is, Jungians) get the rest of the world analytic community to respect what is valid and valuable and significant in Jung's contributions ... Trying to preserve a myth about 'our leader' will not further this effort.[10]

Background information

Although what I write is primarily psychological, ideological and critical – not historical – it may help to provide some background information, which I will discuss throughout the chapters, for those not familiar with Jung's activities in the 1930s. I will also try to summarize, but not at this point critique, some of his ideas about 'Jewish psychology'. These activities and ideas have been the subject of intense argument from the 1930s to the present day. It has to be said that a definitive factual basis for clear-cut opinion is extremely difficult if not impossible to establish. Nevertheless, when lecturing on the topic of Jung, anti-semitism and the Nazis, I have found widespread ignorance, even among Jungian analysts, of what it was that Jung did and said that has caused such a prolonged outcry. Non-Jungian audiences, on the other hand, have often seemed to 'know' definitely that Jung was 'anti-semitic', a 'supporter of Hitler', and so on – but not to be aware of the details.

In 1933 Jung took on the presidency of the General Medical Society for Psychotherapy (GMSP). This was a professional body with members from several countries but nevertheless based in Germany and coming under Nazi control. Jung claimed that he took this post expressly to defend the rights of Jewish psychotherapists and he altered the constitution of the GSMP so that it became a fully and formally international (later, 'supranational') body. The former General Society became the German national member group. Membership was by means of national societies with a special category of individual membership (members-at-large). Jews were already barred from membership of the German national society and so, under Jung's new provision, were enabled to join the Society via membership of the individual section. Jung always maintained that his motives for taking on the presidency were to protect Jewish colleagues in this way and to keep depth psychology alive in Germany. Freud's books were burnt and he was 'banned' in 1933.

Jung also became editor of the *Zentralblatt für Psychotherapie,* the Society's scientific journal. This was one of the leading journals of psychotherapy in central Europe. Jung said that this was a *pro forma* appointment and he was geographically distant from the editorial offices. He said he did not know that pro-Nazi statements of principles would be inserted for general distribution outside, as opposed to inside, Germany by Professor Göring (a cousin of the Reichsmarschall), who had been made President of the (dominant) German section.

Jung's own editorials and articles in the *Zentralblatt,* extracts of which appear below, have also been a main reason why he has been accused of pro-Nazi sympathies and anti-semitism.

According to Geoffrey Cocks in *Psychotherapy in the Third Reich,* Jung's ideas had 'official approval', he visited Nazi Germany to teach on two occasions, and, as a result, 'German psychotherapists did all they could to link Jung's name with their own activities'.[11] Jung's work was cited by German racial theoreticians and appeared in official Nazi bibliographies. Cocks points out that, following Jung's denunciations in 1938–9 of Hitler and the Nazis, his psychology never became the dominant school under the Nazis.

In an interview on Radio Berlin in 1933, Jung commented:

> As Hitler said recently, the leader (*Führer*) must be able to be alone and must have the courage to go his own way. But if he doesn't know himself, how is he to lead others? That is why the true leader is always one who has the courage to be himself, and can look not only others in the eye but above all himself . . . Every movement culminates organically in a leader, who embodies in his whole being the meaning and purpose of the popular movement.[12]

In his paper 'The state of psychotherapy today', published in the *Zentralblatt* in 1934, Jung wrote:

> Freud did not understand the Germanic psyche any more than did his Germanic followers. Has the formidable phenomenon of National Socialism, on which the whole world gazes with astonishment, taught them better? Where was that unparalleled tension and energy while as yet no National Socialism existed? Deep in the Germanic psyche, in a pit that is anything but a garbage-bin of unrealizable infantile wishes and unresolved family resentments.[13]

In the same paragraph, Jung makes the following comments about the Jews: 'The "Aryan" unconscious has a higher potential than the Jewish.' He also states that 'The Jew, who is something of a nomad, has never yet created a cultural form of his own and as far as we can see never will, since all his instincts and talents require a more or less civilised nation to act as frost for their development', and that 'the Jews have this peculiarity with women; being physically weaker, they have to aim at the chinks in the armour of their adversary'.

Finally, Jung warns against 'applying Jewish categories indiscriminately to Germanic and Slavic Christendom'. He says much the same in a footnote to the 1935 edition of *Two Essays on Analytical Psychology:* 'It is a quite unpardonable mistake to accept the conclusions of a Jewish psychology as generally valid.'[14] In a separate *Zentralblatt* editorial he had written in 1933 that 'the differences which actually do exist between Germanic and Jewish psychology and which have been long known to every intelligent person are no longer to be glossed over.'[15]

In a letter to his pupil, Dr Kranefeldt, in 1934, Jung wrote:

> As is known, one cannot do anything against stupidity, but in this instance the Aryan people can point out that with Freud and Adler specifically Jewish points of view are publicly preached, and as can be proven likewise, points of view that have an essentially corrosive character. If the proclamation of this Jewish gospel is agreeable to the government, then so be it. Otherwise there is also the possibility that this would not be agreeable to the government.[16]

Jung was not new to speculations about the Jews. In 1918 he had written that the Jew

> is badly at a loss for that quality in man which roots him to the earth and draws new strength from below. This chthonic quality is to be found in dangerous concentration in the German peoples . . . The Jew has too little of this quality – where has he his own earth underfoot?[17]

However, as we will see in a moment, Jung totally rejected the charge of anti-semitism. He said, in a letter to A. Pupato in 1934, that he 'fought Freud's psychology because of its dogmatic claim to sole validity'.[18]

It is interesting to compare these extracts from Jung's writings with the following:

Freud to Abraham in 1908:

> Please do not forget that it is easier for you than for Jung to follow my ideas, for in the first place you are completely independent, and then you are closer to my intellectual constitution because of racial kinship . . . I nearly said that it was only by his appearance on the scene that psychoanalysis escaped from the danger of becoming a Jewish national affair.[19]

Freud to Ferenczi in 1913:

> Certainly there are great differences between the Jewish and Aryan spirit. We can observe that every day. Hence there would assuredly be here and there differences in outlook on life and art. But there should not be such a thing as Aryan or Jewish science. Results in science must be identical, though the presentation of them may vary.[20]

Attacks and defences: A discussion

Having absorbed the contents of the many attacks on Jung, based on the behaviour and writing outlined in the previous section entitled 'Background information', my attention was stirred by the nature of the equally numerous defences of Jung that have been put forward. I found myself reacting to a psychological similarity between the defences and attacks. Both defenders and attackers of Jung are sitting in judgment on him. Both are looking for a 'final solution' to the Jung problem. Between the cries of 'Let's clear our man once and for all' and 'Let's finish the bastard off' there is a call for a middle way: tot up carefully the competing claims of attackers and defenders so as to reach an apparently balanced point of view. It is said that the matter can never be settled decisively. Though it is tempting to join in this Olympian arbitration between attack and defence, that position can be seen as disengaged, morally supercilious, politically evasive, pseudo-mature and, in any case, as full of a kind of certitude as overt attack or defence! The shadows surrounding Jung are going to linger, for they want us to pay psychological attention to them. In the next section, I will let Jung speak for himself in his own defence.

One particular defence of Jung that is often put forward is that he was only expressing the attitudes of his time. Many other eminent men and women were equally guilty of a kind of *trahison des clercs*. Moreover, it is said that casual, social anti-semitism was apparently so widespread, normal and acceptable in Jung's culture and time that remarks about the Jews, even when couched in scientific language, did not seem *outré*. (Much the same defence has been advanced regarding Eliot, Heidegger and de Man.) Conversely, Jung has been defended by the argument that he should *not* be seen as an important man but rather as just a typical, petit-bourgeois, unthinking, small-minded anti-semitic Swiss burgher. According to Adolf Guggenbühl-Craig, 'the anti-semitism of Jung was a sheer banality of the collective he belonged to'.[21]

But these claims, themselves contradictory, actually *stimulate* a search for evidence that would contradict them and, therefore, there is a risk of undermining the intention of defending Jung. For it seems that there could have been other attitudes available to Jung at the time, other choices that he could have made, other viewpoints possible, particularly given that he was not under direct personal threat. Even in Germany, there were the *Judenfreunde,* 'friends of the Jews' – not just the anecdotal good Germans but people actually prosecuted in the courts by the Gestapo for their attitudes and behaviour. Then there were the *Rassenschänder,* 'race defilers', who were imprisoned for doing what hundreds and thousands had done quite legally before 1933, as the intermarriage statistics show.[22]

We know from a fascinating letter in the London *Times* on November 13, 1988 – from a typical *Times* correspondent, an Anglican (Episcopalian) clergyman of the old school – that problems faced by Jews were openly and frequently discussed in Germany in the late 1930s.[23] Closer to home, there was the public admonition of Jung by Dr Bally in 1934.[24] In 1935 the Dutch section of the International General Medical Society for Psychotherapy refused to host the annual congress on political grounds. Jung was critical of this decision because, he said, it brought politics into science. In 1936, when Jung was invited to speak at the tercentenary celebrations of Harvard University, and to receive an honorary degree, a public row broke out in the pages of the Harvard *Crimson,* the university newspaper, over the appropriateness of inviting Jung. Gordon Allport felt that Jung's 'scientific integrity' had been 'partially stifled under the Nazi thumb'. Henry Murray defended Jung's independence of thought in very strong terms. The point is that, even at the time, Jung's position was not regarded as unproblematic in intellectual circles.[25] Therefore, Adolf Guggenbühl-Craig's point about Jung being a 'collective intellectual' is a very dubious one. To criticize Jung is not a case of 'present-ism', seeing the past from today's vantage point. He was criticized in similar terms at the time, during the 1930s.

Indeed, the *necessity* of deliberately linking politics with 'science' was on the minds of many intellectuals during this period. It follows that Jung's repeated attempts to divorce the two cannot be regarded as absolutely conditioned by the epistemological climate of the day. For instance, the philosopher and critic Walter Benjamin wrote to the Judaic scholar Gershom Scholem in 1937 that he intended to devote a period to an intensive study of Jung's works, not only so as to critique Jung's 'doctrines on archaic images and the collective unconscious', but for openly political reasons. In Benjamin's opinion, Jung had 'leaped to the rescue of the

Aryan soul with a therapy reserved for it alone'. This, Benjamin felt, was an 'auxiliary service to National Socialism [that had] been in the works for some time'. A month later, in the middle of his study period, Benjamin wrote to Scholem that Jung's psychology was 'the devil's work'.[26]

So a result of the claim that the world displayed a universal anti-semitism in the 1920s and 1930s, and that the ideas of Jung and others were just part of that *Zeitgeist,* has been to constellate a counterclaim, one that is potentially damaging to Jung: alternative opinions and ways of thinking did exist. Other non-Jewish analysts, who might also have been expected to reflect 'ordinary' anti-semitism, felt the need to get involved in a different way. D. W. Winnicott, for instance, wrote the following letter to Mrs Neville Chamberlain (sic) in 1938 urging her to question her husband over his silence on the subject of the Jews and Nazi persecution:

> Dear Mrs Chamberlain,
>
> I feel the Prime Minister is too busy to answer questions but I do want to know [something]. Would you try to answer this as many of us are urgently in need of answers that we cannot get . . .
>
> Why does the Prime Minister never mention the Jews. Does he secretly despise them? When in England we say WE, we include Jews who are people like ourselves. I am not asking him to be pro-Jew, but I want to know definitely whether he is or is not secretly anti-Jew . . . at present we seem to be secretly sharing Germany's anti-Jew insanity, and this is not where we want our leaders to lead us.[27]

Many of the articles that appeared in the *Zentralblatt fur Psychotherapie* under the banner of Jung's editorship go well beyond 'ordinary', petit-bourgeois anti-semitism. There are repeated attacks on 'Jewish' mental states and a general lauding of 'northern', Aryan psychology. There is a great deal of praise for Hitler and the Nazi party and, in the opinion of some, even coded messages of support for measures such as the extermination of mental patients. In any event, these articles appeared long after the initial confusion over whether a statement of support for the Nazis was to be printed in the *Zentralblatt* proper for 1933 or only in the German national supplement, due in 1934.[28] Jung claimed that it was because of this confusion that his name appeared attached to such a statement. The question is whether Jung knew of the disgusting (and absurd) nature of these further articles, published in the years 1933–39. He would have heard some of them at conferences. If he did nothing about it, could it have been because he was completely divorced from the editorial policy and activity of the *Zentralblatt?* But we do know that editorial work *was* carried out in Zurich. C. A. Meier, Jung's associate, wrote to James Kirsch that he personally corrected numerous insulting reviews of 'Jewish books and articles'. Jung, on the other hand, did nothing; according to Meier's account, he left everything to Meier.[29]

Here, Meier's memory is at fault. For, in 1937, Jung wrote to Göring as follows:

> Dr Meier has drawn my attention to your short review of Rosenberg's book. For anyone who knows Jewish history, in particular Hasidism, Rosenberg's assertion that the Jews despise mysticism is a highly regrettable error. I would therefore suggest that we pass over this book in silence. I cannot allow my name to be associated with such lapses.[30]

In the same year, the *Zentralblatt* published a paper by Victor Frankl, so it seems that Jewish writers could have their work published.

Our sense of relief and desire to applaud the attempts by Jung and Meier to keep the more egregious parcels of anti-semitic thinking out of the columns of the *Zentralblatt* need to be tempered. For the realization that the power to do this was available to the team in Zurich, even after Göring became joint editor in 1936, raises the uncomfortable question of why it was not exercised more often. Are we to assume that, if Jung could keep out anti-semitic ideas that he did not approve of, the anti-semitic ideas of which he did approve are the ones that remain? I do not think that a simple answer exists. I know from experience how complicated the internal politics of a learned journal can be. It has proved very hard to achieve an accurate portrait of how the *Zentralblatt für Psychotherapie* organized itself in these years but, as we will see in a moment, it is vital to establish the degree of involvement Jung had.

Even if Jung played little or no editorial role on the *Zentralblatt,* surely he at least *read* it? He was sole editor from 1933 to 1936, when Göring became joint editor. If he didn't read it at all, did nobody ever tell him what was in it?

In the *Zentralblatt,* there were a number of pieces co-signed by Jung with others. Some of these troubling little pieces are included in the General Bibliography of Jung's writings but are not included in the *Collected Works* (some pieces are not even in the bibliography). The pattern of exclusion of co-signed pieces from the bibliography and/or published works is not consistent and it has been suggested to me that this might reflect doubt in the minds of the editors of the *Collected Works* over whether Jung wrote some of the pieces signed by him with others. In other words, there would be no need to include these pieces in Jung's corpus because it cannot be established that the articles truly expressed Jung's views. However, as far as I can tell, *Jung never disowned any of these pieces, nor protested that his name had been taken in vain.* We should remember that, for much of this time, he was sole editor of the *Zentralblatt* and we have already seen that he could control the content of the journal when he felt strongly about it. My view is that these pieces, co-signed by Jung and apparently not the subject of intra-editorial dissent at the time, may be taken as expressive of his views. (I must add that it is special pleading to argue that, because these pieces are co-signed, they cannot be connected to Jung. Probably the argument is based on the misunderstandings over the statement of pro-Nazi principles that found its way into the *Zentralblatt,* as mentioned earlier. But that piece was neither signed nor co-signed by Jung; it appeared in a journal of which he was the editor.)

I have recently made a study of one of these co-signed pieces, which was published in 1934 (following the matter of the pro-Nazi statement that appeared in the *Zentralblatt* in 1933). Maybe Jung was taken by surprise once again and his name was used as co-signatory without permission. We simply cannot know for sure but, as stated above, I do not think that such *lèse-majesté* took place for, if it had, Jung or his associates would have done something about it at the time. The contents of this piece make for instructive reading.

The piece is innocuous-looking – a seventieth-birthday greeting to Dr Robert Sommer, one of the co-founders in 1926 of the GMSP, by Matthias Göring and Jung.[31] However, Sommer, according to Geoffrey Cocks, was the 'moving spirit' behind attempts to translate the ideas of 'social and racial hygiene' into the mental health field.[32] Sommer founded an organization in 1923 called *Deutscher Verband für Psychische Hygiene* (German Association for Mental Hygiene). In their birthday tribute, Göring and Jung say of this group that it was a 'comparatively small association before the turning-point, today of extraordinary importance'. The 'turning-point' was, of course, the coming to power of the Nazis.

Göring and Jung go on to praise Sommer's book *Familienforschung, Vererbungs- und Rassenlehre* (which can be effectively translated as Family Studies, Hereditology and Raceology – there are no present-day terms for the last two disciplines). In particular, they praise the new chapter of the book, written in 1927 and added to the existing text of 1907. I wondered why, in 1934, Göring and Jung would go out of their way to praise one particular chapter added in 1927 to a book first published in 1907. Jung certainly knew of Sommer's book, citing it in both the original and the revised versions of a paper on the father (1909 and 1949).[33] But this may have been the first edition. It may not be a *reason,* but we have to recall, as Robert Jay Lifton has pointed out, that from the mid-1930s the Nazi notion of 'life unworthy of life' became firmly established together with the concept of 'medical killing'.[34] (Eugenics fascinated any thinker concerned with equality and we find proposals for the extermination of 'ethnic trash' in the writings of Bernard Shaw and Friedrich Engels.) In the chapter of Sommer's book specifically referred to by Göring and Jung in the *Zentralblatt* we find many statements along the following lines:

> There has been an intrusion of alien blood into the Germanic race.
>
> The morphological differences of human races are in part based on changes in the formation of the skull.
>
> The long-headedness of the so-called Nordic races is of particular importance.
>
> The type of the Nordic race . . . forms a contrast . . . to the backwards sloping forehead of the primitive human races.
>
> Often the formation of the nose is used as a racial criterion in human anthropology. A special emphasis is given to the straight or slightly bow-shaped formation of the nose with regard to . . . Further, a hook-shaped protuberance is regarded as . . .
>
> Recently blood research has become of great importance for raceology.
>
> Practical psychiatry is . . . most closely linked with raceology.
>
> The selection of the gifted has to be performed . . .

There are several possible reasons why – even if he *did* know what was being published in his journal, sometimes over his name – Jung might still have done nothing in contradiction. First, he might have been in full agreement with these views. But, given the Sommer encomium, that would make him an overt Nazi supporter and rabid 'scientific' anti-semite and he denies both of these charges. Second, he might have been playing a long-term political game, continuing his strategy of helping Jewish psychotherapists to go on working. But there is no written or oral evidence that he held back for this reason and, were it the case, I think that there would be some evidence. Third, and I believe this is the answer, Jung's position at the head of the German psychotherapy profession was desirable from the point of view of the development of analytical psychology. The issue here is Jung's leadership. After all, Freud had once written to Jung that psychoanalysis would never find its true status until it had been accepted in Germany. The conquest of Germany was the goal of the psychoanalytic conquistador.[35] History, and Hitler, put that goal within Jung's grasp, and I shall look at Jung as a conquering leader of the field of psychology in the next chapter.

Whether Jung read the *Zentralblatt* or not, contemporary study of that journal is certainly worthwhile. For example, we find an announcement from Jung's co-editor, Matthias Göring, that Jung informed the presidents of the national societies of his intention to resign as President of the IGMSP, which had by this point become an international organization, in 'the summer of 1940'.[36] This is at least one year and maybe two years later than many accounts have hitherto suggested and would place the date of the resignation after the start of the war. Similarly, we find that, as late as 1939, Jung is praising the efforts of Matthias Göring to set up institutions 'where the new generation of psychotherapists can be trained in a spirit and atmosphere that offers the best guarantee for the German people (*das Volk*) to be served by these young doctors in the future.'[37]

Another issue of dating on which the *Zentralblatt* sheds light concerns the time at which Jung became involved with the GMSP (as it then was). It appears that Jung became a participant in 1928 and vice-president in 1930. He was not brought in as a distinguished outsider in 1933 but as a distinguished insider.[38]

Similarly, accounts of the proceedings of the congresses of the IGMSP make it clear that Jung was in attendance and, indeed, actually spoke. Therefore he was present to hear Matthias Göring make the following statement at the 1934 congress in Bad Nauheim. Göring began by saying that he expected all members to have studied *Mein Kampf*, going on as follows:

> Today I say that *Mein Kampf* has to be called a scientific book. Whoever reads the book and the speeches of the Führer and studies his way of being will recognize that he has got something that most of us lack: Jung calls it intuition. It is more important than all science. It is because of that that I demand of all of you that until the next congress, which will take place here in Bad Nauheim once again, you study this book and the speeches of Adolf Hitler thoroughly.[39]

Jung's 'not-ordinary' anti-semitism is further demonstrated by his involvement with Jacob Hauer, a professor of Indology and founder in 1933 of the German Faith Movement. Jung co-led seminars with Hauer on Kundalini Yoga in 1932 and was interested in his work. The German Faith Movement was an attempt to construct a religion more in tune with German history and traditions than Christianity, with its Semitic flavour. The new religion would, according to its founder, be different from Christianity on account of the fact that the 'founder of Christianity and its standard documents have reached us from a different racial and cultural area'. Hauer says he could have as easily called his movement the 'Nordic-Teutonic Faith Movement'. Hauer goes on:

> The German Faith Movement must be understood in close relation with the national movement which led to the formation of the Third Reich. Like the latter, the German Faith Movement is an eruption from the biological and spiritual depths of the German nation . . .
>
> We want the German people to regard its history and territory with religious devotion . . . . We can see God advancing over German soil . . . [40]

The translators say, in their introduction to Hauer's book, that one 'odd note' in a typical service of the German Faith Movement would be the expression in a hymn of undying loyalty to Hitler.

It is hard to assess what Jung really thought about the German Faith Movement. In the relevant passage in 'Wotan', published in 1936, he refers to adherents of the German Faith Movement as 'decent and well-meaning people' but also analyzes them as 'possessed' by the 'god of the Germans' – Wotan. On the other hand, it is no 'disgrace' to know that the God of the Germans is Wotan 'and not the Christian God'. What is clear is that this is in no way a repudiation or condemnation of Hauer; in fact, the passage could be read as an imprimatur for Hauer's group compared to other new religions.[41]

Another defence of Jung is so interesting that I intend to discuss it in some detail. This defence attempts a divorce of Jung's behaviour (including any casually expressed attitudes) from the formal presentation of his ideas in books and articles. These defenders do not excuse Jung's actions but dispute that the true importance of his ideas is affected by them. This defence of Jung can find expression the other way round: though Jung wrote stupid and offensive things about Jews, which he should have corrected, he did not *do* anything that could be regarded as destructive in the real world. The problem with the defence is that, even if one could make such a dissociation between life and work credible in the case of a psychologist, the problem of the influence of the writer's words on the behaviour of others still remains an issue. The use of the writer's words by others has to be considered. Obviously the writer cannot prevent exploitation, but he can protest at it. Did Jung?

I disagree with Geoffrey Cocks who, in his pathbreaking history of psychotherapy in Germany during the Nazi era, offers a version of this defence when he writes that 'Jung conceded more to the Nazis by his words than by his actions'.[42] As noted previously, Cocks himself points out that Jung's analytical psychology had official approval and therefore 'German psychotherapists did almost all they could to link Jung's name with their own activities'. From a political if not a strictly legal standpoint, Jung's professional activities and his psychological theories can be regarded as intertwined. They may not be causally connected in a superficial sense but, if we split them radically, we deny the negative synergy of word and action. If Jung did admit to Rabbi Leo Baeck that he 'slipped up' when they met in Zürich in 1946, then the slip may be understood as referring to this synergy: the influence of thought on action, action on thought. We would not be concerned with Jung's reputation to anything like the same extent if he had merely taken on the presidency of the General Medical Society of Psychotherapy in 1933. Then his efforts to protect the rights of Jewish psychotherapists by altering the constitution of the GMSP (so that it became a fully and formally international body with membership units composed of national societies and a special category of individual membership) would probably seem less controversial. If he had confined himself to the political and institutional arena, then the ingenious way in which his constitutional reforms permitted Jews, barred from the German national society, to practice as individual members would not require justification fifty years later.

But, at exactly the same desperate moment in history, Jung's papers and editorials of the period, dwelling on questions of differing racial and national psychologies and containing disturbing generalizations about Jewish culture and psychology, could easily be misunderstood as supporting Nazi racial ideology. For instance, as we noted earlier, Jews are said 'never to have created a cultural form of their own' but rather to need a 'host nation' for their development. The implication of Jew as 'parasite' (a favourite image of Hitler's) follows on easily (though Jung said he meant something quite specific by the term 'cultural *form*' – see pp. 172–173 below). Similarly, Jews are referred to as 'physically weaker' than others – like women in relation to men. Therefore, like women, they have developed subtle and indirect techniques of attacking and overcoming others. Says Jung, Jews deal with Germans the way women deal with men!

At the very least, the twin presence of action and thought explains why there is such concern today. But I simply cannot persuade myself that the synergy did not exist at the time and is relevant only in terms of our current responses. After all, was not Jung the author of the theory of meaningful coincidences ('synchronicity'), including the idea that the psychic world (his ideas on Jewish psychology, perhaps) and the social world (German politics, perhaps) are acausally intertwined?

Once again, the intended defence is capable of undermining Jung still more.

There are other defences of Jung which exist and, while I do not want to discuss them in as much detail as the two defences already mentioned, I will give a brief account.

Many of those who knew Jung recall that he was also generous and, eventually, protective in his personal behaviour toward Jews. This seems to be the consensus of most colleagues and personal friends.[43] The snag here is that we are all familiar with the 'some of my best friends are Jews' line; it is quite possible to combine good personal relations with a much deeper prejudice. Further, when Jung writes about the Jews he seems to do it as a member of a dominant and 'positive' race. This can be compared with Freud's position as 'the object of racialist concern who uses and projects this difference onto his perceived enemies and friends'.[44]

Actually, there is in existence a considerable amount of testimony that Jung was not always personally well disposed toward Jews. The senior British Jungian analyst Michael Fordham recalls meeting Jung for the first time in 1933 and being treated to a 'harangue' on the Jews and the 'parasitic elements in Jewish psychology'. Jung wondered what the Jews had been feeding on during the forty years in the wilderness. The clear implication was that they were grazing their herds on other people's land. Then Jung said that the Jews were not the same as other races and hence they should wear different clothes so as to emphasize this fact.[45] In a similar vein, Jung apparently told an American student of his not to let her daughter marry a Jew as such marriages never worked.[46]

Perhaps the most interesting material that shows Jung as displaying a personal as opposed to an ideological anti-semitism is to be found in a previously unpublished letter from Jung to Mary Mellon written in 1945, a few months after the end of the war in Europe. Mary Mellon was the inspiration and planner behind the Bollingen Foundation, which was endowed by her and her husband Paul Mellon. The Bollingen Foundation was undoubtedly the means by which Jung's ideas were disseminated widely in the English-speaking world and the Foundation provided financial support for the publication of Jung's *Collected Works* as well as many other scholarly works in the field of collective and cultural psychology. We may suppose that Jung regarded Mary Mellon, who had been a patient of his before the war, as an important person and patron. In the letter, Jung writes:

> You probably have heard the absurd rumor that I am a Nazi. This rumor has been started by Freudian Jews in America. Their hatred of myself went as far as India, where I found falsified photo's [sic] of mine in the Psychological

> Seminar of Calcutta University. It was a photo retouched in such a way as to make me appear as an ugly Jew with a pince-nez! These photo's came from Vienna! This rumor has been spread over the whole world. Even with us it has been picked up with such alacrity, that I am forced to publish all the things I have written about Germany. It is however difficult to mention the anti-christianism of the Jews after the horrible things that have happened in Germany. But Jews are not so damned innocent after all – the role played by the intellectual Jews in pre-war Germany would be an interesting object of investigation.[47]

One thing to note here is Jung's ideational process. It would seem that, in Jung's opinion, the way to ruin a man's reputation is to make him look Jewish and that this tactic was used in an organized way against him by 'Freudian Jews'. It is possible that Jung was temporarily insane or very unbalanced following his heart attack in 1944 but I think we do get an idea of the spleen with which he seems to have regarded Jews.

The second thing to note is the argument in the last two sentences – that it is difficult to discuss the 'anti-christianism' of the Jews and that 'intellectual Jews in pre-war Germany' were not innocent. I wonder what Jung saw as the role of intellectual Jews – is he suggesting some kind of responsibility for the 'horrible things' that he knows were done to them? It is difficult to know what to think but the letter is unsettling, to say the least, and needs to be set alongside the idea that Jung was not anti-Jewish in any personal way.

Sometimes, Jung's work is divided up in such a way that the problematic material is quarantined by detaching it from the main body of his writings, which are not subject to current critical disapproval. It would help these defenders if the contentious passages and behaviour had been the work of extreme youth, say, which they are not. Even so, Jung's work on Judaic themes from, say, 1946 onward is outstanding and can be favourably contrasted with what he had to say on the subject prior to that. But when the problematic material is isolated it is inevitably highlighted. Very little in the way of a defence of Jung is gained by red-lining his work and behaviour between 1933 and 1946.

Finally, Jung may be defended by pointing out that it is only human to make mistakes and that his reputation should therefore remain intact. What is more, there are no absolute standards of good and bad behaviour, and who are we to judge Jung? One's sympathy for this line of argument should be tempered by the reflection that condemning mistakes in another is not anti-human; it is just as human as making mistakes! If you feel critical of Jung, why not express it? It would be tragic if people were to suppress, or be prevented from expressing, their real feelings.

One piece of historical information that was recently made widely available has certainly aroused a good deal of anguished feeling in the Jungian community. In 1944, a secret appendix was added to the by-laws of the Analytical Psychology Club of Zurich, limiting the proportion of Jews who could be members at any one time. The quota for full members was 10 per cent and for guest members 25 per cent. The Club was, at that time, the main forum for the discussion of themes of interest to analytical psychology and it was also an important social centre for those in Zürich to study or analyze with Jung or one of his collaborators. For whatever reason, this appendix was drawn up and signed by the executive committee and it has become unmistakably clear from massive interview testimony that Jung knew of the quota (though the general membership do not seem to have been told officially). Moreover, the quota for Jews was not removed until 1950. It is not surprising that this information has caused a stir.[48]

Jung's self-assessment

In 1934 the Swiss psychotherapist Gustav Bally published his article, critical of Jung's writings and actions, in the *Neue Zürcher Zeitung*. Jung published 'A rejoinder to Dr Bally' in the same periodical a few months later. In this piece (and also, in similar vein, in his letters) Jung defended himself as follows:

> As to the difference between Jewish and 'Aryan-Germanic-Christian-European' psychology, it can of course hardly be seen in the individual products of science as a whole. But we are not so much concerned with these as with the fundamental fact that in psychology the object of knowledge is at the same time the organ of knowledge, which is true of no other science. It has therefore been doubted in all sincerity whether psychology is possible as a science at all. In keeping with this doubt I suggested years ago that every psychological theory should be criticised in the first instance as a subjective confession. For, if the organ of knowledge is its own subject, we have every reason to examine the nature of that organ very closely indeed, since the subjective premise is at once the object of knowledge which is therefore limited from the start. This subjective premise is identical with our psychic idiosyncrasy. The idiosyncrasy is conditioned (1) by the individual, (2) by the family, (3) by the nation, race, climate, locality, and history . . .
>
> May it not therefore be said that there is a Jewish psychology . . . which admits the prejudice of its blood and its history? And may it not be asked wherein lie the peculiar differences between an essentially Jewish and an essentially Christian outlook? Can it really be maintained that I alone among psychologists have a special organ of knowledge with a subjective bias, whereas the Jew is apparently insulted to the core if one assumes him to be a Jew? . . . I must confess my total inability to understand why it should be a crime to speak of 'Jewish' psychology . . .
>
> Are we really to believe that a tribe which has wandered through history for several thousand years as 'God's chosen people' was not put up to such an idea by some quite special psychological peculiarity? If no differences exist, then how do we recognise Jews at all?[49]

In a letter to James Kirsch of 1934, Jung defends himself in a somewhat different manner:

> You ought to know me sufficiently well to realize that an unindividual stupidity like anti-semitism cannot be laid at my door. You know well enough how very much I take the human being as a personality and how I continually endeavor to lift him out of his collective condition and make him an individual.[50]

The question of apology

What did Jung do when he recognized after the war that he might have made a mistake? (Did he recognize it as deeply as all that? is another question.) Why didn't he listen to Drs Bally and Kirsch? Why didn't he retract? Did he try to make amends?

In 1946 Jung published a slim volume which appeared in English in 1947 as *Essays on Contemporary Events*.[51] In it, Jung republished several of his pre-war papers on Germany and the Nazi phenomenon plus a preface, introduction and epilogue that were specially written for the book. Nowhere in this book does Jung explicitly say that he was caught up in the contemporary atmosphere, that he became a devotee of Wotan, that he became so excited by the potential of the Aryan unconscious that he developed a corresponding 'problem' about Jews. He does not retract anything, nor apologize for anything. But, in the preface to the book, he does refer to the 'violence of the impact of world events on the individual analyst'.[52] In the introduction Jung writes of the need to know that 'your worst enemy is right there in your own heart'.[53] Elsewhere, Jung was writing, also in 1946, of the shadow as 'the thing a person has no wish to be' and yet, somehow, is.[54] One could go on to say, as Jung did, that for anything or anyone to have substance and worth, he, she or it would have to possess a shadow.

It is my belief that *Essays on Contemporary Events* represents some sort of attempt on Jung's part to rehabilitate himself. However, I know from talking with many Jungian analysts that the question of an explicit expression of regret by Jung, in a clear, substantial and published form, is a very painful issue.

There is little doubt that Jung minded very much that his reputation and standing had been undermined by what he said and did in the 1930s. Recently available correspondence between Jung and his American supporters between 1947 and 1950 show Jung more-or-less orchestrating a concerted campaign to clear his name. Not for the first time, any notion that Jung could rise 'above' such things as personal reputation has to be dispelled.[55]

Once again, I must part company with Adolf Guggenbühl-Craig. His idealization of Jung is revealed when he asserts that Jung, as a 'genius', '*let* himself be drawn into the collective madness' (emphasis added). I think he was *drawn in,* he did not decide to do it, any more than analysts *decide* to let their patients affect them. Then he failed to comprehend his 'countertransference'.

Certain of Jung's ideas can themselves be explained and clarified and hence made less objectionable. For instance, when he writes that the Jews have no cultural forms of their own, he obviously cannot mean that they have no culture at all. The remark about the Aryan unconscious having a higher potential than the Jewish unconscious can be taken in two ways. The alarming way is to hear Jung as saying that Aryans can go higher and further than Jews. The more reassuring way is to hear Jung as saying that Aryans have a long, long way to go before they reach the level that Jews have reached. But, as Jewish civilization is so much older, Jews may have already fulfilled much of their cultural potential. Is Jung suggesting that we should not expect all that much more from them? Reassurance tips back into alarm.

Finally, there is the question of forgiveness. In 1946, Jung managed to convince Leo Baeck of his bona fides. Baeck, in turn, convinced Gershom Scholem to attend the Eranos conference in 1947 and accept a collegial relation to Jung; the conference was on Jewish mysticism.

Jung and the psychology of the nation

I will argue that the main difficulty with Jung's work in the general area of national psychology is an unwarranted expansion of his psychology, and hence his authority as a leading psychologist, into complicated fields where psychology on its own is an inadequate explanatory tool, especially concepts like the 'collective unconscious'.

To handle the obvious fact of cultural differences in the forms the archetypes of the collective unconscious assume, Jung asserted that there is a 'collective psyche limited to race, tribe, and family over and above the "universal" collective psyche'.[56] This concept of a restrictedly collective level of psyche is depicted in Jolande Jacobi's book *The Psychology of C. G. Jung,* published in 1942 with Jung's express approval, by a 'psychic genealogical tree' (see *Figure 10.1*).

She describes the diagram as follows:

> At the very bottom lies the unfathomable, the central force out of which at one time the individual psyche has been differentiated. This central force goes through all further differentiations and isolations, lives in them all, cuts through them to the individual psyche.

Resting upon this 'unfathomable ground', Jacobi arranges different strata; there are eight in all, arranged like the layers of a cake: the central force, animal ancestors, primitive human ancestors, groups of people, nation, tribe, family, individual. Though Jacobi does not use the word 'race', it is clear from the text as well as from Jung's remarks quoted above that this is what is meant by 'groups of people' (also referred to in the English translation as 'human groups' and in a later, post-war edition as 'ethnic groups' – in the German original, it is *Volksgruppe*).[57]

The hypothesis of a racial layer in Jung's model of the collective psyche has caused as great a furore as his alleged anti-semitism. As a result, a serious charge of racism has been levelled against him and against his psychology. According to most modern definitions, racism involves dividing humankind into distinct and hierarchically gradeable groups on the basis of biological or quasibiological characteristics. A racist is therefore someone who believes that people of a particular race, color or origin are inherently inferior, so that their identity, culture, self-esteem,

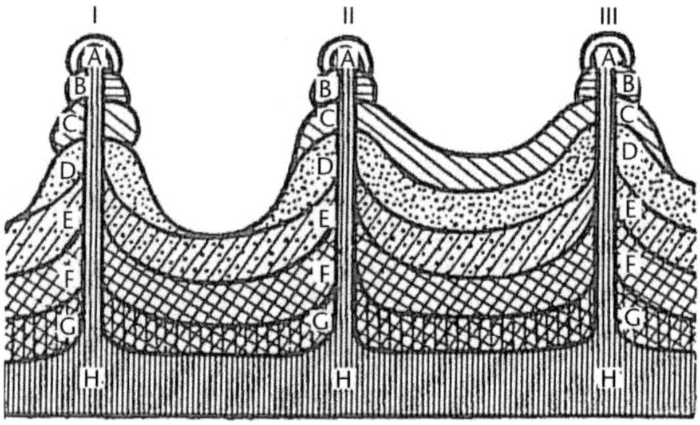

I. Single Nations
II and III. Groups of Nations (e.g., Europe)

A. Individual
B. Family
C. Tribe
D.Nation
E. Groups of People
F. Primitive Human Ancestors
G.Animal Ancestors
H.Central Force

Figure 10.1 Jacobi's 'psychic genealogical tree'

Source: Diagram from Jolande Jacobi, *The Psychology of C. G. Jung* (New Haven: Yale University Press, 1973), diagram XI, p. 34. Copyright @ 1973 by Yale University Press. Reprinted by permission of Yale University Press.

views and feelings are of less value and may be treated as less important than those of the groups believed to be superior.[58]

We have to ask: Does Jung's idea of a racial layer of the psyche conform to this definition?

In a paper entitled 'Jung: A racist', Farhad Dalal thoroughly surveyed Jung's writings, especially on Africa and Africans.[59] He concluded that Jung was indeed a racist in that he thought that blacks were inferior and not just different. Dalal understood Jung to be saying that Africans lack a complete layer of consciousness altogether, that whites are inherently less 'primitive' and that therefore individuation is reserved for them alone, and that it is methodologically correct to use modern Africans to exemplify the psychologist's assertions about the prehistoric human.

Reviewing now the whole question of Jung's racism, I am conscious of an opportunity lost, not only by me in my reply to Dalal,[60] but by Jung himself. As so often with Jung, it is the intuitive cast of his thought which causes the difficulty. Jung's psychological intuitions about the malaise in Western culture were important, but his thinking was handicapped by the means he had available for the communication of his intuitive insights. I certainly do not mean to join in knee-jerk defences of Jung here, but we should recognize that, alongside the unfortunate excursions into racial typology, we can also discern the seeds of a surprisingly modern and constructive attitude to race and ethnicity. For example, in 1935 Jung argued against the imposition of 'the spirit' of one race upon another, referring to a Eurocentric, judgmental approach to other cultures.[61] Here and elsewhere in Jung's writings, there is also a respect for and interest in the evolution of different cultures.

But it is clear that something goes very wrong with Jung's thought when he goes beyond the boundaries of psychology into what has been termed *racial typology*. When Jung's African stays an imaginal African, the African of dreams, or when Jung studies African myth, he makes a creative though politically limited contribution to social thought. But when Jung generalizes about African *character*, and does so from a solely psychological point of view, ignoring economic, social, political and historical factors, then he spoils his own work, inviting the severe criticism he has received. This literalism also plagues his comments about Jews in the 1930s, when the political reality of Jung's own position broke down any possibility of his 'Jews' being safely metaphorical.

What was it that led Jung to spoil his own work, leaving him open to the charge that his theories resemble Nazi ideology? When Jung ceases to serve the psyche and finds a new lodestar in the politics of psychotherapy in Germany, he can scarcely avoid being linked to the Nazis and castigated as an anti-semite. We have to look beyond the general danger of a racial psychology to find an explanation of Jung's behaviour and attitudes in the 1930s. *It is far too vague and facile a conclusion to advance Jung's own racism as the linkage between analytical psychology and Nazi ideology.* There is more in Hitler's theorizing that resembles Jung's than its undeniably racist element. There is also a comprehensive political and historical theory that is hard to disentangle from the racial ideas. The political dogma also uses a *nationalistic* vocabulary and focuses on the idea of the nation.

The key questions that require answers are these: Why did Jung get involved with German political affairs *in the way he did*? Why did he feel *obliged* to publish his thoughts on 'Jewish psychology' at such a sensitive moment? Was there anything in the *structure* of his work that made his active involvement an inevitability? Simply to dismiss Jung as a racist does not help us to address these issues. If we want to know more about Jung, the Nazis, and anti-semitism, then, without in any way minimizing the question of Jung's racism, we have to explore the idea of the nation as it appeared not only in National Socialism, but also in analytical psychology.

Look again at the layers in Jacobi's diagram. Notice that at layer D, 'nation', a quality change has come into the diagram. The introduction of the idea of the nation leads inevitably to the introduction of economic, social, political and historic factors. For the 'national level' of the psyche, unlike levels such as those of the 'animal ancestors', involves an economic, social, political and historical construct of relatively modern origin: the nation. I hope it becomes clearer why I stress that 'race' is too general a theme to serve as an overarching backdrop to the drama which has engulfed Jung. When we look a little more closely at Jung's not-absolutely-collective layer of the collective unconscious, we find that it is not 'race', not 'tribe', and not 'family' that engage Jung, but *nation*. Jung makes numerous references to the 'psychology of the nation' and to the influence of a person's national background, saying that the 'soil of every country holds [a] mystery . . . there is a relationship of body to earth'.[62]

When Jung wrote about America and the Americans in 1918, he introduced the idea that the land in or on which an individual lived influenced the psyche and the psychological development of that individual. 'The mystery of the American earth' was so powerful that, according to him, it had even changed the physiognomy of the citizens. The skull and pelvis measurements of second-generation Americans were becoming 'indianized'.[63] Consideration of this absurd idea shows that Jung is not thinking solely along racial lines, for the immigrants from Europe and the indigenous Indians come from *different* races. No – living in America, living on American soil, *being part of the American nation* all exert profound psychological and, according to Jung, physiological effects. Though the effects may be described along roughly racial lines, they have not been caused by race; it is 'the foreign land' that has 'assimilated the conqueror'.[64] Mary Loomis, a contemporary American Jungian analyst, has written in similar terms about 'the phenomenon of the Native American influence on the psyche' of Americans of European (and presumably African) descent.[65]

There is an important case that Jung wrote about in 1937, a significant date considering the topic of this chapter. A young woman from Europe had been born in Java. As an infant she had a local woman as an *ayah* (which Jung takes to mean a wet-nurse, though the term often describes a nanny). The patient returned to Europe to go to school and quite forgot her childhood, including her one-time fluency in Malay. During the analysis, the patient's dreams included imagery of a marked Indonesian kind. Jung claimed that 'tantric philosophy' (which he read while writing the case up) was most helpful in understanding his patient's dynamics. At one point in the case history, Jung comments that the patient had 'sucked in the local demonology with the *ayah's* milk'.[66] Here again, the argument is not based on race but on the idea that 'earth and native culture constitute the matrix from which we evolve', to use Loomis's words. For Jung, earth plus culture equals nation.

In my view, Jung's account of the relations between a nation and the individuals who are part of it is simplistic. For example, he frequently asserts that 'nations are made up of individuals'[67] or that 'the psychology of the individual is reflected in the psychology of the nation'.[68] Statements like these form the basis for Jung's argument that there is a 'psychology of the nation'.

However, as early as 1921, the writer and critic Robert Musil had pointed out that the idea that 'the will of the nation does not represent the sum of its individuals is nothing new . . . it has been an often-discussed and carefully investigated subject'.[69] In the same paper, entitled '"Nation" as ideal and as reality', Musil makes the observation that what happens is that a style of thinking suitable for addressing an invariant category (such as race) is employed in an unsuitable context of speculation about a highly variable social construct (such as nation).[70] Though 'race' is itself also a culturally constructed category, it is clear what Musil is getting at and we can see the relevance of his point for Jung's thought about national psychology. To the extent that race implies, or has come to mean, something biologically determined, it must be distinguished from concepts such as 'nation'. For, on the level of nation, there are no equivalents to the existence of genetically determined features of race (for example, colour of the skin). Once again, reviewing Musil's ideas, we can see that Jung was not merely 'a man of his time' whom it is silly to contradict with the benefit of hindsight; other thinkers held other views at the time.

Furthermore, nationalism has as its social and political functions the *overriding* of individual distinctions, often including the overriding of so-called racial differences within a single state. Far from being a phenomenon that is somehow secondary to the individual, the nation sets its stamp on her or him through its ideology and power structures – a closely textured web of assumptions about society and the individual's place in it, about morality (what Durkheim called 'collective conscience'), about the rules and concepts of behaviour, about politics, about life itself. Although nationalism requires the equation of state and people, the one is not 'made up' of the other and to say that they are is to fall victim to false consciousness. Of course, we should not forget that defining the differences between 'nation', 'state' and 'people' is still a thorny problem. Germany's divided condition used to be referred to as 'two states, one nation'.

The modern version of 'nation' stems from the late eighteenth and early nineteenth centuries. The idea gradually arose that nationality was a natural possession of everyone and that a person could only participate in civic and political life as part of a nation. It has been argued that it was only when large-scale colonization produced encounters on a mass level with other cultures and colours that the idea of nation came into being – the 'Other' defined the 'Self' as a nation.[71] Just as political allegiance had hitherto not been determined by nationality, so civilization had not been regarded as nationally defined. During the Middle Ages, civilization defined itself religiously and, in the Renaissance and Enlightenment periods, the classical cultures of Greece and Rome became the yardsticks. When civilization started to be defined on the basis of nationality, it was felt for the first time that people should be educated in their own mother tongue, not in the language of other civilizations. Poets and scholars began to emphasize cultural nationalism. They reformed the national language, elevated it to literary status and celebrated the traditional past of their native culture for nationalist ends.

The German nation, as a cultural and political phenomenon, did not exist in these terms before the rise of Prussia at the end of the eighteenth century. German cultural nationalism has been portrayed as stressing instinct over reason, the power of historical tradition over modernization and democracy, the historical differences between nations over their common aspirations.[72] If we analyze typical nationalist ideology (Germany being only one example), we find that much more is involved than emphasis on the geographical unit. We also find an emphasis on some kind of ethical principle, or at least ethical expression, and this is usually couched in comparative (and self-congratulatory) terms: our soldiers are the bravest, the quality of our family life is the finest, we have the best constitution or royal family, we have a special relationship to higher forces, our articles of manufacture are of the highest quality, our upper lips are the stiffest. In other words, *nationalism always involves a form of psychological expression and self-characterization. It follows, therefore, that nationalism elicits the services of psychologists,* who can readily succumb to the notion that this particular cultural project needs their help.

It is my contention that, in C. G. Jung, nationalism found its psychologist and that, in spite of his theoretical concern with the racial unconscious, it is as a psychologist of nationhood that we should also understand Jung and his statements about political problems. He was a psychologist who lent his authority to nationalism, thereby legitimizing ideas of innate, psychological differences between nations. Jung's admittedly problematic pan-psychism,[73] the tendency to see all outer events in terms of inner, usually archetypal dynamics, the neglect in his writing of economic, social, political and historical factors, finds its most extreme reductive expression in the phrase 'the psychology of the nation'. Unfortunately, even among contemporary Jungian analysts, one finds direct echoes of Jung's contempt for everything that is not psychology: 'Nations constitute a powerful phenomenon and, like all important psychological phenomena, they cannot be explained; they can only be approached by mythological images', according to Adolf Guggenbühl-Craig writing in 1991.[74] He goes on to make the following claim, which I see as typical of the arrogant psychological reductionism that ruined Jung's attempts to bring depth psychology to bear on the events of his day: 'All the other explanations, based on economics and sociology, look impoverished compared with the tremendous mythological images by which Jung approached National Socialism.'[75] I regret such statements for they make the much-needed interdisciplinary work on culture, society and politics harder to organize.

With these insights in mind, Jung's offensive generalizations about Jews can be understood more profoundly. There are hardly any references to 'Aryans' in Jung's *Collected Works*. But there are numerous references to Germany and, indeed, to most of the countries of the world. There are also frequent uses of the term 'Germanic', and at first glance it might seem that Jung has made the important distinction between Germany the nation state and Germanic culture, an identifiable, communal and ethnic tradition established over a very long time, to which Jung was committed because it was his chief cultural source. Had Jung consistently made this distinction, we would be able to distinguish clearly the racial from the nationalistic trends in his thought.

Unhappily, the situation is extremely confused and this confusion cannot all be laid at the door of Jung's English translator. In the index to Volume 10 of the *Gesammelte Werke,* under '*Germanisch*', we find '*s. auch Deutschland*'. In 'Wotan', which is the piece of Jung's where the distinction is probably most needed, we find a sentence which has been correctly translated in the following manner: 'Wotan is a *Germanic* datum of first importance, the truest expression and unsurpassed personification of a fundamental quality that is particularly characteristic of the *Germans.*'[76] Later in the same text we find a reference to 'the Germans who were adults in 1914', so it does seem that Jung had a specific historical and geographical entity in mind when he writes of Germans and Germany. At one point, Jung even refers to himself as a 'Germanic', if we attend to the German-language original![77] But, after the war (and even before it), Jung often recalled that he was Swiss, in contradistinction to being German. It follows that modern nations were very much in his mind, as well as large-scale supranational cultural groupings.

Sensing and recasting Jung as the psychologist of nations does not do away with the problem of his racism. But I suggest that his nationalism is the more important factor in understanding the theoretical overlap which occurs, often at a feeling as much as at a thinking level, between Jung and those Nazis whom he so often asserted did not have his political support and whom, in common with other citizens of Western democracies, he came to fear and hate without reservation.

Jung got into trouble less because of Nazi politics than because of his attempt to write a psychology of nations. We have already seen how complex are the historical, economic, political and cultural forces which go into the development of a nation and its nationalism. Jung's mistake was to expand his role as a psychologist to the point where he could seem to regard the nation as an exclusively psychological fact to be observed solely from a psychological point of view. Jung's uncritical psychologizing is illustrated in his favourable response to Count Hermann Keyserling's somewhat eccentric books, two of which he reviewed in the 1920s and 1930s. In these popular works, Keyserling opined that each nation has a definite psychological character and that each contributes one feature to a sort of world personality. In one of these reviews Jung writes that 'the "nation" (like the "state") is a personified concept that corresponds in reality only to a specific nuance of the individual psyche . . . [The nation] is nothing but an inborn character.'[78]

Jung was influenced by C. G. Carus, the German Romantic philosopher of the early nineteenth century, who thought that the relation of the passage of the sun to any given area influenced the character of those living there. According to Carus, one of the first formulators of the idea of the unconscious, new inhabitants of a geographical area acquire the characteristics of its previous, unrelated inhabitants. By this hypothesis, possession of land, central to nationhood, is elevated to a mystical level. Here I would say that Jung followed Carus rather closely, as in his remarks about the 'mystery' to be found in a country's soil. The Germans, according to Carus, acquire and recapitulate the development and achievements of the Caucasians, Persians, Armenians, Semites (sic), Pelasgians, Etruscans, Thracians, Illyrians, Iberians, Romans and Celts. Carus is not advancing a racial theory, for literal biology plays little part in his formulations. For Carus, even though he was a philosopher, and for his follower Jung, the concern is with psychology, not biology.

But Jung went so far in this direction that his ideas about national psychology degenerate into nothing more than a glib typology. His method is to assemble lists of complementary characteristics to serve as stepping stones toward a definition, whether of German or of Jew – exactly the same method that he used to define the psychological attributes of the two sexes.[79] The emphasis is on what a Jew *is,* rather than on what being a Jew is like. Jung's focus is on the predefining of difference via a classification by characteristics. He does not say much about the experience or living out of difference. Just as with the sexes, we find Jung promoting the ethos of complementarity so that any two opposite lists can be combined to produce an absolutely wonderful sounding 'wholeness'. Jew and German seem to constitute two halves of a whole: rational, sophisticated, erudite city-dweller complementing irrational, energetic, earthy peasant-warrior. This fantasy of 'opposites' is presented as something factual, as if revealed by an empirical, psychological method. At no point does Jung admit to being part of a myth-making process, nor does he claim a metaphorical intent, though it is convenient nowadays to claim that Jung's writings on nations were just 'fantasy' and hence only part of his stock-in-trade as a psychologist.

But is what Jung writes really psychology, or is it the use of psychological terminology and Jung's authority as a leading psychologist to convert anecdote, prejudice and desire into definitory, typological statements? I shall return to that question at the end of the next chapter but for now I'd like to ask my readers to hold the idea of Jung as a psychologist of nations in their minds for a while so that I can turn my attention to certain relevant aspects of the political theories of Adolf Hitler. Remember, up to now we have been discussing the hypertrophy of psychology, *its* expansionism, *its* search for *Lebensraum,* 'living space'.

Notes

1 Litvinoff, E. (2008) *Journey Through a Small Planet.* Harmondsworth: Penguin.
2 Adolf Guggenbühl-Craig, 'Jung and anti-semitism'. In Mary Ann Mattoon (ed.), *Personal and Archetypal Dynamics in the Analytical Relationship* (Einsiedeln, Switzerland: Daimon, 1991, p. 495). As the chapter progresses, the reader will become aware of the differences of opinion between Adolf Guggenbühl-Craig and myself.
3 See Reuven Bulka, Editorial, *Journal of Psychology and Judaism,* 6: 2 (1982).
4 See Christopher Hampton, 'George Steiner's *The Portage to San Cristobal of A.H.*' (London: Faber, 1983), pp. 67–84 for a disgustingly inventive depiction of the common processes of Jews and Nazis.
5 For example, Aniela Jaffé, 'C. G. Jung and National Socialism'. In Aniela Jaffé, *Jung's Last Years* (Dallas, TX: Spring Publications, 1971); Geoffrey Cocks, *Psychotherapy in the Third Reich: The Goring Institute* (London and New York: Oxford University Press, 1985).
6 For example, Robert Haymond, 'On Carl Gustav Jung: Psycho-social basis of morality during the Nazi era'. *Journal of Psychology and Judaism,* 6: 2 (1982); Paul Stem, C. G. *Jung: The Haunted Prophet* (New York: Braziller, 1976).
7 For example, Ernest Harms, 'Carl Gustav Jung - defender of Freud and the Jews: A chapter of European psychiatric history under the Nazi yoke'. *Psychiatric Quarterly,* April 1946; James Kirsch, 'Carl Gustav Jung and the Jews'. *Journal of Psychology and Judaism,* 6: 2 (1982).
8 Wolfgang Giegerich, 'Postscript to Cocks'. *Spring,* 1979.
9 I would like to thank Ann Casement for her help in obtaining this material.
10 Eli Weisstub, personal communication, 1990.
11 Geoffrey Cocks, *Psychotherapy in the Third Reich,* p. 129.
12 C. G. Jung, *C. G. Jung Speaking.* Ed. William McGuire (London: Thames and Hudson, 1978), pp. 773–9.
13 C. G. Jung, 'The state of psychotherapy today'. *CW* 10: 354. *CW* refers to the *Collected Works* of C. G. Jung, ed. Herbert Read, Michael Fordham and Gerhard Adler, Trans. R. F. C. Hull (London: Routledge and Kegan Paul; Princeton, NJ: Princeton University Press, 1953–77). References, save where indicated, are by volume and paragraph number.
14 C. G. Jung, *Two Essays on Analytical Psychology. CW* 7: 240n.
15 See *CW* 10: 1014.
16 Published in *International Review of Psycho-Analysis,* 4: 3 (1977).
17 C. G. Jung, 'The role of the unconscious'. *CW* 10: 18.
18 C. G. Jung, *Letters.* Ed. Gerhard Adler (London, Routledge and Kegan Paul, 1973).
19 Sigmund Freud and Karl Abraham, *A Psycho-Analytic Dialogue: The Letters of Sigmund Freud and Karl Abraham 1907–1926* (New York: Basic Books, 1965).
20 Quoted in Ernest Jones, *The Life and Work of Sigmund Freud* (New York: Basic Books, 1955), vol. 2, p. 149.
21 Adolf Guggenbühl-Craig, 'Jung and anti-semitism', p. 495.
22 See Sarah Gordon, *Hitler, Germans and the 'Jewish Question'* (Princeton, NJ: Princeton University Press, 1984).
23 *The Times,* November 13, 1988.

24 See Gustav Bally, 'Deutschstlimmige Psychotherapie?' *Neue Zurcher Zeitung, 343* (1934).
25 I am grateful to Sonu Shamdasani for showing me the relevant Harvard *Crimson.*
26 Gershom Scholem (ed.), *The Correspondence of Walter Benjamin and Gershom Scholem 1932–1940* (New York: Schocken, 1989), pp. 197, 203.
27 See D. W Winnicott, *The Spontaneous Gesture: Selected Letters,* Ed. F. Robert Rodman (Cambridge, MA: Harvard University Press, 1987), p. 4.
28 The story is told most memorably in Aniela Jaffé, 'C. G. Jung and National Socialism'.
29 Quoted in James Kirsch, 'Carl Gustav Jung and the Jews', p. 117.
30 C. G. Jung, *Letters,* vol. 1, p. 238. I am indebted to John Beebe for pointing out this letter and for the information about Victor Frankl.
31 *Zentralblatt für Psychotherapie,* 7: 3 (1934). The GMSP was not formally incorporated until 1928.
32 Geoffrey Cocks, *Psychotherapy in the Third Reich,* p. 46.
33 C. G. Jung, 'The significance of the father in the destiny of the individual'. *CW* 4; Robert Sommer, *Familienforschung, Vererbungs- und Rassenlehre,* 3rd edition ('Dritte durch Rassen- und Stammeslehre vermehrte Ausgabe') (Leipzig: Barth, 1927). The new chapter was entitled 'Raceology and racial history' (pp. 399).
34 See Robert Jay Lifton, *The Nazi Doctors: Medical Killing and the Psychology of Genocide* (New York: Basic Books, 1986). I am deeply indebted to Gottfried Heuer for following up the matter of Sommer, deciding to obtain the second edition of his book, and making the translations that follow. Matthias von der Tann also provided background information for which I am thankful.
35 See C. G. Jung, *Letters,* p. 156; William McGuire (ed.), *The Freud/Jung Letters* (London: Hogarth and Routledge and Kegan Paul, 1974), pp. 13, 38, 126, 166.
36 *Zentralblatt für Psychotherapie, 12*: 3 (1940).
37 *Zentralblatt für Psychotherapie, 11*: 3 (1939). I am grateful to Matthias von der Tann for alerting me to the existence of this piece.
38 See Geoffrey Cocks, *Psychotherapy in the Third Reich,* pp. 46–7. In his book, Cocks paints a picture of the GMSP as being concerned from its beginnings with the 'spiritual' dimension, anti-Freudian, and part of a particular kind of German Protestant movement within the professions. This is important because it contradicts the idea that the GMSP was some kind of consensual umbrella body. In the debates which always characterize the field of psychotherapy, the GMSP was most certainly *parti pris* (see Cocks, pp. 47–9).
39 In Karen Brecht, Volker Friedrich, Ludger M. Hermanns, Isidor J. Kaminer and Dierek H. Juelich (eds.), '*Hier geht das Leben auf eine sehr merkwürdige Weise weiter . . . ':Zur Geschichte der Psychoanalyse in Deutschland* (Hamburg: Kellner, 1985). Published on the occasion of the 34th Congress of the International Psychoanalytic Association held in Hamburg in 1985. This was the first Congress held in Germany since the Holocaust. Gottfried Heuer translates the title as 'Here life continues in a rather strange way'. My thanks to him for providing and translating this material. Jung was definitely present at the meeting in Bad Nauheim in 1934 because his Presidential Address is summarized in the *Zentralblatt für Psychotherapie,* 7: 3 (1934). The Editors of the *Collected Works* believe Jung's address to have been republished as a paper entitled 'Contribution to a discussion on psychotherapy' (in *CW* 10: 1060ff.).
40 Jakob Wilhelm Hauer, Karl Heim and Karl Adam, *Germany's New Religion: The German Faith Movement.* Trans. Scott-Craig and Davies (London: Allen and Unwin, 1937), pp. 18–19, 28–9, 55. I am grateful to Sonu Shamdasani for providing this material.
41 The passage I mention may be found in *CW* 10: 397–8. See William McGuire, *Bollingen: An Adventure in Collecting the Past* (Princeton, NJ: Princeton University Press, 2nd edition, 1989), pp. 26, 39, 46. I think McGuire is wrong to summarize (on p. 26) that 'Jung criticized Hauer in his essay "Wotan"'.
42 Geoffrey Cocks, *Psychotherapy in the Third Reich,* p. 134.
43 Gerhard Adler, Gustav Dreifuss, James Kirsch, personal communications 1977–91.
44 Sandor Gilman, personal conununication, 1992.
45 Michael Fordham, unpublished autobiography.
46 Jung was supposed to have said this to Mary Foote who repeated it to others and put it in her diary. This is the only time in these chapters on Jung and anti-semitism where

I adduce unsubstantiated anecdote. Every other reference is fully sourced or was a direct personal communication.

47 I am grateful to the Jung Estate for permission to publish extracts from this letter and to William McGuire for providing me with a copy of it.

48 See Aryeh Maidenbaum, 'Report from New York'. In Mary Ann Mattoon (ed.), *Personal and Archetypal Dynamics*, pp. 468–70. 48 C. G. Jung, 'A rejoinder to Dr Bally'. CW 10: 1025–8.

49 C. G. Jung, *Letters*, p. 161.

50 Under my editorship, *Essays on Contemporary Events* was reassembled and republished in the *Collected Works* translation of the various constituent pieces (London: Routledge; Princeton, NJ: Princeton University Press, 1988).

51 C. G. Jung, *Essays*, p. xv.

52 C. G. Jung, *Essays*, p. 8.

53 CW 16: 470.

54 Sonu Shamdasani has provided me with copies of numerous letters between Jung and his supporters, and between various supporters, as they put together a public relations campaign to protect his name in the United States. I am grateful to Sonu Shamdasani for sight of this archival material.

55 Adolf Guggenbühl-Craig, 'Jung and anti-semitism', p. 497.

56 C. G. Jung, *The Relations between the Ego and the Unconscious*. CW 7: 235.

57 Jolande Jacobi, *The Psychology of C. G. Jung* (London: Kegan Paul, Trench, Trubner, 1942), p. 33.

58 For example, Ellis Cashmore, *A Dictionary of Race and Ethnic Relations* (London: Routledge, 1984). Also British Government reports such as the Swann Report and the Rampton Report.

59 Farhad Dalal, 'Jung: A racist'. *British Journal of Psychotherapy*, 4: 3, 1988.

60 Andrew Samuels, Reply to Farhad Dalal, 'Jung: A racist'.

61 C. G. Jung, CW *10:* 240n.

62 C. G. Jung, 'The role of the unconscious'. CW 10: 19.

63 Ibid., para. 18.

64 C. G. Jung, 'Mind and earth'. CW 10: 103. Written in 1927.

65 Mary Loomis, 'Balancing the shields: Native American teaching and the individuation process'. *Quadrant*, *21*: 2 (1988).

66 C. G. Jung, 'The realities of practical psychotherapy'. CW 16: 557ff.

67 CW 10: 45.

68 CW 7, p. 4.

69 Robert Musil, '"Nation" as ideal and as reality'. In Burton Pike and David Luft (eds.), *Precision and Soul: Essays and Addresses by Robert Musil* (Chicago, IL: Chicago University Press, 1990), p. 105.

70 Ibid., p. 106.

71 Martin Banton, *The Idea of Race* (London: Tavistock, 1977), p. 13.

72 Henry Kohn, *The Idea of Nationalism* (Oxford: Oxford University Press, 1967).

73 CW 8: 29.

74 Adolf Guggenbühl-Craig, 'Jung and anti-semitism', p. 496.

75 Ibid., p. 497.

76 CW 10: 389, emphasis added.

77 Matthias von der Tann, personal communication, 1989.

78 CW 10: 921.

79 See Andrew Samuels, *The Plural Psyche: Personality, Morality and the Father* (London and New York: Routledge, 1989), pp. 107–22.

CHAPTER 11

NATIONS, LEADERS AND A PSYCHOLOGY OF DIFFERENCE

Retrospective introduction

I don't have much to add the the retrospective introduction to the previous chapter because it is so linked to this one. But I will take the liberty of reproducing here the concluding lines of this chapter in order to make it clear that these matters are of the greatest importance for me and working through them was necessary if I was to stay honest and also make any contribution to thinking about political and social crises.

> My hope is that finding echoes of Jung in Hitler and Hitler in Jung, emotionally wearing though it is, will lead to a decision to try to make a contribution to a contemporary political celebration of difference.
>
> Then depth psychology can joyfully renounce the top table, the level of nation states – for we have seen what a terrible mess it makes when it tries to sit there. But depth psychologists do not need to retreat behind the barricade of 'the clinical'. Depth psychologists can simultaneously go on with an analysis of politics. To do it, I think they need to stand up with the materially disadvantaged and the socially frightened, as well as sit down with educated analysands. They should be engaged when a Law of Return is passed and small ethnic groups gain or regain their lands; hence, they should be engaged when an intifada erupts. They should be concerned with promised lands, as well as with sovereign nation states; with the people as well as with their leaders.
>
> Clinicians may have to question the milieux in which many of them work, for private practice with a privileged clientele is not politically neutral. This mode of working has affected depth psychological thinking. Clinicians may have to question their automatic preference for the inner world and this tendency to make 'inner' and 'outer' or 'private' and 'public' into polar opposites, rejecting multidisciplinary work as 'un-analytical'. As we saw, all images can be read politically.
>
> Before the war, Hitler proclaimed all German modern art to be 'decadent'. Officially approved realistic art was sponsored. Two exhibitions were organized – one of the degenerate and one of the official art. The degenerate exhibition was viewed by two million people, still the world record for any single art exhibition, whereas less than four hundred thousand attended the official exhibition.[39]

In these last two chapters, I have exhibited the decadent and degenerate side of analytical psychology. This has been a cautionary tale for depth psychologists who seek to analyze politics and culture. I tried to show that it was Jung's attempt to establish a culturally sensitive psychology of nations that brought him into the same frame as Nazi anti-semitic ideology. In addition, Jung was absorbed by the question of leadership. Exploring these ideas as thoroughly as possible leads to a kind of reparation, for I think that post-Jungians do have reparation to make. Then it is possible to revalue in more positive terms Jung's overall project. We must couple a less simplistic methodology and a more sensitive set of political values to Jung's intuitions about the centrality of a psychology of cultural difference. If we do so, then analytical psychology has something to offer a depth psychology that is concerned with processes of political and cultural transformation.

Jung, Hitler and the psychology of the nation

It is interesting to note that Hitler did not regard Germany as being composed purely of 'Aryans'. Rather, he hoped to increase the Aryan proportion of the population through genetic selection, deportation and extermination. As I mentioned earlier, throughout Hitler's writings it is clear that there is a pronounced nationalistic as well as a racial component in his thinking. (This is also true of nineteenth- and twentieth-century anti-semitism in general, as the Dreyfus affair showed.[1])

Re-reading Hitler confronts us with a coldly paranoid logic. Hitler regarded all history as consisting of struggles between competing nations for living space and, ultimately, for world domination. The Jews, according to Hitler (who got it from Lueger), are a nation and participate in these struggles with the principal goal of world domination. Hitler thought that this was because the Jews did not possess living space, an identifiable, geographical locality. Therefore, it is the world or nothing for them. In fact, for Hitler, the nationalism of the Jews is 'denationalization, the inter-bastardization of other nations'.[2] The Jewish nation achieves its goal of world domination by denationalizing existing states from within and imposing a homogeneous 'Jewish' character on them – for instance, by its *international* capitalism and by its equally *international* communism. So, in Hitler's thinking, there is a tussle between wholesome nationhood and its corrupting enemy, the Jews. (The question of the nationhood of the Jews is still a pressing problem, especially in the context of Middle Eastern politics, as my Israeli colleague Gustav Dreifuss has reminded me.[3])

Thus, a crucial aspect of *Hitler's* thinking is that the Jews represent a threat to the inevitable and healthy struggle of different nations for world domination. There is an uncomfortable echo to Hitler in *Jung's* view that each nation has a different and identifiable national psychology of its own that is, in some mysterious manner, an innate factor. Merely to juxtapose these two points of view would be distasteful and it is certainly not my intention to make a straightforward comparison of Hitler and Jung, nor to suggest that Hitler influenced Jung. But if we go on to explore *the place of the Jews in Jung's mental ecology*, to try to find out where they are situated in his perspective on the world, then we have to ask whether there is a similarity in the underlying structure of the assumptions about nations, history and culture in these two views. Readers will recall that my intention has been to see whether there is anything in Jung's thinking about the Jews that must lead him to anti-semitism, perhaps forcing honest women and men to give up their interest in analytical psychology.

My perception is that the ideas of nation and of national difference form an interface between the Hitlerian phenomenon and Jung's psychological approach to culture. For, as the psychologist of nations, Jung's theorizing was threatened by the existence of the Jews, this strange nation without land and, hence, in Jung's words of 1918, lacking a chthonic quality, a good relation to the earth.[4] Jung's whole approach to the psychology of the nation was threatened by this nation without cultural forms – that is, without *national* cultural forms – of its own, and hence, in Jung's words of 1933, requiring a 'host nation'.[5]

What threatens Jung in particular can be discovered by inquiring closely into what he means when he describes, as he often does, 'Jewish psychology'. His use of the term is dramatically inconsistent.

First, there is Jewish psychology defined as the typical psychological characteristics to be found in a typical Jewish person and not found in a typical member of another ethnic or racial group. Jung argues that everyone is affected by his or her background and that this leads to all kinds of prejudices and assumptions: 'Every child knows that differences exist.'[6] One can disagree or agree with Jung's views on what the psychology of Jews is like; I have already said that I do not consider such views to be psychological in a professional sense. The observation that there are differences in cultural tradition is not the same as the assertion that there are differences in the actual process of psychological functioning and I do not think Jung manages to validate the latter assertion.

Jung's second use of this term 'Jewish psychology' has a different and even more provocative implication. Here he is referring to systems of psychology developed by Jews like Freud and Adler, systems that claim universal applicability and truth. Such a psychology is a 'levelling psychology' in that it undermines the idea of national differences.[7] Such a psychology has erred in applying 'Jewish categories . . . indiscriminately to German and Slavic Christendom'. We are tempted to make the 'unpardonable mistake [of] accepting the conclusions of a Jewish psychology as generally valid'.[8] It is not Freud's psychoanalysis that is the problem here but *Jewish* psychoanalysis – rather a different thing.

At this point, we have to bring in the fourth group in the drama that has surrounded Jung – Freudians – to add to the Nazis, the Jews and the Jungians. Is Jung saying that the theories of psychoanalysis reflect Jewish psychology, meaning typical Jewish character traits, as exemplified in Freud himself? If so, he surely goes far beyond his habitual position that all psychological theorizing is a 'subjective confession'. Even the prejudice-ridden personal friction between Jung and Freud, which undeniably existed, would not explain why, for Jung, this became his reading of the whole of psychoanalysis. It seems that, for Jung, with his current interest in national psychology, there is an extra ingredient: the Jews as a group, typified by Freudian psychoanalysis, represent a strain of *psychological* denationalization, levelling out all national psychological differences. Psychoanalysis therefore occupies a place in Jung's mind *analogous* to the place occupied in Hitler's mind by capitalism and communism. The great fears are, respectively, of 'levelling' and of 'denationalization'. Jung and Hitler react to the Jews in differing ways of course, but the levelling aim of Jewish psychology and the denationalizing aim of Jewish political and economic activity represent a similar threat to each of them. So each develops a similar theme.

For Hitler, it takes the form of an obsession with a Jewish 'spirit', functioning as a pestilential bacillus, undermining the very idea of nation. For Jung, it takes the form of a depiction of a Jewish psychology, capable of being imposed on all other ethnic groupings and, above all, on all other national psychologies. Jung was afraid that the Jews – Freud and Adler and their followers – would take over psychology, disregarding its rightful soil in German Romantic philosophy. This would be the inevitable cultural carpetbagging of a people without a national land or nationhood of their own.

Jung's ideas that psychoanalysis imposed itself on psychological differences and that this was a specifically Jewish psychological trait appear to have persisted to the end of his life. In 1955, he wrote to Dr Hans Illing that Freud was

> profoundly Jewish to the extent that he never submitted to a personal analysis, which does not prevent him from claiming that his psychoanalytical judgments are valid for everyone else. This corresponds exactly to the Jewish idea of God . . .

Jung's explanation is that there is a 'chosen people complex'.[9]

Jung's psychological expansionism can be seen as counterpointing Hitler's geopolitical expansionism. The former results from Jung's claim that psychology needed rescuing from the danger posed by 'Jewish psychology'. The latter results from Hitler's claim that Europe needed rescuing from the danger posed by Jewish communism or Jewish capitalism.

At one point Jung seems to have had a direct connection in mind between psychoanalysis (his worry) and communism (Hitler's worry). In 1919, in a letter to Sabina Spielrein not yet published in English but available in German, Jung castigates Freud and Lenin in the same sentence as 'disseminators of the rationalistic darkness which might yet extinguish the small lamps of reason'. Jung cannot understand why Spielrein is so upset at the death of Karl Liebknecht, the leader of the communist Spartakusbund in Germany, who, together with Rosa Luxemburg, was murdered in January 1919. Concerning the 'lamps of reason', Jung goes on to say that 'whoever betrays this light to power or cleverness will become a parasite (*Schädling*)'. We might want to ask what Jung has in mind when he writes of the *Schädling* in 1919.[10]

It is in this general area that we may understand the response of those who have picked up on the uncomfortable resonances in Jung's writings to something they have already learned to hate in Hitler. Only when we have understood the basis in the collective mind for the association of Hitler's thinking with Jung's can we begin to explicate the enormous divergences between them. Then we can restore the humanity to Jung's quite dissimilar cultural project.

Regarding the question of the possession of national land, I mentioned earlier that Jung's use of the phrase 'cultural forms' rather than 'culture' is significant. It can be seen that, for Jung, the missing elements in Jewish history and experience that would have made the emergence of Jewish cultural forms possible are those of nation and land. In a letter to C. E. Benda of 1934 he writes:

> Between culture and cultural form there is, as we know, an essential difference. The Swiss, for instance, as you rightly remark, are a people with a culture but no cultural form of their own. For this, you rightly remark, certain conditions are needed, such as the size of a people and its ties to the soil, etc . . . A people with no ties to the soil, having neither land nor homeland, is commonly called nomadic.[11]

Writing to James Kirsch in the same year, Jung once again emphasized the importance of land and nationhood to the creation of cultural forms by pointing out that

Jewish cultural forms might come into being in Palestine. Jung makes the interesting point in this letter that the Jews often become the carriers or even promoters of the culture in which they live, something that was certainly true of pre-war Germany.[12] However, I think many, including Aniella Jaffé, who has otherwise defended Jung, would agree that at this time he did not know enough about Jewish culture to make some of these assertions. Be that as it may, the issue here has been to clarify the nature of the threat the Jews present to Jung's conception of national psychological difference.

It is fascinating to report that Jung's and Hitler's differing but similar fears have, quite recently, entered the academic mainstream. In his book *Black Athena*, Martin Bernal argues that, contrary to conventional wisdom, classical Greek civilization has its deepest roots in Afroasiatic and Semitic cultures.[13] But these influences are usually ignored – according to Bernal – for racist reasons. What is more, Bernal undermines the claim that the Classical Greeks were originally 'Aryans' who moved down from the north. The Greeks, beloved of Freud, Jung, Neumann, Hillman et al., were, putting it crudely, African, Egyptian, Phoenician and Semitic.

From the other end of the intellectual spectrum, genetic researchers have managed to link everyone alive today to a fully human common ancestor – 'a woman who lived in Africa 100,000 to 300,000 years ago'. The theory is known as the 'Noah's Ark' theory. The report I have of this research concludes: 'Whether or not everyone descends from a recent African Eve . . ., [the] Noah's Ark theory suggests that all of today's races are closely related – so closely related that there can only be one 'superior' race: the human one.'[14]

Jung and leadership

I have criticized Jung for using his leadership and authority as a psychologist for non-psychological purposes. I used the words 'Jung's leadership' deliberately to raise the question of where Jung stood as a leader and in relation to the theory and practice of leadership. The whole subject of leadership, as already stated, forms the second overarching backdrop to my material.

That Jung had a desire for leadership and behaved like the leader of a movement is still a contentious claim to make within analytical psychology. Many Jungian analysts, recognizing Jung's exceptional gifts, try to put him beyond a power drive and, therefore, beyond the opportunism to which he is often accused of succumbing in his dealings with the Nazi establishment regulating psychotherapy in Germany in the 1930s. Yet if we look at Jung's earlier career, the part played by his own desire for power in bringing about the break with Freud is often underestimated (and here I *am* engaging psychologically with Jung the man). Jung himself was emphatic that, unlike Freud, he had no ambitions to be a leader and was not interested in forming a school of psychology, in actively spreading his ideas, or taking part in the training of analysts. In *Jung and the Post-Jungians*, I sought to show that Jung displayed many of the features of a typical leader: sometimes maintaining his rule by dividing his followers, selecting individuals for particular support (often by writing forewords for their books), and eventually laying down rather tough academic criteria for the professional training of analysts.[15] In 1935, Jung explicitly claimed Drs Kranefeldt, Heyer and Adler as 'members of my school'.[16] How can we reconcile this skillful dissemination of influence with Jung's claim to be a solitary thinker and his corollary exclamation, 'Thank God I'm Jung and not a Jungian'? Jung's denial that he participated in the making of Jungians is often repeated by those most closely associated with him. I think that Jung's technique was to flatter his followers by maintaining that he did not want disciples; therefore those involved with Jung could never have been mere disciples.

It can be argued that Jung succeeded in relegating his leadership ambitions to his shadow. If so, then we see a projection of something personal in Jung's interest in the *Führer.* But I want to contribute something more profound than the 'wild' assertion or psychological cheap shot that Hitler was Jung's shadow. After all, in what has been described as the 'decade of the dictators', it is certainly not simply a personal issue for Jung. The image of the dictator could fascinate him without its being a projection of unmet needs for recognition and dominance in depth psychology.

In the late 1930s Jung was a prime mover in efforts to unite the psychotherapies behind a common programme and he drew up a list of propositions concerning the theory and practice of psychotherapy.[17] These 'Fourteen Points', also known as 'Views Held in Common', were Jung's attempt to bring unity to depth psychology. We can see now that the seemingly inherent tendency of depth psychology to fragment into warring groups made this a forlorn hope, practically speaking. But we may well wonder at the idealistic and even arrogant aspects of the use of the political catchphrase dating from the time of the formation of the League of Nations to characterize this effort. Was this an attempt to make Jungian analysis the generic psychotherapy? We know that Jung wanted to be the dominant psychological theorist of the day. He regarded his approach to analysis as *subsuming* those of Adler and Freud (for instance, in his paper 'Problems of modern psychotherapy').[18] Any Jungian analysis would include the relevant features of an analysis of each of the other schools, although the vital final stage of analysis known as 'transformation' was said to be possible only in Jung's approach. Had the Fourteen Points caught on, Jung would have become the leading theorist of all psychotherapy.

Bearing these reflections in mind, we can turn our attention to Jung's comments about *political* leadership, for example in the famous interview by Dr Weizsacker on Radio Berlin in 1933. Jung told his listeners, using the key word *Führer,* that 'every great movement culminates in a leader'.[19] Even more interesting is Jung's opinion that the prerequisite for successful leadership is self-knowledge: 'If [the leader] doesn't know himself, how is he to lead others? That is why the true leader is always one who has the courage to be himself.'[20]

Matthias von der Tann has made a careful linguistic analysis of Jung's remarks in this interview.[21] It was only in 1987 that the full German text of the interview once again became available in the public domain, and an important result of von der Tann's research is to highlight how the English translation consistently mutes Jung's imagery, making his remarks altogether more statesmanlike and less inflammatory than they really were.[22] Von der Tann demonstrates that on many occasions Jung uses words and phrases that would have had a particular connotation for German listeners. These words and phrases echo Nazi ideology and propaganda and can be said to constitute a message: Jung is in agreement with what our present leaders are trying to bring about. (Incidentally, the official translation of the English *Collected Works of C. G. Jung* contains several similar examples of sanitization.)

Strangely, we find Jung speaking of Hitler as if Hitler could become a leader conscious of his position, as if Hitler could become an analyzed leader. Where does this idea originate? Jungian analysts-in-training are often reminded that it was Jung who was the first to insist, in 1913, that a prospective analyst be analyzed.[23] Among the many reasons for this requirement is the observation that the patient can go only so far as the analyst has gone, psychologically speaking. So the analyst's neurosis is the brake on the patient's growth – or, as Jung said of the leader, transposing the analytical dictum to the political arena, 'if he doesn't know himself, how is he to lead others?' In the interview, we can hear how Jung reconciles his seeming acceptance of the *Führerprinzip* (the principle of unquestioned leadership) with his lifelong advocacy of Swiss-style democracy. For I really cannot think of a better short definition of individuation than 'having the courage to be oneself'.[24] There seems to be some kind of connection in Jung's mind between the analyst and the political leader. Jung has transposed psychology to the top table, to the world stage.

By 1939 Jung had changed some of his views about leadership. In a letter to an American youth, which came to light via a train of extraordinary coincidences in 1991, Jung responds to the question: 'Can anything good come from a dictatorship?' with the unequivocal statement that 'there is no such thing as a liberal dictatorship'. In this letter, Jung seems rather fatalistic about the political process itself: 'We all ought to be happy if we just happen to have no revolution, no war and no epidemics.' (I do not know how to assess Jung's opinion in this letter that 'if conditions become better, the people become worse'. He might have been thinking of the dangers of mindless affluence – or there might be shards of an anti-democratic tendency in such a view.[25])

With the politics of intellectual endeavour in mind, I would ask if there is anything wrong with a great thinker trying to influence other people, promote his work, and be a leader? Why do Jungians continue to deny that Jung was actively involved in the ideological marketplace – for instance, in 1930s Germany where the banning of Freud left a vacuum in depth psychology? There is obviously some strange investment in sticking to Jung's public version of himself: an unworldly, even other-worldly, poetic genius, naively indifferent to the institutional dynamics of his profession, as well as to politics in general, a man who had almost to be forced to become President of the IGMSP. One has only to read the Freud–Jung letters, in which Jung reveals himself as an enthusiastic psychoanalytic politician, to understand where the naïveté really lies. After all, Jung did not display much hesitation when asked by Freud to become President of the International Psychoanalytical Association.

Jung was certainly not completely dominated by his desire for leadership. He did seem able to value other people's points of view and he had a great capacity to tolerate uncertainty and not knowing. He is believable when he says that 'agreement would only spell one-sidedness and desiccation' and that we need many theories before we get 'even a rough picture of the psyche's complexity'.[26] But Jung's elitism is always just below the surface – nature is, after all, 'aristocratic'.[27] The idea of leadership (like that of the nation) forms part of a psychological backdrop to the interplay of Nazis, Jews, Jungians and Freudians that we have been examining. Indeed, in some form this theme pervades *all* these groups. Nazi claims to leadership result in the installation of the Führer with the final solution; there are time-honored Jewish claims to moral primacy as the chosen people; the Freudian Committee, set up in part to ensure that defectors were not taken seriously, illustrates Freudian desires for hegemony; and Jung tried to organize world psychotherapy under his 'neutral' leadership.

Analytical psychology and renewal

At this point, I would like to restate what, for me, is the key question to ask when considering Jung, anti-semitism and the Nazis. Is there anything in Jung's habitual way of thinking that leads to anti-semitism? I think there is – and it is found in the way Jung employs his ideas of the nation and about leadership. These ideas are ideograms with damaging potential and I have tried to show that Jung deployed them in an insufficiently critical manner.

But what about the future of analytical psychology? Specifically, what about the future of analytical psychology – and depth psychology generally – as a means of developing an analysis or critique of political processes?

Reviewing the troubled and tragic history of psychoanalysis in Germany, Robert Wallerstein, then President of the International Psychoanalytical Association, used these words: 'We need to underline the implicit invitation (nay, demand) that all of us in psychoanalysis reflect together on what this means for our common humanity and where our psychoanalytic identities can fit meaningfully into it.'[28] Similarly, can analytical psychologists employ psychological and critical reflections on Jung, anti-semitism and the Nazis in such a way that some kind of renewal can result? Could this then lead to a more productive engagement of depth psychology with the public sphere?

Since Jung's death in 1961, analytical psychology *has* sought to renew itself from without – through contact with psychoanalysis, religion, classical mythology, even theoretical physics. But what about attending to renewal from within, through seeking those discoveries that come from a self-directed, psychological and critical attitude toward the events and ideas of the past? Can analytical psychology learn from its founder's experiences? I suggest that renewal will not occur until Jungians resolve their work of mourning for Jung. This will lead, eventually, to our giving him up. Jungians are not alone in having problems in disidentifying from the great man who still dominates their discipline. As Wallerstein said, in a presidential address to the Freudian group: 'For so many of us, Sigmund Freud remains our lost object, our unreachable genius, whose passing we have perhaps never properly mourned, at least not in [an] emotional fullness.'[29]

Only when Jung the man, the flawed (and hence overanalyzed) leader, has been mourned can anything be learned from 'Jung' the social and cultural phenomenon. If this could be done, and if we were then to attempt to sketch out a programme of renewal for analytical psychology, what would that programme look like?

Depth psychology, difference and nationalism

To begin with, I think it would help if analysts and therapists (of all persuasions) were to cease expanding the national boundaries of the psychological kingdom and try to work cooperatively with their colleagues in the social sciences. This would mean stopping the abuse of our authority when we advance definitions of the typical psychology of this or that group – whether Jews, Germans, African Americans, homosexuals, women or men. Whether we like it or not, as Jung's experience in the 1930s demonstrates, depth psychology and politics are connected. As a signal of our stopping this abuse, we should consider expressly allying ourselves to so-called marginal and minority groups, for that is the category where we ourselves belong. Such groups are often demoralized and disorganized; sometimes they suffer from a kind of social invisibility (mentally disabled people, for instance). We could contribute our limited but profound expertise to the achievement of their goals. Jung aligned himself with and sought power; we should align ourselves with the powerless. We would do this by using our therapeutic capacity to work with the inexpressible in a clarification of the psychological experience of being Jew, German, African American, homosexual, woman, man. We would assist such groups in getting behind the defensive stereotypes imposed by a threatened dominant culture as we explore the nature of difference itself. Analysts and therapists may even find unnamed cultural groupings, somehow overlooked by social theory.

Some general issues arise from a depth psychological exploration of the psychology of cultural difference. Sometimes, and for some individuals, membership of a minority or marginal group will be of supreme importance, psychologically speaking. At other times, and for other people, it may turn out that the issue is one of sharing in the psychological assumptions and cultural traditions of the majority. It may well be that, on occasions, both of these positions will hold true. Then a pluralistic analysis would suggest that there is a competitive tension between being *alike* (sharing in *one* set of psychological assumptions and cultural traditions) and being unalike (invested in a particular set out of *many* sets of psychological assumptions and cultural traditions).

Refining this point about the competitive tension between identity and difference, as I hinted in Chapter 1 [of this book], it is by no means certain that all the members of a particular group will share in the same psychological experiences. Group homogeneity cannot be assumed. For example, if a psychocultural group is identified by means of a religious background (it could be the Jews), we should not forget the differences introduced into the picture by differences in age, class, sex, geographical origin and so forth. Trying to express this pluralistically brings in that most psychologically pregnant word 'some'. Some Jewish experiences are experienced by all Jews, some are specific to specific kinds of Jews. Moreover, in any one Jew, is there not an inevitable tension between what he or she has in common with other Jews and, still within the experiential area of Jewishness, what he or she does not have in common with other Jews?

Even this point about the 'someness' of cultural experience requires fine tuning. For the groups that I have been discussing have a fragile existence. They are themselves culturally and politically constructed; they are historically contingent entities while, at the same time, having social ontology and psychological reality. (This conundrum for groups is analogous to that faced by the individual, discussed in Chapter 9 [of *The Political Psyche*]. There, I expressed it in terms of a competitive tension between psyche-as-source and person-as-contingent.) The psychological life of a cultural group is, in many respects, strengthened and fostered by the worry that the group itself is evanescent, having no 'real' existence.

The creation of a psychology of difference does not only apply to the social situation of minority or marginal groups; it may also help us to understand the workings of groups that have ample access to the corridors of power and hence can grab a disproportionate share of the cake.

It is subversive work, breaking the contemporary taboo on the discussion of difference (racial, national, ethnic, gender, class). But it has to be done. After all, many of the most convincing objections to Freudian theory rest on a rejection of its supposedly universal generalizations which are in fact suffused by the specific ambience of *fin de siècle* Vienna. Analytical psychology has to free itself from similar cultural blunders rooted in Germanic ideas of Nation and Leadership that obscure other things that we know about nations and leaders. In fact, the entire Eurocentric cast of depth psychology, its own historical and cultural location, will have to be examined. In Chapter 5 [of *The Political Psyche*], I discussed psychological aspects of economic development in the so-called Third World countries and the relevance of depth psychology to non-European political and cultural processes was explored. I agree with those who dispute the universality of the findings of psychoanalysis (for example, the Oedipus complex).

I have not been arguing that there are *no* differences between nations (or between races, or between sexes, or between classes). I am insisting, rather, that it is crucial that these differences not be defined or predefined. It is impossible to classify such differences; they are an unknown. The analyst is not an authority or teacher who has *a priori* knowledge of the psychological implications of the patient's ethnic and cultural background. Rather he or she is a mediator who enables the patient to experience and express his or her *own* difference.[30] When it comes to cultural difference, analysts should privilege individual experience over universal and abstract formulations. As I said earlier, analysts are good at getting people to talk about what they implicitly know but have not yet consciously expressed. Joseph Henderson's refinement of Jung's layers of the collective unconscious, leading to the hypothesis of a 'cultural unconscious', will be helpful here.[31]

However, we still lack an adequate account of the role of collective psychology in a complicated, multifactorial situation. What is more, the cultural unconscious, as an idea, needs further thought. For example, is the cultural unconscious a kind of repository of cultural experience – a storehouse of difference? Or is it the means, already existing as a potential, by which the human psyche gives birth to cultural difference? Or both?

I think that Jung himself was trying, with an inadequate methodology and hence with very mixed results, to do a kind of analysis of cultural difference. In 1934 he wrote to A. Pupato:

> The question that I broached regarding the peculiarities of Jewish psychology does not presuppose any intention on my part to depreciate Jews, but is merely an attempt to single out and formulate the mental idiosyncrasies that distinguish Jews from other people. No sensible person will deny that such differences exist, any more than he will deny that there are essential differences in the mental attitude of Germans and Frenchmen . . . Again, nobody with any experience of the world would deny that the psychology of an American differs in a characteristic and unmistakable way from that of an Englishman.[32]

Jung's focus on the idiosyncrasies that constitute difference led him to speculate on the origins of difference. His most evolved view is that difference stems from: (1) the individual, (2) the family, (3) the nation, race, climate, locality and history. Psychology is one factor among many and hence *the germ of a multidisciplinary approach is here.*

Moving out of the consulting room, depth psychologists could initiate a psychological exploration of a world in which racial strife is as destructive as national strife. Such a world urgently needs a psychological model for practice in which difference is truly valued, in which diversity need not become the reason for schism, and in which competition and bargaining – between race, class, sex, nation – are given a new valency: as normative and as mutually enriching. Moreover, there may even be a distinctly political value in trying to understand difference more profoundly. In the same letter of 1934, Jung wrote to Pupato:

> I would consider it most fortunate if, for example, Germany and France took the trouble to understand each other's characteristic values. But the way things

> are, each explains the other in terms of the assumptions of its own psychology, as you can convince yourself daily by reading the French and German newspapers. That people are also all alike is by this time a familiar fact, but it leads to no end of misunderstandings. These come from the differences, which should therefore be a worthy subject of investigation.[33]

Here we can make *creative* use of that rejection by Jung of the imposition of the psychology of one group upon another.[34]

Alongside the many problems with Jung's ideas about nation and race that we have been tracking, there are also the seeds of a productive and useful approach to difference. Even if Jung's list-making method and his ideology of complementarity are suspect, his intuitions of the importance of exploring differences, preserving them, even celebrating them, remain intact. When I write of the renewal of analytical psychology, I mean just that: reconnecting to Jung's intuition about the importance of difference, but being firm about staying unhindered by excessive dependence on complementarity, on the dogma of 'the opposites', on oppositional thinking and, above all, on essentialism – the argument that things are as they are because it is only natural for them to be that way. It is not enough simply to accept or reject 'the opposites'. We have now to try to make a psychological theory *about* them so as to explain their immense psychopolitical powers. We have to explain how oppositions such as Jew/German, homosexual/heterosexual, black/white, female/male, thinking/feeling actually work on the cultural level. What kind of profound split in humanity and human ideation is being carried by these opposites? What can we learn from fantasies of bringing them together in some kind of conjunction? What political negotiations are possible between the members of the pairs – and then between the pairs themselves, when they are not seen as functioning in isolation? If we make a psychological theory that explains some of these political issues, then we might be better placed to examine, and dispute, what is really meant by 'marginal'. In Chapter 6 [of *The Political Psyche*], I suggested that single parents are performing a kind of cultural laboratory work for everyone in the field of family organization, and in Chapter 3 [of this book] I proposed that Third World industrial strategies have a psychological resonance for cultural processes in the developed world. In Chapter 8 [of *The Political Psyche*] I argued that the gay men's movement has generated forms of social organization and thinking that constitute a critique of existing forms. Becoming less dependent on 'the opposites' enables us to relocate the marginal to the centre of imaginative and progressive political activity. A depth psychological analysis may foster a redrawing of the map of social structure, leading, on the political level, to an urgently needed reallocation of economic resources. For what distinguishes marginality is, in many cases, the absence of economic clout.

As far as differences in national psychology are concerned, we must resist the temptation to indulge in national typology and offer to a multi-disciplinary endeavor *only* what we have learned as depth psychologists. If we do this, then another role for depth psychology emerges. Generalizations about national character and psychology, from all manner of sources, can be interpreted as a form of myth-making crucial to a sense of *Gemeinschaft* (community). National characteristics, or rather what are claimed as national characteristics, are revealed as metaphors and as part of the contemporary quest for *Gemeinschaft*. There is, these days, a yearning for a pre-industrial time, when societal relations seemed to be governed by tradition and agriculture rather than by politics and commerce. The question of the psychological influence of the earth can be tackled psychologically and understood as a group's attempt to express its uniqueness, its own national difference. Even Jung's stress on 'earth' rather than race contains an exceedingly powerful anti-racist potential, making a pluralistic vision of society psychologically viable. For the earth sustains people of different backgrounds, permitting us to realize that the differences that we inherit, culturally and biologically, are of value. Do not modern desires for national identity reflect just that?

It is a matter of the very shape and texture of the countryside: 'the old track fading on the hillside, the tumbled stone of a Saxon steading, winter sunlight on new ploughland, the strip of dark beneath the trees, the names repeating in a country churchyard'.[35] That's one person's vision of England. Or, from a letter written by a Japanese scholar to his Prime Minister: 'The Japanese spirit is to be found in sacred old rocks and pine trees . . . only the Japanese know instinctively how to live in harmony with nature.'[36] The Romantic nature of such nationalistic expressions should not obscure their potentially revolutionary nature or their feel for history. Though clearly in reaction to the evolution of modern societies, there is an aura of renewal and group regeneration that has a political significance; it need not lead inevitably toward fascism.

However, we should recall that there is no such thing as a single, immutable 'pure' national character; a belief in national purity can have only one disastrous outcome. The problem is exemplified in the word 'blood'. When Jung writes that there is a Jewish psychology based on 'blood and history',[37] we need to see through 'blood' to understand it as referring also to the shared history of a connected group of people. But sometimes blood is meant literally, and then the image of purity is bound to arise.

When the idea of national purity is abroad, then we are bound to forget the mutability of nationhood, the ways in which, over time, nations define and redefine themselves. If humanity did begin in one part of Africa, then it is clear that the world as we find it is one station on an unknowably long journey. In Europe, the rise and decline of city states, empires and supranational federations is well documented but, as this mutability is anxiety-provoking, it can easily be set aside. In India and in Africa, patterns of tribal organization and separation often turn out to be of surprisingly recent origin. Nations are ideas: Charles de Gaulle spoke of 'une *certaine idée de la France*'. The mutability of nationhood is another reason why the presence of depth psychologists is required: nation is a coruscating fantasy. But Jung's conception of the role of the psychologist was insufficiently questioning of the apparent fixity of contemporary national arrangements.

I wrote much of this chapter prior to 1989, before the massive political changes in Europe had taken place and before the Baltic and Russian moves to secede from the Soviet Union had got under way. I could not have known then the extent to which discussion of nationalism and issues of national psychology would be in the foreground. For example, the question of German reunification positively reeked of an immense anxiety about the true nature of German national psychology (something that was more-or-less assumed to exist). Though unease about German national psychology is usually admitted to be subjective, difficult to catch in the nets of rationality, it is obviously an exceedingly potent factor in the debate.

Close on the heels of the upsurge of nationalism in Europe comes that classic, perennial parasite on nationalism – anti-semitism. Whether in the rise of Pamyat in the Soviet Union, or the character defamation of the Hungarian Free Democrats as a Jewish party (heavily defeated in the first free elections), or the demonstrations in Poland in 1990 for a Europe 'free of Jews', or the post-revolutionary murmurings in Rumania of getting rid of the Magyars and Jews, or the desecration in 1990 of Bertolt Brecht's tombstone in East Berlin (it was daubed with the words 'Jewish pig' though he was not Jewish) – and not forgetting the wave of anti-semitism in France at the same time or the scarcely disguised blaming of Jews in America for the materialistic excesses of the Reagan era – it is clear that whatever threatens and upsets people about the Jews has upped its work rate once again. There has even been a resurgence of openly expressed anti-semitism in Germany in 1992. I feel that the content of these two chapters, ostensibly about Jung, the Nazis and anti-semitism in the 1930s, takes on a new, wider and more pressing political significance. Could it be that images of the Jews that were active in the 1930s are also the problem today: the nomads with no cultural forms of their own; the Wandering Jews; world citizens; international communists (now, incredibly, reviled for their Marxism in the former Soviet Union and Eastern Europe); wily international capitalists; scholars with a poor relation to the earth but nevertheless protected by their internationally recognized PhDs? Could it be these images of the Jews, the same ones that threatened both Jung and Hitler, these images of the enemies of national differences, that are the problem for today's nationalists?

Whatever the problem really is, there is no use in merely speaking out against nationalism because that would be a simplistic and unrealistic response to such a complicated matter. Rather, we need to make a psychological distinction between different aspects of nationalism, or, putting it another way, between different nationalisms. On the one hand, we have nationalism serving a positive collective psychological function, socially progressive, historically liberalizing and democratizing, reconnecting people to their roots and traditions, celebrating differences in a cornucopia of languages. Nationalism is preferable to world empire or the played-out game of geopolitics dominated by the superpowers. But, on the other hand, we have what could be called 'spiritualized nationalism', the creed of the *Kulturnation,* with the emphasis on kinship, blood, people (*Volk*), earth – the whole mysterious, mystifying Romantic lexicon. Spiritualized nationalism obliterates the social contract, constitutional rights, the political dimensions of life itself. What is collective and held in common is decreed by birth and not by consent. As Saint-Just said, before his execution during the French Revolution, 'There is something terrible about the holy love of one's nation, for it is so excessive that it sacrifices everything to the public interest, without mercy, without fear, without humanity.' We must be careful lest those who possess what is claimed to be a common tongue allow that claim to take precedence over civil rights and constitutional government. This is particularly pressing in the context of the break-up of the Soviet Union. In addition, world economic developments are promoting migration and population movements on such a massive scale that reliable ethnolinguistic homogeneity is ceasing to exist in many areas. Hence, pluralism of language and multi-ethnicity must be accommodated within a nationalistic framework. This requires an agnostic nationalism.

As far as Germany in the 1930s was concerned, nationalism was anything but agnostic. We can see that, without enemies, the *Volk* could not exist. Perhaps this dependence on the Other for national definition was particularly marked in German nationalism dating from the end of the eighteenth century and due to specific features of German political evolution. From a psychological perspective, the creation of an entity other to the nation facilitates the expression of national aggression because the national Other then serves as the object of aggression (what philosophers call an 'intentional object'). The role of plain projection is also important; the Volk-identified nation evacuates what is sensed unconsciously to be its undesirable features into designated enemies (without and, as in the case of

Germany and the German Jews, within). Complementarity plays its usual suspect role so that German virtues are complemented by Jewish vices. Though the *Volk* may sometimes seem all-powerful, it can be, and maybe usually is, manipulated by a leader or leadership class.

The Germany of the 1930s performed a collective psychological function for the rest of the developed world which, in some respects, the Holocaust continues to perform in our time. The great economic depressions of the 1920s and 1930s brought suffering in all the industrialized societies to ruling class and proletariat alike. The kind of national organization Hitler was evolving salved desires for retaliation and rage against the invisible Fates of economic forces on the part of both rulers and ruled. Those classes with aspirations for economic and political leadership saw these brought into concrete form by the alliance of the *Führerprinzip* with German industrial power. Classes with little or no economic power could identify with the world historical role assigned by Hitler to members of his *Volk*. Even the final solution met both these sets of needs.

As Germany was not the only country to suffer economic depression, this argument might also explain the ambivalence of the world community toward Hitler's expansionism; an ambivalence that continues to provoke guilt – a guilt that contributes to a preoccupation with the Holocaust. For the Holocaust was not only the supreme crisis of nationalism, anti-semitism and racism, it was also a crisis for industrialism and for modernity itself.

I can see no alternative to saying that, at the present time, we do not have a satisfyingly full answer to questions of the influence of national (or ethnic, or racial, or class) background upon individual psychology, or the part played by what we call 'psychology' in the formation of what we call 'nation'. Depth psychologists can join with scientists, social scientists and environmentalists in a study of these matters. If they do join up in this way then I think Jung's contribution will prove seminal and valuable: 'Nationalism – disagreeable as it is – is a *sine qua non,* but the individual must not remain stuck in it. On the other hand, in so far as he is a particle in the mass he must not raise himself above it either' (Jung in a letter to James Kirsch written in 1934).[38]

We have to use our judgment and make a distinction. The idea of nationalism, like the idea of race, can lead to paranoia and chauvinism – but it also leads to the undoubtedly healthy and positive desire not to be dominated by something or someone felt as foreign: a foreign suffocating mother, a foreign castrating father, a foreign, disciplinarian super-ego, a foreign, uncomprehending psychological theory. We cannot eliminate competition and division between nations. But why should we? A pluralistic political psychology can demonstrate that competition and division, mediated by bargaining, are productive paths to follow. It may even be that the nation is rather a good milieu for the development of psychological pluralism on the social scale. On one level, the nation contains the various competing interest groups. On another level, the nation itself has to compete politically with all the interest groups that are associated with it. In the spirit of pluralism, the nation has to compete for its special privileges. The nation has a kind of oneness to it – and the nation itself is also part of a kind of manyness.

If certain features of nationalism can be raised to consciousness and identified, leading to a deliberate attempt to counteract them, and if this is done with the knowledge that a degree of failure is inevitable and not totally damning, then we could go beyond the conventional condemnation of nationalism and, by implication, of the idea of the nation. For it would be pointless simply to replace the idealistic approach to nationalism of the 1930s with an overly pessimistic judgment.

If a nation is to function as a locus and as a midwife of psychological pluralism, it has to try to avoid developing a fixed list or classification of what are its psychological characteristics. Or, given that such lists often exist, let us say that they exist as reference points, part of myth-making, things to be seen through. We should certainly see through ideas like Jung's that nations consist of the sum of individuals. Then we become more conscious of the relative autonomy and psychological impact of the form of national organization itself. It follows that psychologists should study constitutions and voice their reactions to them. But psychologists should also take care not to muddle genetic invariants like race with changing social constructs like nations. Frankly, I am not sure that there is anything at all, in either a psychological or a social analysis, that depends on race alone. Therefore, as I hinted earlier, 'race' is itself also a construct. Nevertheless, the temptation that Musil noted in the 1920s, to muddle race and nation, is still with us.

Similarly, we need to be careful not to construct national ideals (for instance, ideals of where the nation is headed) out of what is perceived as the past history of the nation. If we are going to be idealistic, then let us be idealistic in a true sense and not manufacture ideals out of yesterday's arrangements and events. This is not to ignore history, but rather to assign to history a more fruitful role than as the manufactory of ideals that are then converted into spuriously 'eternal' structures (Platonic, archetypal) that are claimed to govern political developments in the future.

Concluding reflections

My hope is that finding echoes of Jung in Hitler and Hitler in Jung, emotionally wearing though it is, will lead to a decision to try to make a contribution to a contemporary political celebration of difference.

Then depth psychology can joyfully renounce the top table, the level of nation states – for we have seen what a terrible mess it makes when it tries to sit there. But depth psychologists do not need to retreat behind the barricade of 'the clinical'. Depth psychologists can simultaneously go on with an analysis of politics. To do it, I think they need to stand up with the materially disadvantaged and the socially frightened, as well as sit down with educated analysands. They should be engaged when a Law of Return is passed and small ethnic groups gain or regain their lands; hence, they should be engaged when an *intifada* erupts. They *should* be concerned with promised lands, as well as with sovereign nation states; with the people as well as with their leaders.

Clinicians may have to question the milieux in which many of them work, for private practice with a privileged clientele is not politically neutral. This mode of working has affected depth psychological thinking. Clinicians may have to question their automatic preference for the inner world, and this tendency to make 'inner' and 'outer' or 'private' and 'public' into polar opposites, rejecting multidisciplinary work as 'un-analytical'. As we saw, all images can be read politically.

Before the war, Hitler proclaimed all German modern art to be 'decadent'. Officially approved realistic art was sponsored. Two exhibitions were organized – one of the degenerate and one of the official art. The degenerate exhibition was viewed by two million people, still the world record for any single art exhibition, whereas less than four hundred thousand attended the official exhibition.[39]

In these last two chapters, I have exhibited the decadent and degenerate side of analytical psychology. This has been a cautionary tale for depth psychologists who seek to analyze politics and culture. I tried to show that it was Jung's attempt to establish a culturally sensitive psychology of nations that brought him into the same frame as Nazi anti-semitic ideology. In addition, Jung was absorbed by the question of leadership. Exploring these ideas as thoroughly as possible leads to a kind of reparation, for I think that post-Jungians do have reparation to make. Then it is possible to revalue in more positive terms Jung's overall project. We must couple a less simplistic methodology and a more sensitive set of political values to Jung's intuitions about the centrality of a psychology of cultural difference. If we do so, then analytical psychology has something to offer a depth psychology that is concerned with processes of political and cultural transformation.

Notes

1 Marcus Marrus, 'Popular anti-semitism'. Catalogue of *The Dreyfus Affair: Art, Truth and Justice*. Exhibition, Jewish Museum, New York (Berkeley, CA: University of California Press, 1987).
2 Sarah Gordon, *Hitler, Germans, and the 'Jewish' Question* (Princeton, NJ: Princeton University Press, 1984), p. 94.
3 Personal communication, 1990.
4 *CW* 10: 18. *Civilization in Transition*. *CW* refers to the *Collected Works* of C. G. Jung, ed. Herbert Read, Michael Fordham and Gerhard Adler, Trans. R. F. C. Hull (London: Routledge and Kegan Paul; Princeton, NJ: Princeton University Press, 1953–77). References, save where indicated, are by volume and paragraph number
5 *CW* 10: 353.
6 *CW* 10: 1029.
7 *CW* 10: 1029.
8 *CW* 7: 240n. *Two Essays on Analytical Psychology*.
9 C. G. Jung, *Letters*. Ed. Gerhard Adler (London, Routledge and Kegan Paul, 1973–4), Vol. 2, p. 48.
10 Aldo Carotenuto, *Sabina Spielrein: Tagebuch einer heimlichen Symmetrie* (Freiburg: Kore, 1986), pp. 222–3. I am grateful to Gottfried Heuer for drawing my attention to the German edition of Carotenuto's book and for making the translation.
11 C. G. Jung, *Letters*.
12 C. G. Jung, *Letters*.
13 Martin Bernal, *Black Athena: The Afroasiatic Roots of Classical Civilisation* (London: Free Association Books, 1987).
14 *The Economist*, August 13, 1988.
15 Andrew Samuels, *Jung and the Post-Jungians* (London and Boston, MA: Routledge and Kegan Paul, 1985), pp. 1–22.
16 *CW* 10: 1060.
17 *CW* 10: 1072.
18 *CW* 16. *The Practice of Psychotherapy*
19 *C. G. Jung Speaking*. Ed. William McGuire (London: Thames and Hudson, 1978), pp. 73–9.
20 Ibid., p. 77.
21 Matthias von der Tann, 'A Jungian perspective on the Berlin Institute for Psychotherapy: A basis for mourning'. *San Francisco Jung Institute Library Journal*, 8: 4 (1989).
22 *C. G. Jung Speaking*, pp. 73–9.
23 *CW* 4: 586–7. *Freud and Psychoanalysis*.
24 See Andrew Samuels, Bani Shorter and Fred Plaut, *A Critical Dictionary of Jungian Analysis* (London and New York: Routledge and Kegan Paul, 1986). Entry on 'individuation'.
25 I was visiting Vancouver and staying with the Jungian analyst John Allan who told me the following story: 'For several years in the early 1980s, I used to co-lead a group

for the University of California at Santa Cruz to the C. G. Jung Institute at Kuznacht. As part of this program, participants would write a brief outline of their objectives and in some cases we would call them to seek clarification at various points.

'In one such case I called a young man and was informed that he would be unable to come. As we talked he asked me if I would like a copy of an old letter of Jung's. He related how he had been hitch-hiking through Kansas and dropped into a bar for a beer. He struck up a conversation with an older man in his late fifties and soon they were chatting about Jung. As it turns out, the older man had written Jung a letter in late 1938 saying that he was an American youth who thought that one answer to the world's problems was for countries to be run by "liberal dictators". What did he (Jung) think? A few months later Jung wrote back. The man in the bar still had a copy of the letter which he gave to the "hitch-hiker" who in turn sent me a copy.'

I suggested to John Allan that the letter be published and we are grateful to the Jung Estate for permission to quote extracts from the letter. (First published in the *Journal of Analytical Psychology, 37*: 2, 1992.)

26 CW 15: 198. *The Spirit in Man, Art, and Literature.*
27 CW 7: 198, 235. CW 17: 343, 345. *The Development of Personality.*
28 Robert Wallerstein, 'Psychoanalysis in Nazi Germany: Historical and psychological lessons'. *Psychoanalysis and Contemporary Thought, 11*: 2 (1987), pp. 360–1.
29 Robert Wallerstein, 'One psychoanalysis or many?' *International Journal of Psycho-Analysis, 69*: 1 (1988), p. 9.
30 Stan Perelman, personal communication, 1989.
31 Joseph Henderson, *Cultural Attitudes in Psychological Perspective* (Toronto: Inner City, 1985).
32 C. G. Jung, *Letters.*
33 Ibid.
34 CW 7: 240n.
35 Quoted in Ian Buruma, 'England, whose England?' *The Spectator*, September 9, 1989.
36 Ibid.
37 CW 10: 10.
38 C. G. Jung, *Letters.*
39 From the catalogue of the exhibition *Stationen der Moderne* (Berlin, 1988).

CHAPTER 12

SCHOOLS OF ANALYTICAL PSYCHOLOGY

Retrospective introduction

This chapter is taken from *Jung and the Post-Jungians,* which was published in 1985. In brief, it was my attempt to understand my entire training and formation as a Jungian analyst, which was characterized by extremely confusing and unsettling polemic and mutual contempt between the warring schools of analytical psychology.

Even today, people refer to the London and Zurich schools which strikes me as ridiculous – for there are 'London' and 'Zurich' analysts all over the world. My more neutral terms (classical, developmental, archetypal) do a better job and make sense to non-Jungians with an interest.

The classification of schools has managed to be both reliable and oft cited – and also quite controversial, mainly because Jungian analysts are highly individualistic and resist being classified.

People often ask me about the title of the book. It had nothing to do with 'post-modern' but was rather a take-off from the title of Brown's book *Freud and the Post-Freudians*.

If I might put in a brief good word for what was my first book, one unsung aspect of it is that every chapter contains a pretty decent summary of Jung's ideas and writings on the topic of the chapter. The topics are: archetype and complex; the ego (including typology); the self and individuation; the development of personality; the analytical process; gender, sex, marriage; dreams; archetypal psychology; case illustration; comparison and evaluation.

So *Jung and the Post-Jungians* is a guide not just to what came after Jung but also to his own works.

To find one's way around in the contemporary Jungian world is not easy. Jung's standing as a psychological thinker and analyst, rather than guru or prophet, is reinforced by analytical psychologists and the writings of the post-Jungians. It no longer rests solely upon Jung's legacy of the twenty volumes of the *Collected Works* and his commensurate charisma. In a way, Jung needs the post-Jungians as much as they need him if his work is to be extended into the future. The prospect for analytical psychology is a shared concern and the inheritance has become a many-stranded skein of thought which has inspired, influenced, challenged and, in some instances, infuriated those who followed.

We should note the extent to which post-Jungians have felt able to challenge or attack Jung's work, often arguing with him on the basis of stringent criticisms from non-Jungians, as well as adapting and integrating parallel developments in other approaches to psychology, and also from completely different disciplines. If I constantly draw attention to the various serious objections that have been made to Jung's work it is because these have had a great impact on post-Jungians. Sometimes Jung anticipates, sometimes he influences, but sometimes he gets it wrong, and sometimes another thinker reaches a broadly similar conclusion but does so in a more coherent or better documented way.

In his book *Jungian Psychotherapy: A Study in Analytical Psychology* (1978), Fordham points out that 'very little has been written on the development of the various schools of analytical psychology that have grown up' (p. 53). I decided to respond to this, bearing in mind Fordham's assertion (ibid., p. ix) that 'analytical psychology is a discipline in its own right . . . its ideas and practices can be assessed without regard to the persons who initiated them.' This has to be a different kind of book from Brown's *Freud and the Post-Freudians* (1961) because, unlike the Freudians, post-Jungians have not yet formed into *officially* recognized schools, though the process has certainly taken place informally. There are schools of analytical psychology in existence with common views, and dogmatism and conflict between these groups has not been avoided. But the reader has less chance of finding out about this from Jungian than from Freudian literature.

Do 'Jungians' exist?

To talk of Jungians, of post-Jungians and of schools of post-Jungians is itself a contentious matter. Jung stated that there simply was *one* Jungian – himself. He eschewed any ambition to start a school of psychology. I imagine he had in mind an attempt to avoid what he considered Freud's excesses of rabbinical authority and the whole painful early history of psychoanalysis, which involved so much personalia. Furthermore, as the ideologue of individuation, with its stress on each person becoming himself and differentiating from others, not to mention his observation that a person's temperament and personal psychology play a part in dictating what he believes, Jung was bound to want to leave it up to the personal capacity of an individual as to how 'Jungian' he would be. However, as Henderson points out, 'there is now a basic Jungian body of knowledge which does not permit unlimited experimentation or theorising.' But he goes on to say that Jung 'abhorred systematisation of any kind and this was a reason why his school took so long to be formed' (1975a, pp. 120–1).

In fact, though, Jung was active throughout his life in the politics of psychology. Reading *The Freud–Jung Letters* (McGuire, 1974), one is struck by the pattern in which it is Jung who is constantly putting forward some idea for a coup or alliance while it is Freud (supposedly the more extraverted of the two) who restrains him, diverting him from excessive character attack. Later, in the 1940s, Jung put forward a proposal designed to unify psychotherapists internationally, consisting of fourteen points around which he felt everyone's ideas could coalesce. Given the extraordinary post-war fragmentation in psychology and the psychotherapies, we can now see that this was a forlorn hope, but the relevance of the episode is that Jung does not fit the image of the solitary genius, indifferent to the real world, even, or especially, to his own profession (and see below, for a further comment on the fourteen points).

Another noteworthy feature of the gradual formation of Jungians into a broad group is the series of forewords that Jung so often wrote for the books of earlier followers. It was obviously important for commercial and other reasons to receive

Jung's imprimatur but, as Fordham has attested (1975, p. 108), Jung seemed to have genuine feelings about doing this. I know of forewords for books by Adler, F. Fordham, M. Fordham, Harding, Hannah, Jacobi, E. Jung, Neumann, von Franz, Wickes, Wilhelm – there are perhaps others.

That suggests that Jung knew perfectly well that for all these writers he functioned as one who introduced them to a wider audience as well as a core or reference point. There is surely nothing shameful or infantilizing about this, but the perpetuation of Jung's denial concerning 'Jungians' does seem harmful.

I did not know Jung and I am not disputing that he was hostile to the *idea* of followers or 'Jungians'. But by all accounts he seems to have had an extraordinarily variegated and multi-faceted personality, as well as a very wide range of knowledge and interests. That is why differing points of view have emerged from his original work. My contention has been that, alongside the contempt for followers, Jung developed many of the more expectable characteristics of a leader especially in his wish that they should 'carry on the work' (Adler, 1979, p. 481). In Shakespeare's *Julius Caesar,* when the conspirators were worried that Caesar might not go to the Capitol, Decius suggests that they leave it up to him; he knows just how to handle Caesar. Among his various techniques for manipulating the great man, Decius continually advises him that flatterers betray:

> But when I tell him he hates flatterers,
> He says he does, being then most flattered.
>
> (Act 2, scene 1)

I am suggesting that we may reverse the proposition: Jung flatters his followers by saying he does not want them. Many post-Jungian books include the by now ritualistic statement that Jung did not want disciples, with the implication that because of this the writer could not possibly be considered a mere follower or disciple. By seeming to eschew his leadership, Jung may have helped maintain it.

In a memoir of Jung to mark the centenary of his birth, Fordham (1975) provided further evidence that Jung was aware of his fatherly role. The analyst members of the Analytical Psychology Club of London, an organization providing a meeting place for all Jungians but not a professional body, were negotiating to separate and found a professional organization, later known as the Society of Analytical Psychology. Presumably some members felt left behind and things were not helped when these people were referred to openly as 'the patients'. But it turned out that Jung had actively promoted this conflict because he felt that any 'family' should have its conflicts. I suppose that in this book [*Jung and the Post-Jungians*] I am charting the course of Jungian family life with its healthy differences.

Training in analytical psychology

This leads us to the question of analytical training and here again we must differentiate what Jung said and what he did. There is no doubt that he had mixed feelings about the institution of formal training programmes, whether in Zürich or anywhere else. When that occurred, he was active in helping to devise a syllabus and insisted that there should be examinations (Hillman, 1962; Fordham, 1978). Jung had bowed to collective standards and permitted changes in the old system, in which vocation, coupled with analysis by himself or a close associate and attendance at his seminars, were all that was required for the formation of an analyst. In this ethos the analysis of the potential analyst was, of course, central. Freud (1912) acknowledged that Jung had been the first to formulate the principle that the analyst should be analysed (Jung 1913, para. 536). However, A.-M. Sandler dates the *institution* of 'training analysis' in psychoanalysis from 1918 (Sandler, 1982, p. 386).

One more subtle development in Zürich (not, as far as I know, copied elsewhere) is that it is possible to attend certain lectures without making the commitment to becoming an analyst. Many are called but few are chosen and there is now a worldwide trend in which problems of selection for training are engaging the attention of Jungian analytic institutes.

These aspects of Jung's position vis à vis training deserve mention because they serve as a counterbalance to an image of Jung as a spontaneous ordinator of analysts. Jung would have been aware of any difficulties earlier students had got into through lack of a professional basis for their work. And a more formal structure may permit greater rather than lesser freedom by providing exposure to a variety of views, though the risk is loss of spontaneity. So Jung's support for examinations and qualifications may paradoxically foster individual professional development as well as assure greater professional mobility and acceptance.

The place of theory

Obviously, we have now to consider the place of theory in analytical psychology. It may be profitable to look at Jung's views on the role of theory and then at what some post-Jungians have to contribute on that subject.

Possibly playfully, at one point Jung expresses a preference for dogma over theory because

> for a certain type of intellectual mediocrity characterised by enlightened rationalism, a scientific theory that simplifies matters is a very good means of defence because of the tremendous faith modern man has in anything which bears the label 'scientific' . . . In itself any scientific theory, no matter how subtle, has, I think, less value from the point of view of psychological truth than religious dogma, for the simple reason that a theory is necessarily highly abstract and exclusively rational, whereas dogma expresses an irrational whole by means of imagery. This guarantees a far better rendering of an irrational fact like the psyche.
>
> (Jung, 1937, para. 81)

Elsewhere, Jung says:

> Theories in psychology are the very devil. It is true that we need certain points of view for their orienting and heuristic value: but they should always be regarded as mere auxiliary concepts that can be laid aside at any time.
>
> (Jung, 1938, p. 7)

What is highlighted is the need to establish where Jung really stood in relation to theory. Many of Jung's writings do not develop a body of theory at all but were written as specific lectures – for Swiss pastors, for the Tavistock Clinic in London, the Terry lectures in the United States, for example.

He was constantly aware that, in psychological research, there is more of an overlap between observer and observed than is usually the case and that personal preferences and constitutional factors play a large part. But Jung's overall approach does suggest the presence of the suspect idea of theory. After theoretical formula has been obtained from 'human material', Jung then applies it in 'my practical work, until it has either been confirmed, modified or else abandoned' (Jung 1913, para. 685). Jung goes on to state that the wealth of comparative, often mythological or anthropological, material serves to introduce, illustrate or amplify the theory – *not* to prove it (ibid.). Thus the theory, derived from observation, exists prior to the listing of the confirming material. I find an awareness of this approach enormously helpful in understanding Jung's work. He begins from the human interaction in analysis or from observation of life, develops a theory, which is then illustrated by comparative material or further observation. Only then could the mass of imagery and data from many sources be organized. The organization itself then helps to understand one aspect or other of human behaviour. Thus the process is circular: human material – theory – illustration – application to human behaviour.

The theoretical entities mentioned in this book do not exist. As L. Stein shows (1958, p. 3), a theoretical entity only exists or is contrived to perform a particular task. He points to the physicists' positron, photon, electron, the biologists' gene, Freud's id, ego and super-ego and Jung's archetypes. Modern scientists use theory not to advance empirical aims or to describe phenomena; they are attempting to indicate what their statements are about, what they *mean*. What is created is a non-empirical entity that can explain facts. The theory is not inferred or deduced from the facts; it may be tested against them. Stein illustrates this in terms of Newton and gravity. Gravity is a totally contrived invention, because no one has ever observed gravity, only that things do or do not fall. The theoretical entity exists only to do a job, which is its 'heuristic value'.

There are two scientific challenges for Jungian psychology. The first is levelled against all depth psychologies which are held to be unscientific because they deal with unprovable areas. In the sense that no one can finally *prove* the existence of, say, the Oedipus complex, this might be so. But Oedipal theory makes sense of such diverse phenomena as a child preferring one parent to the other, the question of the origin of sexual identity, reasons for perversions, hopeless partner choice in marriage, and so on. We may have to conclude that, in part, psychology is not like *other* sciences.

Jung was particularly keen to assert that psychology was a natural science by arguing that its field of reference is not mental *products* but a natural phenomenon, the psyche. My own view is that for those who demand what they consider to be the highest scientific standards, Jungian psychology will always be wanting – although the modern sub-atomic physicist and the student of archetypes share more than a commonsense view would presuppose.

The second scientific challenge comes from the Freudians. In this connection I am reminded of a passage in *Psychoanalysis: The Impossible Profession* in which the journalist author comments ruefully on the way regular Freudians dismiss Kleinian views of the early, internal, infantile world as crazy, fantastic and unprovable 'as if their own reconstructions of the castration complex described perfectly ordinary, everyday events' (Malcolm, 1982, p. 35).

In his *Critical Dictionary of Psychoanalysis* (1972, p. ix), Rycroft observes that he 'suffers from the not uncommon constitutional defect of being incapable of understanding Jung's writings.' And Glover concluded that 'from the point of view of scientific exposition, Jung is at the best of times a confused writer' (1950, p. 69). In subsequent chapters [of *Jung and the Post-Jungians*] I shall be considering these various objections to Jung's ideas but, for all intents and purposes, any attack on depth psychology for being unscientific applies to Freudians as much as it does Jungians.

Dangers of theory

Clarification of Jung's attitude to theory revolves around how far the practitioner can integrate the theory so that it ceases to be an artificial, imposed, technical, external matter and becomes more an expression of personality. Jung warned against a split between the therapist's knowledge of theory and technique and his personality. *Unintegrated knowledge* is the problem. Here we can see how the apparent divergence between Jung the unsystematic sage and Jung the professor who asks for exams can be understood. The theory must be known and then become personal; this is a matter for analysis, self-analysis and introspection. What we should try to avoid is using theory defensively, so that our own feelings are blocked out, or magically, so that only easy answers are sought, or purely logically in terms of arriving at a diagnosis.

Naturally, theory cannot dictate the process of an analysis; there must be adaptations for each case. Provided the material is allowed to emerge and fill out the theory *if* it will, then the danger of over-intellectualizing or over-influencing may be avoided. But it would be an inflated therapist who did not acknowledge the presence of personal influence in therapy as inevitable. Part of the influence must be the therapist's integration of theory. It follows from all this that the cardinal sin is imitation because that would imply predetermined application of theory.

Reification and action language

Language affects understanding and understanding underpins language. The main problem with the language of Jung, and hence to an extent of the post-Jungians, is that one is tempted to reify it – that is to render as concrete, literal and actual that which is shifting, fluid and experiential, for example, *the* unconscious. Reification not only tempts one to apply a predetermined theory but it bypasses the role of the psyche in psychology. Several ways of getting around this problem have been advanced. Lambert (1981) suggests that a distinction should be drawn between metaphorical and scientific language – the language of the imagination and the language of the intellect. The former tends to express itself in visual or auditory imagery; the latter uses rational or conceptual approaches. Jung's terms for these two kinds of thinking were 'fantasy thinking' and 'directed thinking' respectively (Jung 1952, paras 11–46). But, as Jung saw, it is possible to conceive of a complementarity or partnership in which the more rational and logical parts of the mental apparatus go to work on imaginal raw material. However, personal preference for either metaphorical or scientific language means that the goal of having a model in which both languages play a part may be difficult to achieve.

The problem of reification has been taken up by the American psychoanalyst Schafer (1976) who proposes a switch to an 'action language' which would accentuate the dynamic and fluid nature of psychic activity. And Plaut, in a series of personal communications (1981–2), insists on the values of using verbs (usually gerunds) as opposed to nouns. Thus 'thinking' not 'thought', 'resisting' not 'resistance', 'individuating' not 'individuation' and so on.

Uses and abuses of analogy

Jung, like many who approach the psyche, made continual use of analogy. His concept of libido or psychic energy is itself an analogy taken from natural science. In her paper 'Uses and abuses of analogy' (1973), Hubback argues that the making of analogies is a fundamental, imaginative, mental activity; more than simply a tool for understanding. Indeed, images themselves are a form of analogy because they relate to stimuli which are not currently active. But, as she points out, for Jung, the purpose of analogizing is to both make use of and demonstrate the idea that the world may be unitary, the so-called *unus mundus,* a holistic view in which everything connects in some way with everything else. The analogy takes us to a deeper layer of experience of understanding. This is strengthened by the role that hunches, guesses and intuitions play in scientific discovery. An intuition, like an analogy, can bring together two ideas that have not previously been connected.

In analogy, Jung sometimes saw what he did not see before, or saw something from a different angle. Sometimes analogy is closer to psyche than observed reality; often analogy is the opposite of reification. And, I would suggest, analogies with other areas of knowledge may also have had an emotional function for Jung who, like any pioneer, wanted to consolidate his hypotheses.

Hubback quotes Lévi-Strauss: 'By comparison with the natural sciences, we benefit from an advantage and suffer an inconvenience; we find our experiments already prepared but they are uncontrollable. It is therefore understandable that we attempt to replace them with models' (ibid., p. 95). This can be set against an attack on Jung quoted in *Freud and the Post-Freudians:* 'Jung's method . . . is to argue that because A is somewhat like B and B can, under certain circumstances, share something with C, and C has been known on occasion to have been suspected of being related to D, the conclusion in full-fledged logical form is that A=D. As the language of *science* this is meaningless' (Brown, 1961, p. 45).

Hubback's conclusion was that abuse of analogy occurs if there is not mutual agreement concerning the meaning of words used and, above all, the area being focused upon. Analogies can be used defensively to deny differences and hence avoid anxiety. I would say that the primitivity of the analogy is both its strength and its weakness – we are grabbed emotionally but may overstate our case. Nevertheless, effective use of analogy can transform opacity into a wider appreciation.

For example, returning to Jung's use of the terms *libido* and *psychic energy,* the analogy enables Jung to refer to differences in psychological intensity or to express evaluations of psychological experiences. The concepts may be used to communicate about what is experiential or subjective. Energy is not perceived as a force in a mechanical sense.

Diagrams are a special case of analogy, bringing in their wake all the dangers of reification. Their usefulness seems to vary according to the aptitudes and preferences of the observer. One advantage is that the psychological diagram engages us at a more than intellectual level. The conventions of the dividing line between phases of development, or the line which encircles parts, making of them a whole, bring in the risk of oversimplification. Attempts have been made to overcome the hard-edged problems by use of overlapping circles which permit an acknowledgment of blurring and hence correspond more closely to reality (e.g. Lambert, 1981, p. 194).

Additional problems are shown clearly in, for example, Jacobi's *The Psychology of C.G. Jung* (1942) in which one diagram of the psyche places the ego *at the centre*, relating outwards, first to the personal and then to the the collective unconscious. Another diagram places the collective unconscious, and specifically that part of it that can never be brought to consciousness, at the centre with the ego *on the periphery*. Of course, both points of view are valid, but the inevitable weakness of the single perspective diagram is that we miss the quality of experience in which sometimes our self-awareness is central and sometimes our basic drives or unconscious motivations take over.

Metapsychology

This term was invented by Freud as a counterpart to 'metaphysics'. It refers to the most theoretical view of psychology and involves a linking of concepts removed from the empirical base which was relevant at one point in their evolution. Earlier, we discussed the idea that theoretical entities do not exist; metapsychology attempts to treat them as if they did.

Freud sub-divided his own metapsychology into its dynamic, topographical and economic aspects. Let us consider what this implies for analytical psychology.

The notion that the psyche is dynamic rather than static is fundamental to Freudian, Jungian and post-Jungian psychology. What is conceived of is an interplay of forces, often instinctual, and the idea of conflict between opposing forces. For Freud, unresolved and unregenerate conflict is the wellspring of neurosis whilst Jung regarded the coming together of apparently irreconcilable psychic contents as the basis of healthy development, providing a new position from which the individual can proceed. Perhaps the major dynamic conflict (and Freud and Jung would agree on this even if afterwards variance sets in) is that between consciousness and unconsciousness. This is enhanced in the Jungian view by the proposition that there is also a self-regulatory function within the unconscious. For the moment, the main element we can descry in the dynamic aspect of metapsychology is that parts of the psyche can move together and, conversely, apart. This rhythm of combining and uniting on the one hand, and on the other, separating, differentiating and discriminating, turns out to be an important theme in Jung and a vital one for the post-Jungians in their approaches to the development of personality and to individuating and individuation.

To talk of the topography of the psyche involves identifying sub-systems and placing them either spatially (as Freud did at first) or structurally (as he did later). The roots of the topographical approach lie in anatomy and physiology in which the various parts of the human body have their own location and are connected to other areas and organs. More specifically, attempts continue to be made to locate the place where fantasies originate and so on. The whole notion of the unconscious implies that much is hidden – rather like the foundations of a building – but is operating all the same, particularly in psychopathology. Both Freud and Jung perform a dissection of the psyche as a whole to reveal its parts and sub-systems. Topography permits the mode of functioning and main characteristics of a particular sub-system to be looked at in relative isolation, as in the analysis of a complex.

The economic approach has been touched on earlier in relation to analogy. As regards metapsychology, the hypothesis is that psychological activity can be expressed in terms of the energy available for any potential process and that this can vary. Perhaps this can best be illustrated from clinical practice. Patients with obsessional symptoms may find themselves unable to cease the symptomatic activity by way of conscious striving. Economically, more energy is invested in the symptom than is available for attempts to overcome it. When we come to consider the interaction of the complexes we shall constantly be making use of this hypothesis.

There is little place in metapsychology for discussion of what is innate or constitutional in personality and what stems from interaction with the environment.

Unknowing Jungians

Where interest in Jung has swung away from the arcane and esoteric aspects to an examination of the clinical applicability of his ideas, he is revealed as a surprisingly modern thinker and psychotherapist, who anticipated in a most striking manner many of the ways in which psychoanalytic and other psychological thinking has developed. As Roazen said, in his monumental study *Freud and his Followers:*

> Few responsible figures in psychoanalysis would be disturbed today if an analyst were to present views identical to Jung's in 1913.
>
> (1976, p. 272)

And the same may be said for many of Jung's later formulations.

A list of the ways in which post-Jungian analytical psychology is in tune with various developments in psychoanalysis suggests that not only is Jung in the therapeutic mainstream but that there is a sense in which analysis and psychotherapy today are in fact 'Jungian'. We really need a new category – *unknowing Jungians.* During the course of this book we shall look at the interplay between Jung, post-Jungians and unknowing Jungians, mainly in psychoanalysis. We shall, in effect, be providing a detailed substantiation of Roazen's insight (not to mention other, more general, claims on Jung's behalf). Sometimes an idea from analytical psychology can help with a thorny problem in psychoanalytic theory, and vice versa.

My intention is not, as it were, to claim that Jung invented the wheel, or adopt the posture of a fanatical supporter of Jung (there are too many objections to Jung's ideas in this book for that). But my teaching experience and contact with psychoanalytic colleagues suggests that Jung is not yet perceived as a trustworthy figure; there is a credibility gap. By showing that much of modern analysis and psychotherapy has a pronounced Jungian flavour I hope to do something about this credibility gap and interest the reader to explore further those aspects of analytical psychology which he had been prone to dismiss.

I give here a list of the changes and developments in psychoanalysis with which I shall be concerned throughout and which reflect this 'Jungian' reorientation, together with the names of the theorists with whom they are most closely connected:

- Stress on early pre-oedipal experience of attachment to, and separation from, mother (*Klein,* the British School of object relations theorists: *Fairbairn, Guntrip, Winnicott, Balint.* Also *Bowlby*).
- A vital part is played in psychological life by innate psychic structures (archetypes) (*Klein, Bowlby, Spitz, Lacan, Bion*).
- There is a creative, purposive, non-destructive aspect to the unconscious (*Milner, Rycroft, Winnicott* on play, and cf. *Maslow* and humanistic psychology).
- Symptoms should not be looked at solely in a causal-reductive manner but in terms of their meaning for the patient (*Rycroft* and existential analysis).

- A move in analytic theory away from patriarchal, male-dominated and phallocentric approaches; attention is paid to the feminine (feminist psychology and psychotherapy, *[Juliet] Mitchell, Stoller, Lacan*).
- Stress on the clinical *use* of countertransference (most analysts today – e.g. *Searles, Langs, Racker, Little, Winnicott*).
- The idea that analysis is a mutually transforming interaction and hence that the analyst's personality and his experience of the analysis are of central importance (*Langs, Searles, Lomas,* interactionalism).
- The idea that regression in analysis may be helpful and useful, and can be worked with (*Balint, Kris*).
- Analysis should be concerned with the self as much, if not more, than the ego; the self is understood as a cohesive expression of the person rather than as one of a number of representations in the ego (*Kohut, Winnicott*).
- There are sub-divisions of personality (complexes) with which an analyst can work (*Winnicott's* true and false-selves, and cf. Gestalt therapy, transactional analysis).
- Incestuous fantasy is symbolic (*Bion, Lacan, Mitchell, Winnicott*).
- That issues of personal integration (individuation) are more central than 'sanity' or 'genitality' (*Erikson, Milner*).
- The idea that schizophrenic phenomena have meaning (*Laing* and his colleagues).
- Expansion of analytic interest into the second half of life (*Levinson, Parkes, Erikson, Kübler-Ross*).
- The idea that problems between parents find expression in children (family therapy).

Schools of analytical psychology

We now turn our attention to the question of the various schools of post-Jungian analytical psychology. It may be regrettable that these divisions exist or it may be healthily inevitable, but they cannot be ignored. This is because theoretical differences do lead to differences in analytical and therapeutic practice, determine which parts of the patient's material get attention, and contribute to the meaning inherent in the material.

I describe three existing classifications of post-Jungian schools, then my own classification and conclude with a consideration of how broad a spectrum Jungian psychology could or should encompass, with a discussion on eclecticism.

Adler's classification

Adler's system was the first of the three classifications to be published (1967). He felt that it was necessary for analytical psychology to change and develop in much the same way that Jung's own ideas underwent modification; even though this was bound to lead to some confusion, it could not be avoided. Adler describes a continuum ranging from an 'orthodox' to an 'unorthodox' attitude. The orthodox group continue to use Jung's concepts and approaches in more or less the form and manner in which he left them. Clinically, this implies a stress on elucidation of archetypal patterns which give meaning and, via amplification with comparative data, or by the use of active imagination, into consciousness purposive and teleological elements in the psychic material.

The notion of amplification is a highly developed form of analogy in which the content or story of an already known myth, fairy tale or ritualistic practice is used to elucidate or 'make ample' what might be but a clinical fragment – a single word or dream image or bodily sensation. If the clinical fragment triggers off in analyst or patient the knowledge already possessed then sense can be made of the material. For example, a woman who cannot understand why she does not get on with her mother may dream of meeting a man in an underground place. Amplification may make use of a mythologem of the collective unconscious, i.e. Demeter and Persephone, and thereby accentuate or make apparent sexual rivalry and ambivalent feelings towards the other's sexuality as the reason for the mother-daughter rift. Apart from assisting in the bringing to consciousness of this dynamic, amplification helps the patient to see that she is not alone in her problem, that it is 'typical'.

The idea of active imagination derives from Jung's discovery that the unconscious has an independent symbol-producing capacity. Jung found that this could be used analytically and designated working with such material *active* imagination to distinguish it from passive fantasizing and also to emphasize that the patient may have to make choices based on the outcome of his active imagination. Active imagination is a channel for 'messages' from the unconscious by any means; for example, by media such as painting, modelling or writing. These products are not viewed aesthetically but valued for the information they contain about pre-subjective areas of the psyche. Active imagination is therefore a special type of fantasy involving the participation of the ego and with the goal of a connection to internal, objective reality. The ego will hold a psychic fragment, as in the example above, in a contemplative manner and then:

> It is as if imagination begins to stir and a dream of the unconscious begins to unfold. Generally the ego is included in the drama, moving through the scene or asking questions. So with an attitude which acknowledges the reality of the psyche, a conversation begins between conscious and unconscious, and thus one enters the dialectic method which allows the psyche freedom of expression.
>
> (Weaver, 1964, p. 4)

The timing of active imagination in the course of an analysis and the type of person for whom it is appropriate are important questions that are entered into in Chapter 6 [of *Jung and the Post-Jungians*], which is concerned with the analytical process.

Both amplification and active imagination rest on a trust in the dynamic activity of the self, which can be repressed just as much as aggression or sexuality can be repressed. If the analysis facilitates the removal of the repression, then initiating the process just outlined will lead to movement.

At the other end of his spectrum, Adler places a second group, the 'neo-Jungians'. This group have modified Jung's ideas by attempting to integrate psychoanalytic concepts (in America from Erikson, in England from Klein and Winnicott). This leads to a departure from Jung's forward-looking approach to interpretation, away from amplification and active imagination in analysis to favour what Adler designates as 'reductive' interpretation. It implies a far greater stress on infantile material, the repetition of infantile patterns in adult life and the historic child in the adult. Working with infantile material in analysis and therapy virtually forces a concentration on the interaction between analyst and patient because the transference, composed in part of infantile wishes, impulses and forms of psychic mechanisms such as primitive defences, provides the only channel for this material.

Adler's third element in his spectrum is a central group that attempts to combine the two rather different approaches just mentioned and of which he regards himself a member. Adler distinguishes this 'middle group' from the neo-Jungians by asserting that, for this group, the analysis of transference is only one of several instruments available to the analyst. 'Equally, *if not more important* to him, will be the interpretation of dreams (and to a lesser degree the more specialised method of active imagination)' (1967, p. 349, emphasis added). Adler stresses that his conception of transference is far wider than that derived from psychoanalysis, because in addition to the infantile angle is added the possibility of projecting into the analyst unconscious potentials not yet lived.

Fordham's classification

Fordham, too, perceives that the various post-Jungian schools lay differing emphasis on differing aspects of Jung's work (1978, p. 50). Fordham does not feel that Adler's use of transference is more than a minor concession (ibid., p. 16) and therefore his classification is at variance with Adler's. His approach is based on geography. For example, he feels that at the C. G. Jung Institute in Zürich it is Jung's later style which is being offered to the students. According to Fordham, this led Jung 'more and more away from analysis and towards studying the possibilities he could discern in the unconscious' (ibid., p. 50). I think that what excites Fordham's criticism is that the teaching in Zürich is not only based on an exaggeration of Jung's later orientation, but that it overlooks the fact that this was never intended by Jung to *replace* his earlier, often more clinical, interests.

Because Jung's own work with patients developed into something highly idiosyncratic and personal to him, very little has been written about what actually happens in 'Zurich-style' analysis. Fordham is also interested and puzzled by the practice of multiple analysis said to be in use in Zürich, meaning either a patient seeing more than one analyst at a time or a process of consecutive analyses with analysts chosen for specific reasons such as sex or psychological type. Fordham sees the Zürich style of analysis as a cultural phenomenon strengthened by the peculiar position of the Institute in Zürich at the centre of a Jungian sub-culture that is not exclusively (or even primarily) clinical. In Fordham's view, the whole emphasis of this school is laid on revealing the myth-like characteristics of the patient's material and applying to the material an already-existing model of the psyche. Thus the material ends up being assigned to one particular slot or other.

Fordham, continuing his geographical survey, comes to London, where, he says, post-Jungians pay attention to transference in a way that differs from the Zürich model so radically that Fordham is prepared to speak of a 'London School'. This roughly corresponds with Adler's 'neo-Jungians'. The London School developed partly because early members were interested in what actually transpired between patient and analyst and partly because Jung's account of maturation in infancy and childhood was felt to be inadequate. Fordham notes that a good deal of interaction with psychoanalysts took place and that 'in particular the Kleinian school, with its emphasis on unconscious phantasy and countertransference, made a fertile interchange possible' (ibid., p. 53).

Rounding off his classification, Fordham notes that similar interchanges with psychoanalysts have taken place in San Francisco and in Germany. But he feels that the use of typological theory in San Francisco is a special feature of post-Jungian work there, whilst in Germany interesting work is being done on counter-transference. It should be noted that Fordham's London–Zürich differentiation is more than something conveniently contained by those two centres, and this is a weakness of his classification. It is possible to see 'London' and 'Zürich' influences in many other Jungian centres.

Fordham faced the London–Zürich conflict of his time openly and acknowledged that dogmatism and reaction formation had set in. The situation has been further complicated in London where a second group has emerged with its own organization and training with the stated objective of 'teaching Jung's psychology in an undiluted form' (Adler, 1979, p. 117). We shall turn in a moment to a consideration of factors that are relevant to this split but I want to continue to discuss previous attempts to classify post-Jungians.

Goldenberg's classification

The third classification system is that of Goldenberg (1975). She felt that Jungians had not yet formed into schools, thus differing from Fordham and Adler. There is therefore no tradition of self-criticism or evaluation from within – other than interaction between individual analysts. She feels that scholars in other disciplines, such as herself, would have freer access to Jungian concepts and post-Jungian developments, and also that Jungians would be able to communicate with each other and clarify their ideas if some classification were to be made.

Goldenberg divides post-Jungians into two groupings – the second and third generations. She means generations in intellectual history and in relation to Jung as an epistemological core rather than anything to do with the actual age of the contributor. She considers a person a member of the second generation if 'he sees himself as a disciple or teacher of Jung and has tried, in one way or another, to present a coherent account' (p. 203). Goldenberg points out that the terms 'second generation' and 'coherent account' were first used by Jung himself in the foreword to Neumann's *Origins and History of Consciousness* (1954). Goldenberg has therefore also picked up the importance of these forewords in charting the evolution of the post-Jungian mind or, in certain cases, laying the mantle upon the writer.

It is clear that Jung valued attempts to organize his work and to communicate it. And certainly works by second-generation Jungians are extremely popular (perhaps even more popular than Jung's books) because, without expressing any significant disagreement with Jung, they render his ideas into simpler form or express things more clearly than he did. However, Goldenberg would see *both* Fordham and Adler as second generation. She reserves the title of third generation for the school of analysts who define themselves as 'archetypal psychologists'. For Goldenberg, this is the first generation of people who do not feel any responsibility to Jung personally although they recognize his influence. I think that this last point is the salient feature of this classification. The question of 'responsibility to Jung' may really be what distinguishes second from third generation post-Jungians.

Comment

It is clear that these classifications are mutually exclusive – for instance Goldenberg's third generation are simply not noticed in the other two classifications (though Adler might claim that archetypal psychology was not a force in the late 1960s).

And Fordham disputes Adler's claim to the middle ground, while Adler seems almost ready for the neo-Jungians to depart the fold. It is a confusing and unpleasant state of affairs and one which perplexes students and current practitioners alike. I am indebted to Clark (personal communication, 1982) for an anecdote concerning a series of seminars he gave for trainee Jungian psychotherapists on the strands in modern Jungian psychology. The students felt these issues so deeply that on occasion tears attested to the anxiety that diversity and schism can cause. The positive side of the story is that the students valued the chance to undertake comparative work.

A new classification

In formulating my own classification I have wanted above all to provide a model that will allow for individual differences whilst describing post-Jungian schools with sufficient coherence and coalescence to be of use in the twin aims summarized by Goldenberg – to provide access into post-Jungian developments for outsiders and to enable a higher degree of structuring, ordering and mutual reflection in internal debate.

My hypothesis is that there are indeed three main schools. We can call these the *Classical School,* the *Developmental School* and the *Archetypal School.* My method is to select three aspects of theoretical discussion and three of clinical practice to which all analytical psychologists relate. I hope to demonstrate that it is the *ordering and weighting* of these that underpin the evolution of the schools.

The three theoretical areas are:

(1) the definition of archetypal;
(2) the concept of self;
(3) the development of personality.

The three clinical aspects are:

(1) the analysis of transference–countertransference;
(2) emphasis upon symbolic experiences of the self;
(3) examination of highly differentiated imagery.

With regard to theory, I think the Classical School would weight the possibilities in the order 2, 1, 3. That is, the integrating and individuating self would be most important, other archetypal imagery and potentials would come close behind and the early experience of the individual would be seen as of somewhat lesser importance. (I imagine this to represent, in general terms, Jung's own ordering of priorities, hence the use of the word 'Classical'.) The Developmental School would weight these possibilities in the order 3, 2, 1. Importance would be given to the personal development of the individual, which would then involve a consideration of the self, seen as generating its archetypal potentialities and imagery over a lifetime. The Archetypal School would consider archetypal imagery first, the self second, and development would receive less emphasis. Thus the ordering would be 1, 2, 3.

Turning to clinical practice, the Classical School would weight the possibilites 2, 3, 1 or perhaps 2, 1, 3. I am not sure whether transference–countertransference or a pursuit of particularized imagery would come second to the search for the self. The Developmental School would order its clinical priorities 1, 2, 3, or possibly 1, 3, 2. Here again, I am sure that transference–countertransference would be considered a most important aspect, but I am not certain whether experience of the self or an examination of imagery would rate second position. The Archetypal School would probably function in the order 3, 2, 1. That is, particularized imagery would be regarded as more useful than symbolic experiences of the self and both would be more central than transference–countertransference.

Of course there is overlap with the earlier classifications. My Classical School is Similar to Adler's 'orthodoxy' and Fordham's 'Zürich School'. My Developmental School bears resemblance to Adler's 'neo-Jungians' and to Fordham's 'London School'. My Archetypal School is termed by Goldenberg 'third generation Jungians'.

I did not select the six themes by accident – theorists of all three schools have reinforced the emphases I have suggested. For example, Adler (Classical School), in a 'personal statement' (unpublished, 1975) wrote:

> We put the main emphasis on symbolic transformation. I would like to quote what Jung says in a letter to P. W. Martin (20/8/45): 'The main interest of my work is with the approach to the numinous . . . but the fact is that the numinous is the real therapy.'

As far as the Developmental School is concerned, the editorial introduction to a collection of their papers (Fordham et al., 1974) states that

> the recognition of transference as such was the first subject to become a central one for clinical preoccupation . . . Then, as anxiety about this began to diminish with the acquisition of increased skill and experience, countertransference became a subject that could be tackled. Finally . . . the transaction involved is most suitably termed transference/countertransference.
>
> (p. x)

That introduction went on to discuss whether the term 'interpretation' has any analytic meaning if unlinked with the past development of the patient. Hillman, speaking for the Archetypal School, asserts:

> At the most basic level of psychic reality are fantasy images. These images are the primary activity of consciousness . . . *Images are the only reality we apprehend directly,*

and in the same paper he refers to the 'primacy of images' (1975, p. 174).

It has been suggested to me (Lambert, personal communication, 1982) that the six elements could be constituted in a grid, similar to that drawn up in psychoanalysis by Bion (1963). This is shown in *Figure 12.1*. Bion's grid is designed to help an analyst reflect on problems that arise in analytic practice; it is a method of recording in an abstract manner what he and the patient have been doing, ranging from the most simple to the most elaborate interactions. In fact, I would not suggest that my grid is in any way comparable to Bion's monumental edifice with its forty-eight categories. But the use to which this grid may be put is similar: as part of the professional self-analysis of the analyst, an exploration of the analyst's professional inner world. Even more important, readers of this book may use the grid to orientate themselves in the various post-Jungian debates.

	Transference–countertransference	Symbolic experiences of the self	Examination of highly differentiated imagery
Definition of archetypal			
The concept of self			
The development of personality			

Figure 12.1

Any classification is, to an extent, a creative falsehood in that there are unlikely to be many individuals who exactly fit the descriptions. For some temperaments, classification is seen as of little value or even as destructive to individuality. Classification is itself suspect as each writer, secretly or openly, favours the group he knows best. But on the other hand, the very existence of classifications such as those of Adler, Fordham and Goldenberg is significant, not to mention catch-phrases such as Plaut's 'Klein-Jungian hybrid' (1962) or Hillman's invention of the term 'archetypal psychology' (1975, pp. 138–47).

I have not presented my classifications in an either/or way; I have made it a central feature that *all* analytical psychologists are likely to use *all* these theories and are interested in *all* these clinical areas at some time and with some patients. Taken altogether, the six headings constitute a large part of the discipline of analytical psychology as a whole – this is the common core or base derived from Jung with all subsequent additions. Following Bion (1965), we may call this the *post-Jungian vertex,* implying an overall point of view or perspective. What defines an analytical psychologist will be whether he relates actively to debates which arise from the differing emphases which may be given to the six headings. Such emphasis, weighting and preference, together with the choices made by individual analysts, constitute the schools. So a classification into schools, carried out in this way, can tell us *as much about what is held in common* as about differences of opinion.

Further, we should expect to find in the schools of analytical psychology more than a common tradition. We may discover something in common in the developments within the various schools, a common ideological and practical future. In Chapter 11 [of *Jung and the Post-Jungians*] I draw together elements of such a future, but the attempt to do so is a thread running through the book.

I am sure the schools have a 'contra-ideological' component. For example, Hubback has shown how, even in the Developmental School, questions of amplification and active imagination (not usually associated with that school) have been given attention (1980). She comments that it is often a patient, or a group of patients, who provides the stimulus for interest in a particular topic; hence the need for a classificatory approach based on priorities rather than exclusivities.

I mentioned earlier that the schools of psychoanalysis have over time taken on a more formal structure than those of analytical psychology. It is reasonable to suggest that a similar process will take place in analytical psychology and that this has already begun. Thus any temptation to ignore the existence of schools or to minimize their importance is historically unsound, or may hark back nostalgically to an earlier, more unified, period.

In this context we may note what Segal (1979) has to say about the way in which the British Psychoanalytical Society came to organize its training to take account of the reality of differences between schools of psychoanalysis – the 'B Group' composed of Anna Freud and her followers, and the 'A Group' composed of both the Kleinians and what later became known separately as the 'Middle Group' of uncommitted analysts. Segal believes that, after the earlier acrimony during the 1940s, as differences were worked on, things settled down, and that the organization of the training to take account of the groups not only gives students a firm base in their chosen path but 'also an acquaintance with divergent points of view' (ibid., p. 111).

Segal's account is also interesting for the light it sheds on the way in which the warring factions related to Freud: 'both sides of the controversy quoted Freud repeatedly, but the quotations were different. One could say, Which Freud? Whose Freud?' (ibid., p. 95). And because a key issue was whether Melanie Klein *was* a Freudian, it will not come as a surprise to analytical psychologists (who have, as may be seen throughout this book, their own version of this problem) to hear that

> to the end of her life [Klein] felt a little bewildered and deeply hurt by Freud's coolness towards her and her work, which she saw as being close to his. Believing that she had developed it in the same ethos and further than any other living analyst, she found it very difficult to bear that he did not see it that way.
>
> (ibid., p. 171)

Perhaps polemic is inevitable. Heraclitus tells us that *polemos,* meaning strife or conflict, is the 'father of all, the king of all'. In addition to ideological factors, the schools of analytical psychology radiate emotional reality and that may be seen as a necessity for an emerging profession.

One complicating factor is that post-Jungian groups have tended to cluster round strong leader figures. I do not think this results from *conscious* fostering, but the erection of leaders, no doubt stemming from a desire to avoid the anomalous and to have ideas arranged in a hierarchy of acceptability, has personalized some of the differences between the schools (cf. Samuels, 1981).

What is more, the schools are bound to become more, rather than less, powerful in that the various founders are likely to select as trainees those who will be sympathetic to whatever consensus may exist in a particular school.

Returning to my own classification for a moment, a further way to avoid rigidity is to see the schools as overlapping to some extent. That not only allows for individuals who fall between schools but also demonstrates differences within schools. This is shown in *Figure 12.2*; the names are arranged alphabetically to facilitate the reader's returning to this chart as he progresses through the book, and the presence of names in the same column implies theoretical similarity rather than a public alliance (though this may exist). Of course there are numerous thinkers on whose work I am not commenting, or with which I am not familiar, or who do not write books and papers; their names cannot appear.

CLASSICAL					
DEVELOPMENTAL				ARCHETYPAL	
Carvalho	Abenheimer	Blum	Adler	Guggenbühl	Avens
Davidson	Blomeyer	Bradway	Binswanger	Shorter	Berry
Fordham	Clark	Detloff	Castillejo	R. Stein	Casey
Gordon	Dieckmann	Edinger	Fierz		Corbin
Jackson	Fiumara	Hall	Frey-Rohn		Giegerich
Kay	Goodheart	McCurdy	Groesbeck		Grinnell
Lambert	Hobson	Neumann	Hannah		Hillman
Ledermann	Hubback	Perry	Harding		Lopez-Pedraza
Lyons	Jacoby	Schwartz	Henderson		Miller
Maduro	Newton	Ulanov	Humbert		M. Stein
Plaut	Moore	Whitmont	Jacobi		
L. Stein	Redfearn	Willeford	Jaffé		
Strauss	Samuels		E. Jung		
Zinkin	Seligman		Mattoon		
	Williams		Laughlin		
			Layard		
			Meier		
			Perera		
			Singer		
			Stevens		
			von der Heydt		
			von Franz		
			Weaver		
			Wheelwright		
			Wolff		
			Woodman		

Figure 12.2

The limits of analytical psychology

I have used the term *post-Jungian* in preference to *Jungian* to indicate both connectedness to Jung and distance from him. The questions that will inevitably be asked are: how broad a community should analytical psychology be? Is it possible, or even desirable, that the multiplicity of viewpoints with which we shall be engaged be given *any* common designation? How fluid can practice be with regard to a particular patient before it becomes professionally responsible to refer him to another analyst or even to another kind of practitioner?

Henderson, whom I would think of as a member of the Classical School, touches on these questions when reviewing the collections of papers which have been put out by the Developmental School. He says:

> What readers missed in these papers as they appeared . . . was the sense of adventure to which they were accustomed by the inclusion of large philosophic ideas and the amplification of archetypal images with reference to religion, alchemy and primitive myths such as are to be found in Jungian literature from the pens of such writers as Neumann, von Franz, Adler, Hillman and others.
>
> Now . . . we can see why it was wrong to expect them to be different from what they are. They do not pretend to add much to Jung's teleological (i.e. forward-*looking*) method, with its strong reliance on the language of religious symbolism . . . It is a part of Fordham's stated claim that Jungian analysis is not incompatible with Freudian analysis, and I think that in certain significant respects . . . this claim has been justified.
>
> (1975b, p. 203)

Henderson reminds us that it is pointless to expect something to do more than it is designed to do or to criticize something for not being what it was never intended to be. Accepting diversity means accepting limitations in ourselves and others. However, the idea that Freudian and Jungian analysis may be compatible is, for some Jungians and Freudians, quite unacceptable.

Here, as so often, extremists from both the Freudian and the Jungian camps find themselves in the same bed. In psychoanalysis, Glover attacks any notion of compromise, quoting John Morley:

> At the bottom of the advocacy of a dual doctrine slumbers the idea that there is no harm in men being mistaken, or at least only so little harm as is more than compensated for by the marked tranquility in which their mistake wraps them.
>
> (Glover, 1950, p. 187)

Glover goes on to attack eclecticism which claims to be a commonsense, objective way of going about things. He rejects any gentleman's agreement between opponents. In this he is joined by Adler who objects strongly to Fordham's statement in his obituary of Jung that Jung's personal incompatibility with Freud and the resultant separation appears a disaster from which analytical psychology and psychoanalysis both suffer and will continue to suffer until the damage is repaired. Adler feels that one must accept that we have to make a choice and live with the sacrifice involved (Adler, 1971, p. 114). Adler is speaking both of his rejection of Freudian-Jungian synthesis and of his attitude to internal Jungian diversity – his insistence upon 'undiluted' Jung as mentioned earlier.

Adler is therefore at peace with the idea that Jungian psychology might lose 'on the side of understanding physical phenomena, object relations and some actual therapeutic insights' (ibid., p. 117). The danger for post-Jungians, as Adler sees it, is that, with so much diversity, they will be assimilated and so lose their original point of view. As we have just seen, it is now a matter of concern as to what *is* involved in the Jungian view.

In his book *The Art of Psychotherapy* (1979), Storr takes a different attitude to Adler's altogether. He prophesies that soon psychological schools will cease to exist as separate entities because theoretical disputes are storms in teacups which disguise the basic similarity of what analysts and therapists actually do. From an Olympian standpoint, it is possible that similarities outweigh differences, but this proposition may turn out to be more of a hoped-for programme as there are no signs that the schools of depth psychology are losing their appeal (that is, the schools still exert an attraction even though there has been a swing away from analytical approaches in general).

If Storr means that cross-fertilization is taking place to an unprecedented degree then I am in complete agreement. I would also concur that unbridled devotion to one idea or one man can be destructive. But it is surely necessary for an analyst or therapist to work with conviction, even passion. If this is lacking then something may be lost.

Research material showing that therapists of all persuasions get similar results does not mean, and should not be taken as implying, that it does not matter what you believe. I cannot simply adopt a Gestalt technique – it would be inauthentic and ridiculous for me to do so, given my orientation and training. It follows that choice, arising out of character and conviction, will have to be exercised and we may conclude that questioning and critical acknowledgment of a tradition is a virtue; becoming acquainted with that tradition is then an obligation. However, the requirement of critical choice is not an easy one to fulfil in a complicated and conflict-ridden field.

Conflict and choice

Where does the reader with an interest in Jungian ideas and a desire to update that knowledge go? Popper once said that the place for any beginning seeker after knowledge to go is *where the disagreements are*. If you acknowledge that psychological theory and practice develop organically, by the way of a process, then the point where current practitioners disagree reflects the state of the art. Here you can be sure of being in the presence of the best minds and talents and the most contemporary viewpoints or syntheses of what has gone before and predictions of what might happen next (Popper, 1972).

This notion opposes the apparently more sensible and customary view that we should start with what is known and agreed, and when that has been mastered or at least understood, engage in the grown-up disagreements. Of course the arena where experienced people differ is a heady place to enter, dizzymaking, frightening, fragmentary, but basing a quest for knowledge on *conflict* rather than *consensus* has its points. I have developed these ideas at length elsewhere (Samuels, 1981), but here I would like to suggest that the main advantage of conflict-oriented rather than consensus-oriented study is that the former continually puts the reader in an *active*, problem-solving situation. He has to decide which of several views is more reliable and suits him best. He will himself be at the tip of a line of inquiry stretching back to Jung and beyond but his first task will be to look into the conflict and then to choose.

Popper says 'we do not know how or where to start an analysis of this world. There is no wisdom to tell us. Even the scientific tradition doesn't tell us. It only tells us where other people started and where they got to' (Popper, 1972, p. 129). So instead of studying the works of Freud, Jung, Klein, Neumann in a 'sensible' order, one might start with Hillman's attack on the developmental approach (1975, pp. 5–48) or Fordham's attack on Neumann's views on childhood (Fordham 1981). There you have two excellent minds at work; what turns them on, energizes them, is worth noticing. Such arcane conflicts are supposed to be too much for the non-specialist to bear. It does not matter if some aspects of the disputes I am chronicling are beyond the grasp of some readers; more will be understood in time and *starting at the beginning is no guarantee of comprehension.*

A pragmatic colouring can be put on most of this. William James said that 'ideas become true just so far as they help us get into satisfactory relations with other parts of our experience' (James, 1911, p. xii). So, for example, the psychological theories we are discussing are not to be seen as *answers* to questions of human nature but as *instruments* to guide future action and practice. Pragmatism involves a type of democratic procedure in which a person is free to decide which of various conflicting hypotheses to accept. If his rational examination of the alternatives cannot help him make a decision then he is free simply to follow his own inclination.

One final note on the schools. Those readers whose knowledge of analytical psychology is not extensive should use the classification, grid and lists to orient themselves and find meaning in what follows [in *Jung and the Post-Jungians*]. Those more *au fait* with the field may, in addition, want to entertain the idea that the schools can also be seen as separate strands existing in the mind of an analyst, sometimes competing and sometimes synthesizing. To both groups of readers I would say that the book [*Jung and the Post-Jungians*] is, in some sense, in tune with Jung's own thinking when he urged that opposites have to be discriminated before they can be brought together. The schools represent such a discrimination, and the notion that the schools taken together define the discipline represents the combination, the *conjunctio.*

References

Adler, G. (1967) 'Methods of treatment in analytical psychology'. In B. Wolman (ed.) *Psychoanalytical Techniques.* New York: Basic Books.

Adler, G. (1971) 'Analytical psychology and the principle of complementarity'. In J. Wheelwright (ed.) *The Analytic Process.* New York: Putnam.

Adler, G. (1979) *Dynamics of the Self.* London: Coventure.

Bion, W. (1963) 'Elements of psychoanalysis'. In *Seven Servants.* New York: Jason Aronson, 1977.

Bion, W. (1965) 'Transformations'. In *Seven Servants.* New York: Jason Aronson, 1977.

Brown, J. (1961) *Freud and the Post-Freudians.* Harmondsworth: Penguin.

Fordham, M. (1975) 'Memories and thoughts about C. G. Jung'. *Journal of Analytical Psychology, 20*: 2, 102–13.

Fordham, M. (1978) *Jungian Psychotherapy: A Study in Analytical Psychology.* Chichester: Wiley.

Fordham, M. (1981) 'Neumann and childhood'. *Journal of Analytical Psychology, 26*: 2, 99–122.

Fordham, M., Gordon, R., Hubback, J., Lambert, K. and Williams, M. (1974) Editors' Introduction to *Technique in Jungian Analysis.* London: Heinemann.

Freud, S. (1912) 'Recommendations to physicians'. Std Edn 12. London: Hogarth.

Glover, E. (1950) *Freud or Jung.* London: Allen & Unwin.

Goldenberg, N. (1975) 'Archetypal theory after Jung'. *Spring*.
Henderson, J. (1975a) 'C. G. Jung: A reminiscent picture of his method'. *Journal of Analytical Psychology, 20*: 2, 114–21.
Henderson, J. (1975b) Review of *Analytical Psychology: A Modern Science* (M. Fordham, ed.) and *Technique in Jungian Analysis* (M. Fordham, R. Gordon and J. Hubback, eds). *Psychological Perspectives, 6*: 2, 197–203.
Hillman, J. (1962) 'Training and the C. G. Jung Institute, Zurich'. *Journal of Analytical Psychology, 7*: 1, 3–19.
Hillman, J. (1975) *Loose Ends*. Dallas, TX: Spring.
Hubback, J. (1973) 'Uses and abuses of analogy'. *Journal of Analytical Psychology, 18*: 2, 91–104.
Hubback, J. (1980) 'Developments and similarities, 1935–1980'. *Journal of Analytical Psychology, 25*: 3, 219–36.
Jacobi, J. (1942) *The Psychology of C. G. Jung*. London: Kegan Paul, Trench, Trubner; New Haven, CT: Yale University Press.
James, W. (1911) *Pragmatism*. London: Fontana, 1962.
Jung, C. G. (1913) 'General aspects of psychoanalysis'. *CW* 4. *Freud and Psychoanalysis*.
Jung, C.G. (1937) *Psychology and Religion*. *CW* 11.
Jung, C.G. (1938) Preface to the Third Edition of 'Psychic conflicts in a child'. *CW* 17. *The Development of Personality*.
Jung, C. G. (1952) *Symbols of Transformation*. *CW* 5.
Lambert, K. (1981) *Analysis, Repair and Individuation*. London: Academic Press.
McGuire, W. (1974) (ed.) *The Freud–Jung Letters*. London: Hogarth and Routledge and Kegan Paul; Princeton, NJ: Princeton University Press.
Malcolm, J. (1982) *Psychoanalysis: The Impossible Profession*. London: Pan.
Neumann, E. (1954) *The Origins and History of Consciousness*. London: Routledge and Kegan Paul.
Plaut, A. (1962) 'Some reflections on the Klein-Junian hybrid'. Unpublished.
Popper, K. (1972) *Conjectures and Refutations: The Growth of Scientific Knowledge*. London: Routledge and Kegan Paul.
Roazen, P. (1976) *Freud and His Followers*. London: Penguin.
Rycroft, C. (1972) *A Critical Dictionary of Psychoanalysis*. London: Penguin.
Stein, L. (1958) 'Analytical psychology: A modern science'. In M. Fordham, R. Gordon, J. Hubback, K. Lambert and M. Williams (eds.), *Analytical Psychology: A Modern Science*. London: Heinemann, 1973.
Samuels, A. (1981) 'Fragmentary vision: A central training aim'. *Spring*.
Sandler, A.-M. (1982) 'The selecton and function of the training analyst in Europe'. *International Review of Psychoanalysis*, 9: 4, pp. 386–97.
Schafer, R. (1976) *A New Language for Psychoanalysis*. New Haven, CT: Yale University Press.
Segal, H. (1979) *Klein*. London: Fontana.
Storr, A. (1979) *The Art of Psychotherapy*. London: Heinemann.
Weaver, R. (1964) *The Old Wise Woman*. London: Vincent Stuart.

CHAPTER 13

NEW DEVELOPMENTS IN THE POST-JUNGIAN FIELD

Retrospective introduction

This chapter was commissioned by Polly Young-Eisendrath and Terence Dawson for the second edition (2008) of their edited *Cambridge Companion to Jung*. I had also written an introductory chapter for the first edition in 1998 but took the chance to completely update the classification of the schools of post-Jungian analytical psychology. Hence what you find here more or less replaces what you have read in the previous chapter in terms of where I am with it now.

However, this second and later classification is much more polemical and hence less reliable and, in general, though people have noted what I think nowadays about the schools, they continue to use and refer to the original 1985 classification and I am happy with this.

I was trying in this version to make a comment on the state of the Jungian clinical field today. I felt that the classical school had spawned an extreme version of itself that I called the fundamentalist school. The developmental school had also generated an extreme version of itself that I called the psychoanalytic school. I felt that, as a distinct clinical entity, the archetypal school had been absorbed into the classical school.

So the first classification of developmental-classical-archetypal got replaced by psychoanalytic-developmental-classical-fundamentalist.

I also used the chapter to address significant problems in the reception of Jung in our culture, in academia and in clinical circles.

In university settings, it is my habit to begin lectures on analytical psychology, especially to those not taking degrees in Jungian psychology, by asking those present to do a simple association exercise to the word 'Jung'. I ask them to record the first three things that come to mind. From the (by now) 1,000+ responses, I have found that the most frequently cited themes, words, concepts or images have (in order) to do with (a) Freud, (b) psychoanalysis and (c) the Freud–Jung split. The next most frequently cited association concerns (d) Jung's anti-semitism and alleged Nazi sympathies. Other matters raised include (e) archetypes, (f) mysticism/philosophy/religion and (g) animus and anima.

Obviously, this is not properly empirical research. But if we 'associate to' the associations, we can see that there *is* a lingering doubt about the intellectual, scholarly and ethical viability of taking an interest in Jung. Even so, in these pages, I shall argue that there is more to the question of Jung and Freud's psychoanalysis than the oft-repeated story of two wrestling men.

Over the past decade, there has been increasing clinical and academic interest in analytical psychology in non-Jungian circles, in spite of the fact that its core texts are not effectively represented on official reading lists and curriculum descriptions. Outside of this interest, though, Jung is mentioned primarily as an important schismatic in the history of psychoanalysis and not as a contributor worthy of sustained and systematic study in his own right. Although many psychoanalysts pass over his name in silence, many therapists – and not just Jungian – have 'discovered' Jung to have been a major contributor to what appears now as cutting-edge new developments in clinical work. In this chapter, I shall suggest that Jung's ideas merit a place in their own right in general clinical training in psychotherapy and in the contemporary academy. I shall also explain how I see the overall shape of the post-Jungian field via two classifications of the field into schools of analytical psychology. The first of these summarizes the proposal I made back in 1985 in *Jung and the Post-Jungians;* the second is more contemporary and more provocative.

The 'Jung' problem

It is impossible to make this argument without first exploring the cultural and intellectual contexts in which it is mounted. Until recently, Jung has been 'banished comprehensively' from academic life, to borrow a phrase used by the distinguished psychologist Liam Hudson (1983) in a review of a collection of Jung's writings. Let us try to understand why it is so.

First, the secret 'committee' set up by Freud and Jones in 1912 to defend the cause of 'true' psychoanalysis spent a good deal of time and energy on disparaging Jung. The fall-out from this historical moment has taken a very long time to evaporate and has meant that Jung's ideas have been slow to penetrate psychoanalytic circles and hence have not been welcomed in the academy, whose preferred depth psychology – certainly in the humanities and social sciences – has been Freudian and post-Freudian psychoanalysis.

Second, Jung's anti-semitic writings and misguided involvements in the professional politics of psychotherapy in Germany in the 1930s have, understandably in my view, made it almost impossible for Holocaust-aware psychologists – both Jewish and non-Jewish – to generate a positive attitude to his theories. Some portions of the early Jungian community refused to acknowledge that there was any substance to the charges held against Jung, and even withheld information that they deemed unsuitable for the public domain. Such evasions only served to prolong a problem which must be faced squarely. Present-day Jungians are now addressing the issue, and assessing it both in the context of his time and in relation to his work as a whole.[1]

Third, Jung's attitudes to women, blacks, so-called 'primitive' cultures and so forth are now outmoded and unacceptable. It is not sufficient to assert that he intended them to be taken metaphorically – not least because this may not have been how he intended his writing to be taken! We can now see how Jung converted prejudice into theory and translated his perception of what was current into something supposed to be eternally valid. Here, too, it has turned out to be the work of the post-Jungians that has discovered these mistakes and contradictions and corrected Jung's faulty or amateur methods. When these corrections are made, one can see that Jung had a remarkable capacity to intuit the themes and areas with which late twentieth-century and early twenty-first-century psychology would be concerned: gender; race; nationalism; cultural analysis; the perseverance, reappearance and socio-political power of religious mentality in an apparently irreligious epoch; the unending search for meaning – all of these have turned out to be the problematics with which psychology has had to concern itself. Recognizing the soundness of Jung's intuitive vision facilitates a more interested but no less critical return to his texts. This is what is meant by 'post-Jungian': correction of Jung's work and also critical distance from it.

Jung and Freud

The break in relations between Jung and Freud is usually presented in introductory and even in more advanced texts as stemming from a father–son power struggle and Jung's inability to come to terms with what is involved in human psychosexuality. On the surface of the Oedipus myth, the father's son-complex is not nearly as easy to access as the son's father-complex. It is tempting to forget Laius' infanticidal impulses and so we do not see much analysis-at-a-distance of Freud's motives. And yet I believe that Freud's actions and intentions toward Jung played at least as large a role as did Jung's toward Freud in bringing about their split and subsequent rivalry.

As far as Jung's angle on sexuality is concerned, the fact that much of the content of his 1912 breakaway book *Wandlungen und Symbolen der Libido* – originally translated as *Psychology of the Unconscious* (*CW* B) – concerns an interpretation of the incest motif and of incest fantasy is usually overlooked. The book is highly pertinent to an understanding of family process and the way in which events in the outer family cohere into what might be called an inner family. In other words, the book now called *Symbols of Transformation* (Jung, 1952) is not an experience-distant text. It asks: how do humans grow, from a psychological point of view? It answers that they grow by internalizing – that is, 'taking inside themselves' – qualities, attributes and styles of life that they have not yet managed to master on their own. From where does this new stuff come? From the parents or other caretakers, of course. But how does it happen? Characteristic of the human sexual drive is the impossibility for any person to remain indifferent to another who is the recipient of sexual fantasy or the source of desire. Incest-fuelled desire is implicated in the kind of human love that healthy family process cannot do without. A degree of sexualized interest between parents and children that is *not* acted out – and which must remain on the level of incest *fantasy* – is necessary for the two individuals in a situation where each cannot avoid the other. 'Kinship libido', as Jung named this interest, is a necessity for internalizing the good experiences of early life.

This account of Jung's early interest in family incest themes challenges the assumption of a vast difference between Jung and Freud's foci. The scene is then set for a linkage of Jungian ideas with other critically important psychoanalytic notions, such as Jean Laplanche's (1989) theory of the centrality of seduction in early development. In a more clinical vein, Jung's incest theory leads us to understand child sexual abuse as a damaging *degeneration* of a healthy and necessary engagement with 'incest fantasy'. Situating child sexual abuse on a spectrum of expectable human behaviour in this way helps to reduce the understandable moral panic that inhibits constructive thinking about the topic and opens the way for its troubling ubiquity to be investigated.

Jung's contribution to psychoanalysis and psychotherapy

Most contemporary psychotherapists accept the idea that Freud's ideas and theories undergird modern practices. However, post-Freudian psychoanalysis has gone on to revise, repudiate and extend a great many of Freud's seminal ideas. Ironically, as a result of these critiques, many positions of contemporary psychoanalysis are reminiscent of those taken by Jung in earlier years. This is not to say that Jung himself is responsible for what is most interesting about contemporary psychoanalysis, or that he worked these things out in as much detail as the psychoanalytic thinkers concerned. But, as Paul Roazen (1976, p. 272) has pointed out, 'Few responsible figures in psychoanalysis would be disturbed today if an analyst were to present views identical to Jung's in 1913.' To explicate this claim, I explain twelve vital psychoanalytic issues in which Jung can be seen as a precursor of recent developments of 'post-Freudian' psychoanalysis. The list that follows culminates in an extended discussion of Jung's pioneering role in what is now known as Relational Psychoanalysis.

(1) While Freud's Oedipal psychology is father-centered and is not relevant to a period earlier than about the age of four, Jung provided a mother-based psychology in which influence is often traced back much earlier, even to prenatal events. For this reason, he may be seen as a precursor of the work of Melanie Klein, of the British School of object relations theorists such as Fairbairn, Winnicott, Guntrip and Balint, and, given the theory of archetypes (of which more in a moment), of Bowlby's ethologically inspired work on attachment. Post-Jungians such as Knox (2003) and Wilkinson (2006) have shown how Jungian archetypal theory anticipates and expands neuroscientific research into the centrality of early relationships. Jung's theories are useful also for re-conceptualizing psychotherapy from a neuroscientific perspective.

(2) In Freud's view, the unconscious is created by repression, a personal process derived from lived experience. In Jung's view, the unconscious has a collective base, which means that innate structures greatly affect, and perhaps determine, its contents. Not only post-Jungians are concerned with such innate unconscious structures. In the work of psychoanalysts such as Klein, Lacan, Spitz and Bowlby one finds the same emphasis on pre-structuralization of the unconscious. That the unconscious is structured like a language (Lacan's view) could easily have been stated by Jung. A nuanced post-Jungian review of these ideas is carried out by Hogenson (2004).

(3) Freud's view of human psychology is a bleak one and, given the history of the twentieth century, it seems reasonable. But Jung's early insistence that there is a creative, purposive, non-destructive core of the human psyche finds echoes and resonances in the work of psychoanalytic writers like Milner and Rycroft, and in Winnicott's work on play. Similar links can be made with the great pioneers of humanistic psychology such as Rogers and Maslow. Jung's argument that the psyche has knowledge of what is good for it, a capacity to regulate itself, and even to heal itself, takes us to the heart of contemporary expositions of the 'true self' such as that found in Bollas's recent work, to give only one example. Stein (1996) offers a good example of a post-Jungian perspective on meaning and purpose.

(4) Jung's attitude to psychological symptoms was that they should be looked at not exclusively in a causal-reductive manner but also in terms of their hidden meanings for the patient – even in terms of what the symptom is 'for'.[2] This anticipates the school of existential analysis and the work of some British psychoanalysts such as Rycroft and Home. Cambray (2004) offers a fascinating post-Jungian view of non-causal approaches to psychopathology.

(5) In contemporary psychoanalysis, there has been a move away from what are called male-dominated, patriarchal and phallocentric approaches; in psychology and psychotherapy alike, more attention is being paid to the 'feminine' (whatever might be meant by this). In the past two decades, feminist psychoanalysis and psychotherapy have come into being. There is little doubt that Jung's 'feminine' is a *man's* 'feminine', but parallels between feminist-influenced psychoanalysis and gender-sensitive Jungian and post-Jungian analytical psychology may be drawn (see Kast, 2006, for an up-to-date account of animus/anima theory).

(6) The ego has been moved away from the centre of the theoretical and the therapeutic projects of psychoanalysis. Lacan's decentering of the ego exposes as delusive the fantasy of mastery and unification of the personality, and Kohut's working out of a bipolar self also extends well beyond the confines of rational, orderly ego-hood. The recognition of a non-ego integration of dissociated states is anticipated by Jung's theory of Self: the totality of psychic processes, somehow 'bigger' than ego and carrying humanity's apparatus of aspiration and imagination. Corbett (1996) offers a well-researched and argued account of Jung's notion of Self.

(7) The deposing of the ego has also created a space for what might be called 'sub-personalities'. Jung's theory of complexes, which he referred to as 'splinter psyches', fills out contemporary models of dissociation (Samuels, Shorter and Plaut, 1986, pp. 33–35). We can compare Jung's tendency to personify the inner divisions of the psyche with Winnicott's true and false selves and with Eric Berne's 'transactional analysis' wherein ego, id and superego are understood as relatively autonomous. Guided fantasy, Gestalt work and visualization would be scarcely conceivable without Jung's contribution: 'active imagination' describes a temporary suspension of ego control, a 'dropping down' into the unconscious, and a careful notation of what one finds, whether by reflection or some kind of artistic self-expression.

(8) Many contemporary psychoanalysts hold a strong distinction between ideas like 'mental health', 'sanity' and 'genitality', on the one hand, and, on the other, the idea of 'individuation'. The difference is between psychological norms of adaptation, themselves a microcosm of societal values, and an ethic which prizes individual variation more highly than adherence to the norm. Although Jung's cultural values have sometimes been criticized as elitist, he is *the* great writer on individuation. Psychoanalytic writers on these themes include Winnicott, Milner and Erikson. Fierz (1991) shows the relevance of these perspectives to contemporary psychiatry and psychotherapy.

(9) Jung was a psychiatrist and retained an interest in psychosis all his life. From his earliest clinical work with patients at the Burghölzli hospital in Zurich, he argued that schizophrenic phenomena have meanings which a sensitive therapist can elucidate. In this regard, he anticipates R. D. Laing and the anti-psychiatry movement of the 1960s. Jung's final position on schizophrenia, in 1958, was that there may be some kind of biochemical 'toxin' involved in the serious psychoses that would suggest a genetic element. However, Jung felt that this genetic element would do no more than give an individual a predisposition with which life's events would interact leading to a favourable or unfavourable outcome. Here, we see an anticipation of today's psycho-bio-social approach to schizophrenia and borderline personality disorder.

(10) Until recently very few psychoanalysts have created a whole-of-life psychology, one that would include the fulcrum events of mid-life, old age

and impending death. Jung did. Developmentalists like Levinson, as well as those who explore the psychology of death and dying (such as Kübler-Ross and Parkes), all acknowledge Jung's very prescient contribution.

(11) Finally, although Jung thought that children have distinct personalities from birth, his idea that problems in childhood may be traced to the 'unlived psychological life of the parents' (Jung, 1918, p. 25) anticipates many findings of family therapy.

(12) This much longer concluding section concerns Jung's approach to clinical work. Relational Psychoanalysis emphasizes a two-person psychology and intersubjective influences on unconscious relating. Historians of this relatively new and increasingly influential school have begun to acknowledge Jung as a pioneering influence (e.g. Altman, 2005). Ironically, however, there has been little direct contact between Relationalists and Jungians, probably due to the fall-out from the Freud–Jung split. Contemporary post-Jungian analysts (e.g. Samuels et al., 2000) have little difficulty in resonating with many of the ideas and practices evolving within the evolving tradition of relational psychoanalysis.

Jung asserted that analysis was a 'dialectical process', intending to highlight the fact that two people are involved in a relationship, that emotionally charged interactions between them are two-way and that, in the deepest sense, they are to be conceived of as equals (Jung, 1929, p. 8). Analysis, Jung goes on to say, is 'an encounter, a discussion between two psychic wholes in which knowledge is used only as a tool.' The analyst is a 'fellow participant in the analysis.' Jung's focus was often on 'the real relationship' (cf. the psychoanalytic text by Greenson, 1967), making his point in very challenging terms: 'In reality everything depends on the man [*sic*] and little on the method' (Jung 1968, p. 7).

Jung's perspectives have encouraged post-Jungian analysts to explore the extent to which they themselves are 'wounded healers', bringing their strengths and weaknesses to the therapy situation (see Samuels, 1985, pp. 173–206).

As early as 1929, Jung was arguing for the clinical usefulness of what has come to be called the 'countertransference' – the analyst's subjective response to the analysand. 'You can exert no influence if you are not subject to influence,' he wrote, and 'the countertransference is an important organ of information' (Jung, 1929, pp. 70–72). Clinicians reading this chapter with a knowledge of psychoanalysis will know how contemporary psychoanalysis has rejected Freud's overly harsh assessment in 1910 (Freud, 1910, pp. 139–151) of the countertransference. Freud claimed it was 'the analyst's own complexes and internal resistances' and hence something to be got rid of. Jung is, in contradistinction, one of the important pioneers of the clinical use of countertransference, along with Heimann, Little, Mitchell, Winnicott, Sandler, Searles, Langs and Casement.

The clinical interaction of analyst and analysand, once regarded as the analyst's objective or neutral perceptions and the analysand's subjective ones, is now regarded primarily as a mutually transforming interaction. The analyst's personality and ethical position are no less involved in the process than his or her professional technique. The real relationship and the therapeutic alliance weave in and out of the transference/countertransference dynamics. The term for this is 'intersubjectivity' and Jung's alchemical model for the analytical process is an intersubjective one.[3] In this area, Jung's ideas share common ground with the diverse views of Atwood and Stolorow, Benjamin, Greenson, Kohut, Lomas, Mitchell and Alice Miller.

Let me restate the intention of providing this *catalogue raisonnée* of Jung's role as a pioneering figure in contemporary psychotherapy. Recall that Jung has been called a charlatan and a markedly inferior thinker to Freud. It is by now reasonable to claim that it is clearly time that the disciplines of psychiatry, psychotherapy and psychoanalysis recognized Jung's valuable contributions. A major aim of this volume is to situate his ideas squarely within the mainstream of contemporary psychoanalysis without losing their specificity.

The post-Jungians

What does the term 'post-Jungian' mean and what is the state of the field? Since Jung's death in 1961 there has been an explosion of creative professional activity in analytical psychology. In 1985 (Samuels, 1985) I coined the term 'post-Jungian'. I did not have post-modernism in mind at all. I was borrowing from a (then) well-known book called *Freud and the Post-Freudians* (Brown, 1961). I meant to indicate a connection to, and a critical distance from, Jung. The key word is 'critical'. If I were to write my book again I would include 'critical' in the title to emphasize the distance I intended alongside the overt membership of the Jungian world.

I needed to find a way of describing analytical psychology because the then current classifications were so problematic. People referred to two schools of analytical psychology as the 'London' and 'Zurich' schools after the cities of their origins. But geography was useless as a means of classifying what was going on. Even in the 1980s, and certainly in the 1990s, there were London school analysts and Zurich school analysts all over the world who had never been anywhere near London or Zurich. Moreover, as there are four Jungian societies in the city of London, to refer to what goes on in all of them as 'London' was inaccurate and, to some, offensive – for they display huge differences of outlook and practice, which is one reason why there are four of them.

Another belief that was prevalent in the 1980s and 1990s was that there was a divide between 'symbolic' and 'clinical' approaches to analytical psychology. This divide, as Zinkin (personal communication, 1983) wisely pointed out, was undermining of the field because no self-respecting Jungian was going to say that he or she did not work symbolically and no clinician could not be clinical! And so this troubling distinction needed to be amended into a useful set of categories. What I did in *Jung and the Post-Jungians* (Samuels, 1985) was to assume that all of the schools of analytical psychology knew about and made use of all the ideas and practices available through Jungian psychology. I emphasized key prioritizing and weighting within each of three rather different schools, which are connected by virtue of the fact that they are, to some degree, competitive with each other.

I admitted openly that the schools are creative fictions, that there is a huge amount of overlapping and that in many respects it was the patients who had constructed the schools as much as the analysts.

To summarize: I sorted analytical psychology into three schools: (1) the *classical school,* consciously working in Jung's tradition, with a focus on the self and individuation. I made the point that one should not equate classical with stuck or rigid. There can easily be evolutions within something classical; (2) the *developmental school,* which has a specific focus on the effects of infancy and childhood on the evolution of adult personality, and an equally stringent emphasis on the analysis of transference/countertransference dynamics in clinical work. The developmental school maintains a close relationship with object relations psychoanalysis (although the rapprochement is mostly one-way, with an indifference towards the Jungians); and (3) the *archetypal school* plays (in the most profound sense) with and explores images in therapy, paying the greatest respect to images just as they are without seeking an interpretive conclusion. The notion of *soul,* developed by the archetypal school, suggests the deepening that permits a mere event to become a significant experience.

This classification was, in fact, prompted by my own confusion as a then beginner in a field that seemed utterly chaotic and without maps, aids or companions as the various groups fell out, split and, in some cases, split again. I intended to indicate some connection to Jung and the traditions of thought and practice that had grown up around his name, and also some distance or differentiation. In order to delineate 'post-Jungian' analytical psychology, I adopted a pluralistic methodology in which *dispute* rather than consensus would define the field. Analytical psychology could then be defined by the debates and arguments and not by the core of commonly agreed ideas. A post-Jungian could thus be interested in and energized by the various debates on the basis of clinical interests, intellectual exploration, or a combination of these.

My threefold classification arose from a detailed examination of statements and articles written by post-Jungians which had a self-defining intent. Such polemical articles reveal more clearly than most what the lines of disagreement are within the Jungian and post-Jungian community. I have suggested elsewhere (Samuels, 1989a) that argument and competition are more often than not the case in psychoanalysis and depth psychology.[4] The history of psychoanalysis, especially the new, revisionist histories now appearing, show this tendency rather clearly.

For example, the following comes from Gerhard Adler, whom I regard as an exponent of the classical school:

> We put the main emphasis on symbolic transformation. I would like to quote what Jung says in a letter to P. W. Martin (20/8/45): 'The main interest in my work is with the approach to the numinous . . . but the fact is that the numinous is the real therapy.'[5]

Next is an extract from an editorial introduction to a group of papers published in London by members of the developmental school:

> The recognition of transference as such was the first subject to become a central one for clinical preoccupation . . . Then, as anxiety about this began to diminish with the acquisition of increased skill and experience, countertransference became a subject that could be tackled. Finally . . . the transaction involved is most suitably termed transference/countertransference.
>
> (Fordham et al., 1974, p. x)

And, finally, here is a statement from Hillman, speaking for the archetypal school of which he is the founder:

> At the most basic level of reality are fantasy images. These images are the primary activity of consciousness . . . *Images are the only reality we apprehend directly.*
>
> (Hillman, 1975, p. 174)

Arising from the process of competition and bargaining, weighting and prioritizing, those distinct and opposing claims should – we may imagine an analyst or therapist who can hold in mind all these views – be used in different contexts or on different occasions with different patients. In other words, it is possible to regard the schools metaphorically, as presences potentially able to co-exist in the mind of any post-Jungian analyst. Moreover, we should bear in mind that there are now more than 2,500 Jungian analysts worldwide in twenty-eight countries and probably an additional 10,000 psychotherapists and counsellors who are Jungian in orientation or heavily influenced by analytical psychology. Debates have been going on explicitly for fifty years and implicitly for perhaps seventy. Many practitioners will have by now internalized the debates themselves and feel perfectly capable of functioning as either a classical or a developmental or an archetypal analytical psychologist according to the needs of the individual analysand. Or the analyst may regard his or her orientation as primarily classical, for example, but with a flourishing developmental component, or some other combination.

A new classification of the schools of analytical psychology

The classification of the post-Jungian scene into the above three schools has been generally regarded as useful, though, given the weddedness of Jungians to individualism as the highest value, the very existence of a classification has been experienced by some as irritating. After all, everyone is unique, aren't they? To this unwitting provocation of the individualists, I will now add yet another classification of the field of analytical psychology into four schools.

The developmental and classical schools stand as they were in 1985. But the third school, the archetypal school, seems to me to have been integrated into the classical or even eliminated as a clinical perspective. However, as I see it, there are now two new schools to consider, each of which is an extremist version of one of the existing schools. The extremist version of the classical school I call the 'fundamentalist school' and the extremist version of the developmental school I call the 'psychoanalytic school'. The resultant four schools could be presented as a simple spectrum: *fundamentalist–classical–developmental–psychoanalytic.*

Like all fundamentalisms, Jungian fundamentalism desires to control who or what is in or out. Hence it tends to be stigmatizing. One hears this sometimes in assessment for training: 'He or she is not psychologically minded,' it can be said. Or people or training candidates are typed, even stereotyped, according to Jungian typology in an authoritarian way. Intellectual women may be termed 'animus-ridden'. As a fundamentalism, this form of analytical psychology attempts to be purist and above the marketplace, denying the financial or commercial aspect of doing therapy and claiming a direct connection to the work and life of Jung. Jung is regarded as a prophet, divinely inspired and perhaps even a new religious leader. He is imitated in how he lived his life – sometimes called the 'Jungian way'.

The positive aspect of Jungian fundamentalism is that there is something good and worthwhile in the idea of living in accord with psychological principles and striving for authenticity, perhaps against the odds in the contemporary world (cf. Christopher and Solomon, 2000). And yet, this kind of fundamentalism exaggerates and exploits our undeniable needs for order, pattern, meaning and a presiding myth. Psychologies that express evanescent, shifting, anti-foundational, anti-essentialist, playful natures cannot find a place in the Jungian fundamentalist *Weltanschauung*. The fundamentalists – remaining pure – ignore everything else that is going on in psychotherapy and even in the worlds of ideas, politics, the arts or religion.

On the other end of the spectrum, I would make a similar critique of the Jungian psychoanalytic school. I wish to emphasize that I am not against the use of psychoanalytic ideas and practices as I have indicated in my understanding of the developmental school. I am, however, deeply concerned about what can become an elimination of a Jungian perspective so that it seems not to exist. How has this come about? I think it has often been based on something exceedingly personal among Jungians who had earlier classical or developmental analyses that were not satisfying or transformative. Sometimes, these defects are attributed to the analysis having been insufficiently 'psychoanalytic' – not enough attention paid to infancy and to transference. Their espousal of a Jungian merger with psychoanalysis may be based on anger and on a transferential idealization of the psychoanalyses many of them went on to have. We hear a massive congratulation to psychoanalysis for its possession of exquisite analytic skills as if Jungian analysts were utterly devoid of them.

These psychoanalytic Jungians overlook Jung's clinical contributions and become alienated from their own birthright, displaying all the unsettling zeal of a convert. They seem to forget that clinical material comes alive not because of theory, but because of the way in which meaning emerges in the therapeutic relationship, as past traumas and difficulties are recognized in the analysis.

Psychoanalytic Jungians elevate the analytic frame over the analytic relationship and emphasize the analytic process over the contents of the psyche that become manifest during such process. The therapeutic relationship becomes 'mammocentric', as I call it. It is understood mainly in terms of the infant–mother dyad; the mouth and the breast are regarded as an almost exclusive paradigm for what is happening intersubjectively between the analytic couple, reducing all other complex insights or wisdom to this one metaphor.

To reprise my argument: I believe that the classical and developmental schools have spawned extremist versions of themselves. For different reasons, I am very concerned about these extreme expressions of competition and debate within analytical psychology. The fundamentalists may undermine the field through their radical purity while the psychoanalytic Jungians erase the originality and refinement of Jung's approach.

Jung in the academy

I conclude here by referring briefly to the situation regarding Jung in universities. Currently, in universities of many countries, there is a considerable interest in Jungian studies. Central to this is a historical revaluation of the origins of Jung's ideas and practices, and of the break with Freud. Literary and art criticism influenced by analytical psychology (even though still often based on somewhat mechanistic and out-of-date applications of Jungian theory) are beginning to flourish. Film studies is a particularly fertile discipline for Jungian thinking (see Hauke and Alister, 2001). Anthropological, social and political studies explore Jung's intuitions about directions for the future. Jung's influence on religious studies continues, as it has for a long time.

In some universities, psychoanalytic studies are much more established, whereas Jungian studies are really just getting off the ground. There could be some advantages to being a generation behind: it might be possible – and I would stress the word 'might' – for analytical psychology to avoid some of the damaging gaps between clinical work and academic applications.

If this kind of alienation is to be avoided in Jungian studies, then both the academic and the clinical camps will have to better interact with one another. A struggle between competing groups to 'appropriate' analytical psychology is neither desirable nor necessary. Each side can learn from the other. In the last thirty years, analytical psychology has become a healthily pluralistic discipline, although burdened by the extremes of fundamentalist and psychoanalytic narrowness. It is time for it to become more consciously interdisciplinary and to actively claim its proper place in the larger socio-cultural debates.

Notes

1 See Chapter 10 [of this book] for a full discussion of my views on Jung's anti-semitism, his alleged collaboration with the Nazis and the response of the Jungian community to the allegations.
2 See the Introduction to Samuels (ed.) (1989b) pp. 1–22 for a fuller account of Jung's ideas about the 'teleology' of symptoms and about psychopathology generally.
3 See Samuels (1989a, pp. 175–193) for a fuller account of Jung's alchemical metaphor for the analytical process.
4 For my theory about pluralism in depth psychology, see Samuels (1989a).
5 Gerhard Adler, unpublished public statement at the time of a major institutional split in the Jungian world in London.

References

Altman, N. (2005) 'Relational perspectives on the therapeutic action of psychoanalysis.' In J. Ryan, *How Does Psychotherapy Work?* London: Karnac Books.
Brown, J. (1961) *Freud and the Post-Freudians.* Harmondsworth: Penguin.
Cambray, J. (2004) 'Synchronicity as emergence.' In J. Cambray and L. Carter (eds.), *Analytical Psychology: Contemporary Perspectives in Jungian Analysis.* London and New York: Routledge.
Christopher, E. and Solomon, H. (2000) *Jungian Thought in the Modern World.* London: Free Association Books.
Corbett, L. (1996) *The Religious Function of the Psyche.* London and New York: Routledge.
Fierz, H. (1991) *Jungian Psychiatry.* Einsiedeln: Daimon.
Fordham, M., Hubback, J., Gordon, R. and Lambert, K. (eds.) (1974). *Technique in Jungian Analysis.* London: Heinemann.
Freud, S. (1910) 'The Future Prospects of Psycho-analytic Therapy.' In J. Strachey (ed.), *The Standard Edition of the Complete Psychological Works of Sigmund Freud,* 24 vols. London: The Hogarth Press, 1953–1974, vol. 11.
Greenson, R. (1967) *The Technique and Practice of Psychoanalysis.* London: Hogarth.
Hauke, C. and Alister, I. (2001) *Jung & Film: Post-Jungian Takes on the Moving Image.* London and New York: Routledge.
Hillman, J. (1975) *Loose Ends.* Dallas, TX: Spring Publications.
Hogenson, G. (2004) 'Archetypes: Emergence and the psyche's deep structure.' In J. Cambray and L. Carter (eds.), *Analytical Psychology: Contemporary Perspectives in Jungian Analysis.* London and New York: Routledge.
Hudson, L. (1983) 'Review of Storr (ed.), *Jung: Selected Writings.' Sunday Times,* March 13, 1983.
Jung, C. G. (1912) *Psychology of the Unconscious: A Study of the Transformations and Symbolisms of the Libido* (B. Hinkle, Trans.). *CW* B (W. McGuire, Ed.), 1984. Princeton, NJ: Princeton University Press; London: Routledge & Kegan Paul.
Jung, C. G. (1918) 'The Role of the Unconscious.' *CW* 10. *Civilization in Transition.*
Jung, C. G. (1929) 'Problems of modern psychotherapy.' *CW* 16. *The Practice of Psychotherapy.*
Jung, C. G. (1952) *Symbols of Transformation. CW* 5.
Jung, C. G. (1968) *Alchemical Studies. CW* 13.

Kast, V. (2006) 'Anima/animus.' In R. Papadopoulos (ed.), *The Handbook of Jungian Psychology*. London and New York: Routledge.

Knox, J. (2003) *Archetype, Attachment, Analysis: Jungian Psychology and the Nascent Mind*. London and New York: Routledge.

Laplanche, J. (1989) *New Foundations for Psychoanalysis* (D. Macey, Trans.). Oxford: Blackwell.

Roazen, P. (1976) *Freud and His Followers*. London: Penguin.

Samuels, A. (1985) *Jung and the Post-Jungians*. London and Boston, MA: Routledge & Kegan Paul.

Samuels, A. (1989a) *The Plural Psyche: Personality, Morality and the Father*. London and New York: Routledge.

Samuels, A. (ed.) (1989b) *Psychopathology: Contemporary Jungian Perspectives*. London: Karnac.

Samuels, A. et al. (2000) 'Analytical psychology after Jung with clinical case material from Stephen Mitchell's *Influence and Autonomy in Psychoanalysis*.' *Psychoanalytic Dialogues, 10*: 3.

Samuels, A., Shorter, B. and Plaut, F. (1986). *A Critical Dictionary of Jungian Analysis*. London and Boston, MA: Routledge & Kegan Paul.

Stein, M. (1996) *Practicing Wholeness*. New York: Continuum.

Wilkinson, M. (2006) *Coming Into Mind: The Mind–Brain Relationship: A Jungian Clinical Perspective*. London & New York: Routledge.

INDEX

When the text is within a figure, the number span is in bold.
Eg, Hubback, J. 194, 203, **205**
When the text is within a note, this is indicated by page number, 'n', note number.
Eg, GMSP 149, 154, 156, 157, 169n38

www.ingramcontent.com/pod-product-compliance
Ingram Content Group UK Ltd.
Pitfield, Milton Keynes, MK11 3LW, UK
UKHW022020180926
475701UK00005B/953

9781138818811